Lecture Notes on Mathematical Modelling in the Life Sciences

Series Editors
Angela Stevens
Michael C. Mackey

For further volumes:
http://www.springer.com/series/10049

Anita T. Layton • Aurélie Edwards

Mathematical Modeling in Renal Physiology

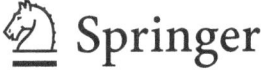 Springer

Anita T. Layton
Department of Mathematics
Duke University
Durham, North Carolina
USA

Aurélie Edwards
Centre de Recherche des Cordeliers
ERL 8228, UMRS 1138 Equipe 3
Paris, France

ISSN 2193-4789 ISSN 2193-4797 (electronic)
ISBN 978-3-642-27366-7 ISBN 978-3-642-27367-4 (eBook)
DOI 10.1007/978-3-642-27367-4
Springer Heidelberg New York Dordrecht London

Library of Congress Control Number: 2014945102

© Springer-Verlag Berlin Heidelberg 2014
This work is subject to copyright. All rights are reserved by the Publisher, whether the whole or part of the material is concerned, specifically the rights of translation, reprinting, reuse of illustrations, recitation, broadcasting, reproduction on microfilms or in any other physical way, and transmission or information storage and retrieval, electronic adaptation, computer software, or by similar or dissimilar methodology now known or hereafter developed. Exempted from this legal reservation are brief excerpts in connection with reviews or scholarly analysis or material supplied specifically for the purpose of being entered and executed on a computer system, for exclusive use by the purchaser of the work. Duplication of this publication or parts thereof is permitted only under the provisions of the Copyright Law of the Publisher's location, in its current version, and permission for use must always be obtained from Springer. Permissions for use may be obtained through RightsLink at the Copyright Clearance Center. Violations are liable to prosecution under the respective Copyright Law.
The use of general descriptive names, registered names, trademarks, service marks, etc. in this publication does not imply, even in the absence of a specific statement, that such names are exempt from the relevant protective laws and regulations and therefore free for general use.
While the advice and information in this book are believed to be true and accurate at the date of publication, neither the authors nor the editors nor the publisher can accept any legal responsibility for any errors or omissions that may be made. The publisher makes no warranty, express or implied, with respect to the material contained herein.

Printed on acid-free paper

Springer is part of Springer Science+Business Media (www.springer.com)

Contents

1	**Introduction: Basics of Kidney Physiology**	1
	1.1 Basic Kidney Anatomy and Blood Supply	1
	1.2 The Nephron	2
	1.3 Further Reading	5
	References	5
2	**Glomerular Filtration**	7
	2.1 Background	7
	2.2 Structure of Glomerular Capillaries	8
	2.2.1 Assessment of Glomerular Function	9
	2.2.2 Model Purpose and Validation	10
	2.3 Material Balance Equations	12
	2.3.1 Fluid Filtration	12
	2.3.2 Solute Filtration	16
	2.3.3 Protein Plasma Concentration Profile	19
	2.3.4 Fundamental Equations of Glomerular Filtration	20
	2.4 Isoporous Model	21
	2.4.1 General Assumptions	21
	2.4.2 Hindrance Factors	23
	2.4.3 Ultrafiltration Coefficient	23
	2.4.4 Fitting the Model to Experimental Data	24
	2.4.5 Isoporous Model Limitations	25
	2.5 Heteroporous Models	25
	2.5.1 Model Formulation	25
	2.5.2 Continuous Pore Size Distributions	27
	2.5.3 Discrete Pore Size Distributions	28
	2.5.4 Approximate Integration of Mass Balance Equations	29
	2.5.5 Heteroporous Model Performance	31
	2.5.6 Heteroporous Model Limitations	32

	2.6	Ultrastructural Model of Glomerular Filtration	33
		2.6.1 Water Filtration	34
		2.6.2 Filtration of Macromolecules	37
		2.6.3 Current Limitations	38
	2.7	Problems	39
		References	40
3	**Urine Concentration**		**43**
	3.1	Biological Background: How Does an Animal Produce a Concentrated Urine?	43
	3.2	Modeling Flow Along a Renal Tubule	44
		3.2.1 Mass Conservation Equations	44
		3.2.2 Water Fluxes	46
		3.2.3 Solute Fluxes	47
	3.3	Countercurrent Multiplication in a Loop	48
	3.4	Countercurrent Multiplication in a Loop, Revisited	50
		3.4.1 Model Assumptions	50
		3.4.2 Model Solution	51
	3.5	The Central Core Model	53
		3.5.1 Model Assumptions	54
		3.5.2 Model Solution	54
	3.6	The Distributed-Loop Model	57
	3.7	Current State of Affairs	59
	3.8	Problems	60
		References	61
4	**Counter-Current Exchange Across Vasa Recta**		**63**
	4.1	The Renal Medullary Microcirculation	63
		4.1.1 Background	63
		4.1.2 Anatomy of the Medullary Microcirculation	64
	4.2	Counter-Current Exchange	66
		4.2.1 Purpose	66
		4.2.2 Determinants of Counter-Current Exchange Efficiency	66
	4.3	Conservation Equations in Vasa Recta	69
	4.4	Water Transport Across Vas Rectum Walls	71
		4.4.1 Descending Vasa Recta	72
		4.4.2 Ascending Vasa Recta	73
	4.5	Solute Transport Across Vas Rectum Walls	74
	4.6	Transport Across Red Blood Cells	75
		4.6.1 Water and Non-reactive Solutes	75
		4.6.2 Oxygen Transport	75
	4.7	Full Model Specification	78
		4.7.1 Interstitial Values	79
		4.7.2 Varying Number of Vasa Recta	79
		4.7.3 Boundary Conditions	80
	4.8	Problems	81
		References	82

Contents

5 Tubuloglomerular Feedback 85
  5.1 A Negative Feedback Loop 85
  5.2 Brief Introduction to Delay-Differential Equations 87
    5.2.1 A Simple Example 87
    5.2.2 Stability Analysis 89
  5.3 A Partial Differential Equation Model with Delayed Feedback 90
    5.3.1 Solute Conservation Along the Thick Ascending Limb 90
    5.3.2 Tubuloglomerular Feedback Response 92
  5.4 Numerical Solution and Limit-Cycle Oscillatory Behaviors 92
    5.4.1 Time-Independent Steady-State Solution 92
    5.4.2 Limit-Cycle Oscillations 94
  5.5 Characteristic Equation 96
  5.6 Bifurcation Analysis 98
    5.6.1 A Model with Zero Chloride Permeability 98
    5.6.2 A Model with Nonzero Chloride Permeability 100
  5.7 Modeling Coupled TGF Systems 103
  5.8 Problems 105
  References 106

6 Electrophysiology of Renal Vascular Smooth Muscle Cells 107
  6.1 Background 107
  6.2 Overview of Cell Electrophysiology 108
    6.2.1 Electrical Circuit Model of the Cell Membrane 108
    6.2.2 Nernst Equilibrium Potential 109
    6.2.3 Ion Conservation Equations 111
  6.3 Ion Channels 112
    6.3.1 Current-Voltage Relationship of a Single Open Channel 113
    6.3.2 Channel Gating 115
    6.3.3 Current Across a Population of Channels 116
  6.4 Calcium Signaling 118
    6.4.1 Plasma Membrane Ca^{2+} Transporters 119
    6.4.2 Calcium Buffers 124
    6.4.3 Sarcoplamic Reticulum Calcium Stores 126
    6.4.4 Temporal Variations in Calcium Concentration 131
  6.5 Kinetic Model for Cellular Contraction 135
  6.6 Problems 138
  References 139

7 Vasomotion and Myogenic Response of the Afferent Arteriole 141
  7.1 The Afferent Arteriole 141
  7.2 Nonlinear ODEs 142
  7.3 The Morris-Lecar Model 144
    7.3.1 Model Equations 145
    7.3.2 Simulations, Nullclines 146
  7.4 Spontaneous Vasomotion 148
  7.5 Myogenic Response 151

	7.6	Problems	153
		References	154
8	**Transport Across Tubular Epithelia**	155
	8.1	Fundamental Aspects of Transepithelial Transport	155
		8.1.1	Paracellular and Transcellular Pathways	156
		8.1.2	Passive and Active Transport	158
		8.1.3	Acid-Base Balance	159
	8.2	Principal Classes of Transepithelial Transporters	160
		8.2.1	Aquaporins	160
		8.2.2	Na,K-ATPase Pumps	161
		8.2.3	An Antiport System: The Na^+/H^+ Exchanger	163
		8.2.4	A Symport System: The Na^+-Cl^- Cotransporter	165
		8.2.5	Non-equilibrium Thermodynamic Formalism	167
	8.3	Fundamental Equations of Epithelial Models	169
		8.3.1	Morphological Properties	169
		8.3.2	Time-Dependent Conservation Equations for Water and Solute	169
		8.3.3	Rate of Solute Generation and Proton Conservation	173
		8.3.4	Conservation of Electric Charge	174
	8.4	Full Model Specification	175
		8.4.1	Determinants of Volume Flux	175
		8.4.2	Determinants of Solute Flux	176
		8.4.3	Numerical Solution	177
		8.4.4	A Simple Cell Model	177
		8.4.5	Current Limitations	181
	8.5	Problems	182
		References	183
9	**Solutions to Problem Sets**	185
		References	218
Index		219

Chapter 1
Introduction: Basics of Kidney Physiology

Abstract The kidney not only filters metabolic wastes and toxins from the body, but it also regulates the body's water balance, electrolyte balance, and acid-base balance, blood pressure, and blood flow. This chapter introduces basic kidney anatomy, with a focus on the nephron and the renal microcirculation.

1.1 Basic Kidney Anatomy and Blood Supply

The kidneys are organs that serve a number of essential regulatory roles. Most of us know that our kidneys function as filters, removing metabolic wastes and toxins from the blood and excreting them through the urine. But the kidneys also serve other essential functions. Through a number of regulatory mechanisms, the kidneys help maintain the body's water balance, electrolyte balance, and acid-base balance. Additionally, the kidneys produce or activate hormones that are involved in erythrogenesis, calcium metabolism, and the regulation of blood flow.

In humans the kidneys are located in the abdominal cavity, with one kidney on each side of the spine. Each kidney is a bean-like structure that consists of two regions; the outer region is the cortex, and the inner region is the medulla. The cortex contains glomeruli, which are clusters of capillaries, and convoluted segments of tubules, whereas the medulla contains almost parallel arrangement of tubules and vessels.

Despite their relatively small size ($\sim 0.5\%$ of total body weight), the kidneys receive $\sim 20\%$ of cardiac output. The kidneys receive blood from the renal arteries, which divide into anterior and posterior branches, which then in turn branch into interlobar arteries and then arcuate arteries. (The renal artery and interlobar artery are shown in Fig. 1.1, with labels 3 and 2, respectively. The anatomy of the renal microcirculation is also shown in Fig. 4.1.) The arcuate arteries traverse through the boundary of the cortex and the medulla, branch into interlobular arteries and give rise to the afferent arterioles that supply the glomeruli. (Two mechanisms by which the afferent arteriole regulates downstream blood pressure and tubular

Fig. 1.1 Schematic diagram of a kidney (Obtained from Wikimedia Commons. *1*: Renal pyramid, *2*: Interlobar artery, *3*: Renal artery, *4*: Renal vein, *5*: Renal hylum, *6*: Renal pelvis, *7*: Ureter, *8*: Minor calyx, *9*: Renal capsule; *10*: Inferior extremity, *11*: Superior extremity, *12*: Interlobar vein, *13*: Nephron, *14*: Renal sinus, *15*: Major calyx, *16*: Renal papilla, *17*: Renal column)

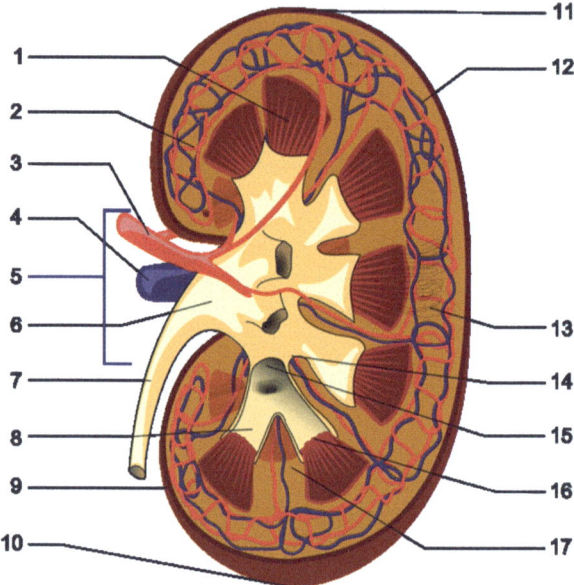

reabsorption are discussed in Chaps. 5 and 7.) The glomerular capillaries rejoin to form efferent arterioles, some of which supply the dense peritubular capillary network that feeds the tubules in the cortex, whereas others descend into the medulla to form hairpin-shaped vessels called the vasa recta, which supply the capillary network in the medulla. The delivery of oxygen and nutrients to tissues and the removal of water and other solutes from the medulla by counter-current exchange across vasa recta is discussed in Chap. 4. Like the vascular smooth muscle cells of the afferent arterioles, the descending vasa recta pericytes can control blood flow supply to the renal medulla, a process that is discussed in Chap. 6.

1.2 The Nephron

The functional unit of the kidney is the nephron. Each human kidney is populated by about a million nephrons. An old illustration of a nephron, reproduced from *Gray's Anatomy* (Gray, 1918), by English anatomist and surgeon Henry Gray (1827–1861), is shown in Fig. 1.2. One anatomical error in that illustration is that it fails to depict the passage of the cortical ascending limb by the glomerulus before becoming the distal convoluted tubule. That was not known in 1918, but is shown in a relatively more recent, but still decades old, drawing by Kriz et al. (1972), Fig. 1.3.

Each nephron consists of an initial filtering component called the renal corpuscle and a renal tubule specialized for reabsorption and secretion. The renal corpuscle is the site of formation of the glomerular filtrate, and is composed of a glomerulus and

1.2 The Nephron

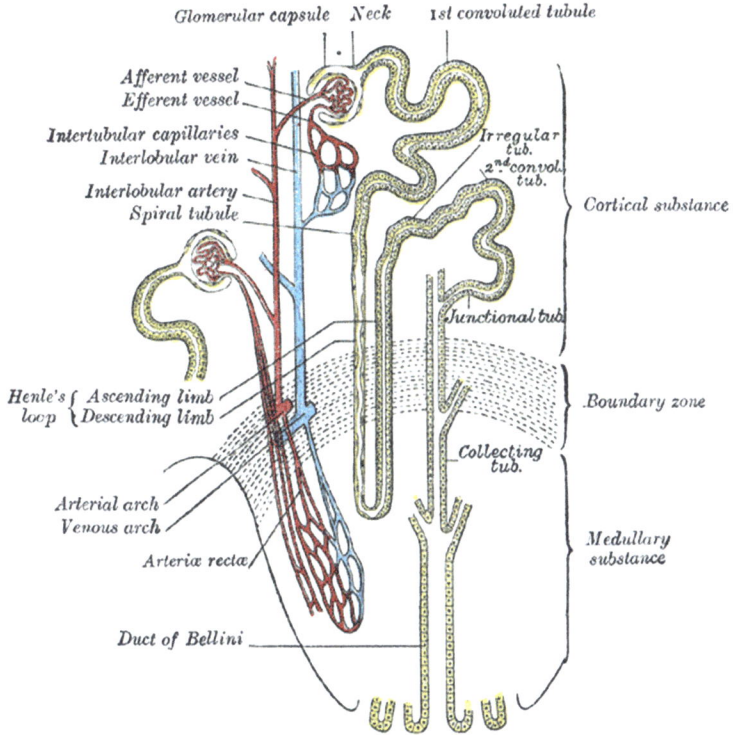

Fig. 1.2 A faithful reproduction of a lithograph plate from *Gray's Anatomy* (Obtained from Wikimedia Commons)

Bowman's capsule. Recall that a glomerulus is a tufts of capillaries arising from the afferent arterioles. A fraction of the water and solutes in the blood supplied by the afferent arteriole is driven by pressure gradients into the space formed by Bowman's capsule. Glomerular filtration is discussed in Chap. 2. The remainder of the blood flows into the efferent arteriole.

The renal tubule is the portion of the nephron in which the tubular fluid filtered through the glomerulus circulates before being excreted as urine. The role of the renal tubule is to adjust the composition of the filtrate. This adjustment takes place as the filtrate flows along the tubules, where reabsorption (i.e., removal from the filtrate, back into the interstitium, and then into the circulation) of water and some solutes and secretion (i.e., addition into the tubular fluid) of other solutes occurs. The composition of the final urine is adjusted so that daily intake roughly equals urinary excretion.

The renal tubular system consists of many segments, including (given in an order consistent with fluid flow direction)

Fig. 1.3 An illustration of three nephrons, together with their glomeruli (Adapted from Kriz et al. 1972)

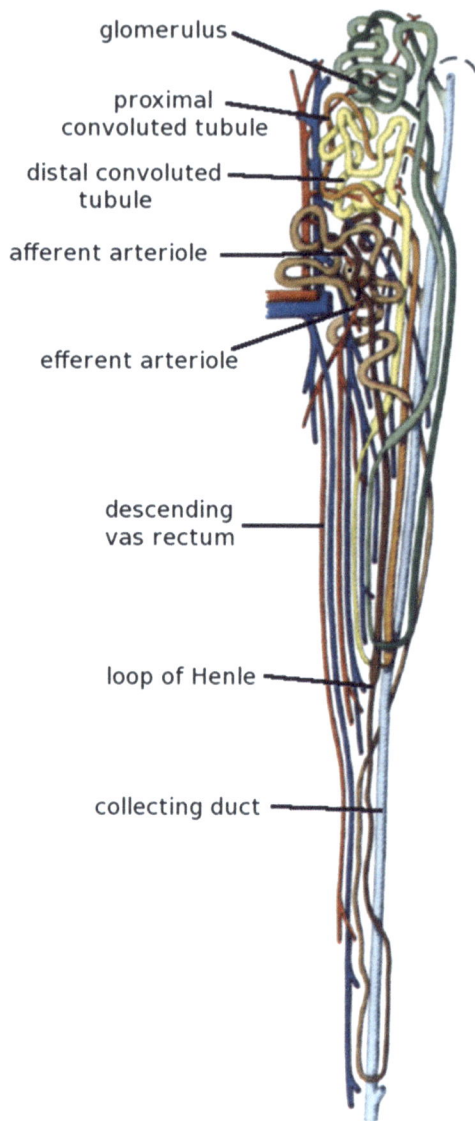

- The proximal tubule, which consists of two segments: the proximal convoluted tubule that lies within the cortex, and the proximal straight tubule (those that are associated with the long loops are actually quite tortuous) that lies within the outer stripe of the outer medulla;
- The loop of Henle, a hairpin-like tubule that lies mostly in the medulla; the loop of Henle in turn consists of a descending limb and an ascending limb;
- The distal convoluted tubule, which lies within the cortex;

- The connecting tubule, which also lies within the cortex;
- The collecting duct, which spans the cortex and the medulla.

The tubular segments are lined by an epithelial cell barrier, which mediates water and solute exchanges between the tubular lumen and the surrounding interstitium. The structure of the epithelial cells varies widely among the different tubular segments. For instance, the ascending limb cells in the cortex and medulla are "thick," whereas the descending limb cells have few mitochondria and little cell membrane amplification. The function (or transport) properties also vary among different tubular segments.

Since the kidneys receive about one-fifth of the total cardiac output, and filter a significant fraction ($\sim 20\%$) of the blood they receive, the main function of the renal tubules is to recover most of the glomerular filtrate. Otherwise, we would lose all our blood plasma in less than half an hour! The proximal tubule reabsorbs the largest fraction of the glomerular filtrate, including about two-thirds of the water and NaCl, as well as filtered nutrients like glucose and amino acids. The loop of Henle that follows participates in the formation of concentrated or diluted urine. (The formation of a concentrated urine is discussed in Chap. 3.) That is accomplished, in part, by the thick ascending limb actively pumping NaCl into the interstitium of the medulla, without water following. As a result, the fluid that reaches the distal tubule is dilute relative to blood plasma. The collecting duct exploits this hypotonicity by, depending on the requirements of the body, either allowing or not water to flow, via osmosis, into the surrounding interstitium. Epithelial transport processes are discussed in Chap. 8.

1.3 Further Reading

This very brief introduction to kidney physiology highlights the aspects of the kidney anatomy and function that a reader should be familiar with before proceeding to the modeling chapters, but it certainly does not do justice to the many and very complicated functions performed by the kidney. For those who are interested in learning more about kidney physiology, we recommend *Vander's Renal Physiology*, by Douglas Eaton and John Pooler (2004).

References

Eaton, D.C., Pooler, J.P.: Vander's Renal Physiology, 6th edn. McGraw-Hill Medical, New York (2004)
Gray, H.: Anatomy of the Human Body, 20th edn. Lear & Febriger, Philadelphia/New York (1918)
Kriz, W., Schnermann, J., Koepsell, H.: The position of short and long loops of Henle in the rat kidney. Z Anat Entwickl-Gesch **138**, 301–319 (1972)

Chapter 2
Glomerular Filtration

Abstract The formation of urine begins with the filtration of blood by glomerular capillaries. In this chapter, we introduce mathematical models of glomerular filtration. These models seek to relate the filtration properties of the capillary wall to its structure, so as to better understand the underlying causes of changes in glomerular selectivity. We first describe the general equations that govern filtration across a porous, size-selective membrane. We then examine three different model representations of the capillary wall, in order of increased sophistication, and provide examples of their clinical applications.

2.1 Background

The first step in the formation of urine is the filtration of blood by glomerular capillaries. The filtrate is collected into Bowman's capsule and subsequently flows through the tubular system where it undergoes major changes in volume and composition. The glomerulus has been described as a "very refined ultrafiltration device, capable of filtering large volumes of plasma while efficiently retaining proteins within the circulation" (Deen et al. 2001). Indeed, in a typical person, each kidney filters about 90 l a day; yet, the Bowman space-to-plasma ratio of albumin concentration is thought to be <0.001. These unusual permeability properties originate from the very specific ultrastructure of the glomerular capillary wall, as described below.

The size and number of glomeruli in mammalian kidneys are roughly proportional to body and kidney size. The number of glomeruli per kidney is approximately 10,000 in mice, 30,000 in rats, 200,000 in rabbits, and 1,000,000 in humans.

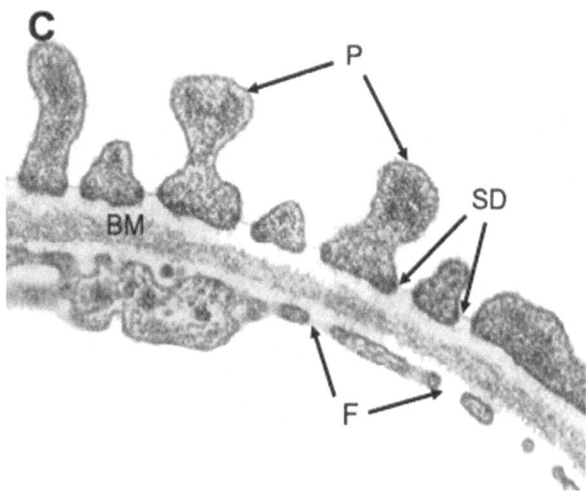

Fig. 2.1 Transmission electron micrograph of a transverse section through the glomerular capillary wall of a normal rat. *P* podocyte foot process, *SD* slit diaphragm, *BM* basement membrane, *F* endothelial fenestration. Magnification: approximately ×48,000 (Adapted from Pavenstadt et al. (2003))

2.2 Structure of Glomerular Capillaries

The glomerular capillary wall is composed of three layers, as shown in Fig. 2.1: a fenestrated endothelium, a basement membrane, and the foot processes of epithelial cells (which are known as podocytes). These foot processes (or projections) wrap around the capillaries and are separated by slit diaphragms, through which filtration occurs. Together, the three layers constitute a size- and charge-selective barrier that filters large amounts of fluid and small solutes while preventing the passage of large proteins and cells into the urine.

The fenestrations of glomerular endothelial cells are trans-cytoplasmic holes of 60–80 nm diameter. The endothelial cells are covered by a surface coat known as the glycocalyx, which is essentially composed of proteoglycans and sialoproteins. This coat extends over the glomerular endothelial fenestrations, where it plays an important role in restricting the passage of proteins.

The glomerular basement membrane is a gel-like material which serves to anchor endothelial cells and podocytes on either side. Its principal components are type IV collagen, laminin, proteoglycans and nidogen. Type IV collagen forms an interconnected network of fibers within the membrane that is thought to provide tensile strength to the capillary wall. Laminins also constitute a network that is highly crosslinked to the type IV collagen network. Heparan sulfate proteoglycans impart anionic charge to the membrane, but their contribution to the overall charge-selectivity of the capillary wall remains uncertain. Nidogen (or entactin) is a sulfated glycoprotein that may be important in binding all the components of the glomerular basement membrane together.

Foot processes from adjacent podocytes are linked by a specialized cell–cell junction known as the slit diaphragm. The configuration of the slit diaphragm is not entirely elucidated. Some investigators have described a zipper-like structure

2.2 Structure of Glomerular Capillaries

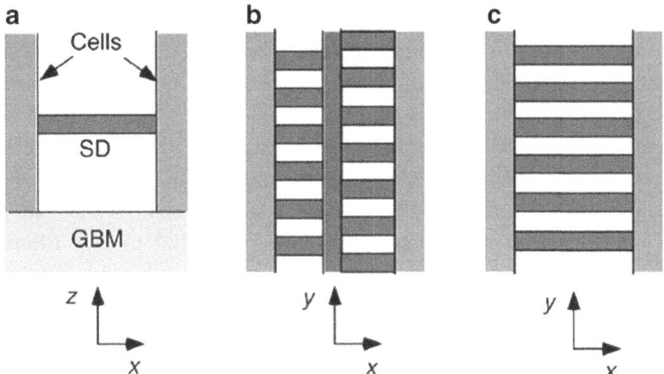

Fig. 2.2 Representation of the slit diaphragm (*SD*) between two podocytes, atop the glomerular basement membrane (GBM). (**a**) View from the same orientation as in Fig. 2.1. (**b**) Perpendicular view of the zipper-like structure. (**c**) Perpendicular view of the ladder-like structure (Reproduced from Deen et al. (2001))

in which regularly spaced cross-bridges, alternating from side to side, extend from podocyte plasma membranes to a central filament that is parallel to, and equidistant, from the cell membranes (Rodewald and Karnovsky 1974). Others have observed instead a ladder-like structure, consisting in equidistant cross-bridges connecting podocyte membranes (Hora et al. 1990). Both representations are depicted in Fig. 2.2.

2.2.1 Assessment of Glomerular Function

How do we measure kidney function, and more specifically glomerular function, in animals and humans? Can these measurements be interpreted using mathematical models to gain insight into the underlying causes of glomerular injury? In this section, we describe routine markers of glomerular function.

The standard measure of the ability of the kidney to excrete a given solute S is the *renal plasma clearance* of S, that is, the volume of plasma that is completely cleared of solute S per unit time. It is calculated as:

$$cl_S = \frac{C_S^U F_V^U}{C_S^P}, \qquad (2.1)$$

where C_S^P and C_S^U are the plasma and urine concentration of solute S, and F_V^U is the urine flow. Clearance measurements are used to determine renal plasma flow as well as the glomerular filtration rate.

If the solute being considered is completely cleared from plasma during a single pass through the kidney, then its molar flow rate in urine (i.e., the product $C_S^U F_V^U$)

is equal to that entering the kidney in plasma. The renal plasma clearance of that solute is therefore equal to the *renal plasma flow* (RPF). Such is almost the case for PAH (para-aminohippurate), the clearance of which is used to determine RPF. Note that in reality, not all PAH is removed from the renal circulation during one pass; the venous plasma concentration of PAH is about 10 % of its arterial plasma concentration. The clearance of PAH therefore underestimates RPF by about 10 %.

If the solute being considered is neither reabsorbed nor secreted along the tubules, then the amount of that solute in urine is equal to that filtered by the glomerular capillaries. If, in addition, the solute is freely filtered by the glomerular capillary wall, its clearance is then equal to the *glomerular filtration rate* (GFR). Inulin satisfies both conditions, and its clearance therefore provides an accurate measure of GFR. However, inulin is an exogenous substance, and measuring its clearance is difficult to do in routine clinical practice. Endogenous markers, such as creatinine, are thus preferred. However, small amounts of creatinine are secreted by proximal tubular cells. Unless drugs that inhibit this secretion (such as cimetidine) are administered, the creatinine clearance can overestimate GFR by 10–30 % in normal individuals, and more in patients with chronic kidney disease.

The ratio of the glomerular filtration rate-to-plasma flow is known as the mean *filtration fraction* (FF). Typical values for RPF and GFR in healthy humans, normalized by the standard body surface area (1.73 m^2), are 600 and 120 ml/min/(1.73 m^2), respectively. Thus, the filtration fraction is about 20 %. RPF, GFR, and/or FF are required inputs for mathematical models of glomerular filtration. Another useful input is the concentration of plasma proteins (essentially albumin and IgG) in afferent plasma, which can be determined by techniques such as immunodiffusion.

The *fractional clearance*, or *sieving coefficient*, of solute S (denoted θ_S) is defined as the fraction of filtered solute that is excreted in urine. It is therefore equal to the renal plasma clearance of the solute divided by GFR. In practice, θ_S is often calculated as the solute-to-inulin clearance ratio:

$$\theta_S = \frac{cl_S}{cl_{inulin}} = \frac{C_S^U C_{inulin}^P}{C_S^P C_{inulin}^U}. \tag{2.2}$$

Note that the fractional clearance of a solute that is neither reabsorbed nor secreted along the tubule is equal to its Bowman space-to-plasma concentration ratio. Thus, the sieving coefficient of such solutes directly reflects the selectivity of the glomerular capillary wall. Dextran and Ficoll are polysaccharides with those properties, and are often used to assess glomerular function, as shown in Fig. 2.3.

2.2.2 Model Purpose and Validation

The first quantitative analysis of glomerular function dates back to 1899, when the British physiologist Ernest Starling showed that the forces governing fluid transport across capillary walls could explain the formation of the glomerular ultrafiltrate

2.2 Structure of Glomerular Capillaries

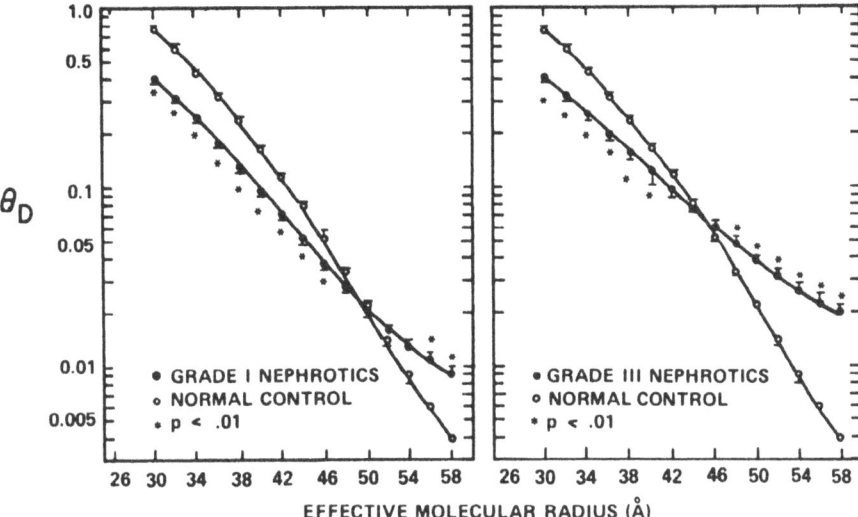

Fig. 2.3 Dextran sieving curves. The fractional clearance of dextrans with varying molecular weight is plotted as a function of their molecular radius. Results for healthy controls and nephrotic patients are compared. The latter are divided into several groups, depending on their IgG clearance (<0.001 for grade I, >0.01 for grade III). The progression of disease is associated with an increase in the filtration of large dextrans (Reproduced from Deen et al. (1985))

(Starling 1899) – Starling is also known for his discovery, with his brother-in-law Sir William Bayliss, of peristalsis and of the first hormone, secretin. However, it wasn't until the early 1970s that progress in experimental techniques (such as micropuncture) and newly available data made it possible to launch a major renal modeling effort. Investigators such as B.M. Brenner, C. R. Robertson, W.M. Deen, and their colleagues then began to build a series of increasingly sophisticated models of glomerular filtration (Brenner et al. 1971; Deen et al. 1972; Chang et al. 1975). Until the 1990s, these models represented the capillary wall as a homogeneous membrane, generally characterized by one or several populations of pores. In the last decade or so, William Deen, a chemical engineering professor at the Massachusetts Institute of Technology, has led the effort to develop models of glomerular filtration that take into account the specific ultrastructure described above. The early "pore" models are described in detail below, as they illustrate general and important concepts in fluid and solute filtration, whereas later models are described much more succinctly.

The principal objective of mathematical models of glomerular function is to relate the filtration properties of the capillary wall to its (presumed) ultrastructure: the resulting structure-function relationship serves to examine the underlying structural causes of changes in glomerular selectivity (e.g., in clearance data), and to better understand pathophysiological mechanisms.

Whatever their representation of the barrier, models of glomerular filtration are characterized by sets of parameters, several of which cannot be experimentally determined and must therefore be adjusted. The value of these unknown parameters is determined by fitting model predictions to experimental data, typically to sieving curves. Optimized parameter values are obtained by minimizing the sum of squared errors:

$$SSE = \sum_S \left(\theta_S^{calc}/\theta_S^{meas} - 1\right)^2, \qquad (2.3)$$

where the superscripts "calc" and "meas" refer to calculated and measured values respectively. Note that SSE values can also be used to compare different models; the lower SSE, the better the "goodness of fit" of the model.

The next section describes the general equations governing filtration across a porous, size-selective membrane. The following sections illustrate three different representations of the capillary wall, in order of increased sophistication, and provide examples of their clinical applications.

2.3 Material Balance Equations

2.3.1 Fluid Filtration

Fluid Conservation Equation

In spite of their actual tortuosity, glomerular capillaries are idealized as a network of identical, parallel capillaries with homogeneous properties along their entire length. The capillaries are represented as rigid cylinders of radius r and length L, as shown in Fig. 2.4.

Let P denote the plasma compartment, and Q^P the volumetric rate of plasma flow in a capillary. At a given position x along the capillary, a portion of the flow can be reabsorbed into (or secreted from) the surrounding medium via a transversal flux across the capillary wall. Assuming that the capillaries are rigid, there is no accumulation of fluid within the plasma compartment. Thus, a material balance for volume over the portion of capillary comprised between x_1 and x_2 can be written as:

$$Q^P(x_2) = Q^P(x_1) - \int_{x_1}^{x_2} 2\pi \, r \, J_V(s) \, ds, \qquad (2.4)$$

where J_V is the plasma volume flux, expressed as a flow per unit capillary area and taken as positive if outwardly directed. Equation (2.4) may be written in differential form:

2.3 Material Balance Equations

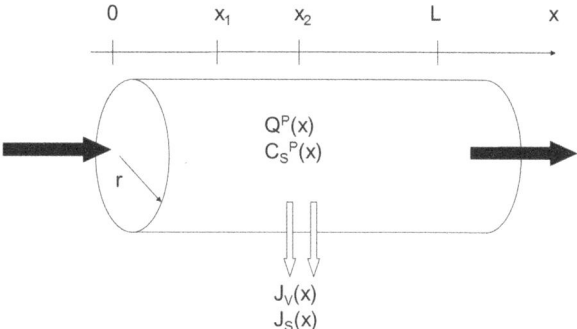

Fig. 2.4 Schematic representation of plasma and solute flow within a glomerular capillary of length L. Q^P is the volumetric rate of plasma flow, and C_S^P is the plasma concentration of solute S. J_V and J_S denote the transversal fluxes of plasma volume and solute S across the capillary wall

$$\frac{dQ^P}{dx} = -2\pi\, r\, J_V, \tag{2.5}$$

where we have omitted the spatial dependence of the variables for simplicity. Equation (2.5) was derived for a single capillary. Assuming that r remains constant, it can apply equally to one glomerulus, or to all the glomeruli of one or two kidneys, if it is re-written as:

$$\frac{dQ^P}{dx} = -\frac{S^P}{L}J_V, \tag{2.6}$$

where the definitions of plasma flow rate (Q^P) and capillary surface area (S^P) are adjusted accordingly, and L is the capillary length.

What are typical values of renal flow? In healthy humans, the kidneys receive 1/5th of the cardiac output, or roughly 1 l/min in an adult of average size. Systemic hematocrit is ∼40 %, which yields a renal plasma flow of about 600 ml/min. Clinicians typically normalize the renal flow by the body surface area, to account for variations due to size. The average body surface area is estimated as 1.73 m², thus the normalized renal plasma flow is about 600 ml/min/(1.73 m²). This means that in a male of body surface area equal to 1.9 m², a normal RPF is ∼600 (1.9/1.73) = 660 ml/min, and the afferent Q^P is approximately 330 ml/min per kidney, or ∼5.5 nl/s per glomerulus, assuming 1,000,000 nephrons per kidney. About 1/5th of this flow is in turn filtered by the glomeruli (Fig. 2.5).

Volume Flux

To integrate Eq. (2.6), we must specify the flux J_V. Fluid flow across a semi-permeable membrane such as the capillary wall is driven by transmembrane hydraulic and osmotic pressure differences. The osmotic pressure is the pressure that must be applied to a fluid to stop the inflow of water across a water-permeable membrane, as described in more detail in Chap. 3.

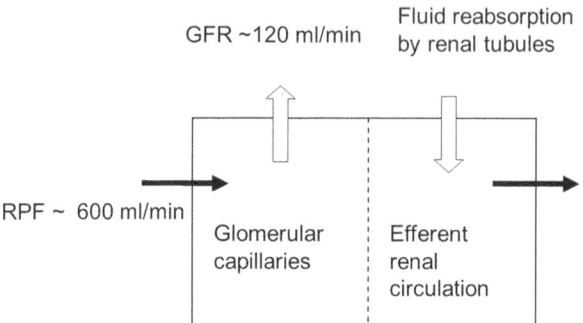

Fig. 2.5 Filtration of plasma flow by the glomerular capillary network. In humans, both kidneys receive about 1 l/min, 60 % of which is plasma, i.e., the renal plasma flow (RPF) is about 600 ml/min, and the plasma flow entering each glomerulus (Q^P) equals ~5 nl/s. The filtration fraction, defined as the ratio of the glomerular filtration rate (GFR) to RPF is normally about 20 %, so that GFR is ~120 ml/min. Most of the filtered flow is reabsorbed downstream by the renal tubules

Much of the seminal work on fluid and solute transport across biological membranes was done in the 1950s by Katchalsky and colleagues, based upon non-equilibrium thermodynamics. The practical phenomenological equations that Kedem and Katchalsky developed for volume and solute fluxes are still commonly used by biophysicists and physiologists, particularly when the membrane is viewed as a "black-box". The generalized form of the *Kedem–Katchalsky (KK) equation* for the volume flux across a homogeneous membrane (Eq. 39 in Kedem and Katchalsky (1958)) can be written as:

$$J_V = L_p \left(\Delta P - \sum_S \sigma_S \Delta \Pi_S \right), \tag{2.7}$$

where L_p is the hydraulic conductivity of the membrane, ΔP is the transmembrane difference in hydraulic pressure, $\Delta \Pi_S$ represents the contribution of solute S to the osmotic pressure difference, and σ_S denotes the osmotic reflection coefficient of the membrane to solute S, which varies between zero and unity. If the solute is non-penetrating, σ equals 1; conversely, if the solute is freely filtered, σ equals zero. L_p and σ_S are both phenomenological coefficients.

In practice, the contribution of small, permeable solutes to the osmotic pressure is often approximated as $RT\sigma C$, where R is the gas constant and T is the absolute temperature. The volume flux is therefore calculated as:

$$J_V = L_p \left(\Delta P - \Delta \Pi_{np} - RT \sum_{\text{small solute } ss} \sigma_{ss} \Delta C_{ss} \right), \tag{2.8}$$

2.3 Material Balance Equations

where $\Delta\Pi_{np}$ represents the contribution of non-penetrating solutes (such as proteins) to the osmotic pressure difference. The pressure exerted by plasma proteins is known as the oncotic pressure; thus, when Eq. (2.8) is applied to blood flow, the $\Delta\Pi_{np}$ term is referred to as the oncotic pressure difference.

The contribution of each of the three pressure terms on the right-hand side of Eq. (2.8) varies considerably depending on the barrier. In renal tubules, the hydraulic and oncotic pressure differences are negligible relative to the last term (see Chap. 3). Conversely, across the glomerular capillary wall, ΔP and $\Delta\Pi_{np}$ are quite large, and because the wall is non-selective with respect to small solutes such as sodium and urea (i.e., $\sigma_{ss} = 0$), the last term is zero. Since protein concentration in Bowman's space is negligible, the volume flux across the glomerular capillary wall is determined as:

$$J_V = L_p \left(P^P - P^B - \Pi_{pr}^P \right), \tag{2.9}$$

where the superscript "B" denotes Bowman's space, and the subscript "pr" refers to proteins. The product of the hydraulic conductivity (L_p) and capillary surface area (S^P) is known as the *ultrafiltration coefficient* (K_f):

$$K_f \equiv L_p S^P. \tag{2.10}$$

If we consider the entire kidney, the product of the volume flux and the capillary surface area equals the glomerular filtration rate. Hence, integrating Eq. (2.9) over the whole kidney yields:

$$GFR = K_f \left(<\Delta P> - <\Pi_{pr}^P> \right) = K_f <P_{UF}>, \tag{2.11}$$

where $<>$ denotes an average value over the whole kidney, and P_{UF} is the net ultrafiltration pressure.

In healthy males, the total GFR for both kidneys is $\sim$125 ml/min, which means that the kidneys filter about 180 l a day. As illustrated in Fig. 2.6, the oncotic pressure in plasma is about 20–30 mmHg, and the hydraulic pressure difference ΔP is about 30–50 mmHg. Hence, $<P_{UF}>$ is on the order of 10 mmHg, and K_f on the order 12.5 ml/min/mmHg.

For inter-organ comparisons, it is helpful to express K_f per unit weight. The weight of a human kidney averages 125–150 g, so K_f is $\sim$4.5 ml/min/mmHg/100 g kidney. In other capillary beds, K_f is 2–3 orders of magnitude smaller. In the intestine for example, K_f is only about 0.08 ml/min/mmHg/100 g, that is, 50 times lower. The high K_f of the glomerular capillaries, which allows for the rapid filtration of blood, results from the combination of a high surface area for exchange and a large hydraulic conductivity.

Fig. 2.6 Hydraulic and oncotic pressure differences across the glomerular capillary wall

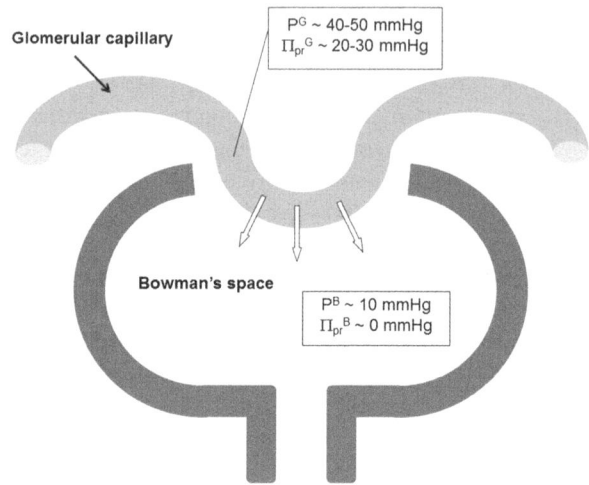

2.3.2 Solute Filtration

Solute Conservation Equation

Let's now consider the fate of a solute S present in plasma. The plasma molar flow rate of S (in moles per unit time) is given by the product of its plasma concentration C_S^P and the plasma flow rate Q^P. As the solute flows along the capillary, some fraction is reabsorbed into (or secreted from) the surrounding medium. If the solute is non-reacting, the overall number of moles of S remains constant. In addition, there is no accumulation of solute within the capillary lumen at steady state. Thus, a material balance for a non-reacting solute S over the plasma volume element comprised between x_1 and x_2 at steady state yields:

$$Q^P(x_2) C_S^P(x_2) = Q^P(x_1) C_S^P(x_1) - 2\pi r \int_{x_1}^{x_2} J_S(s)\, ds, \quad (2.12)$$

where J_S is the plasma flux of solute S, expressed as a molar flow per unit capillary area. The differential form of Eq. (2.12) can be written as:

$$\frac{d\left(Q^P C_S^P\right)}{dx} = -2\pi r\, J_S. \quad (2.13)$$

Some proteins such as albumin are highly concentrated in plasma ($\sim$1–10 g/dl), and thus exert a significant oncotic pressure therein, which opposes fluid filtration across the capillary wall, as described below. Because such plasma proteins play an important role in glomerular filtration, we consider them separately from other

2.3 Material Balance Equations

solutes. In healthy kidneys, the fraction of plasma proteins that is filtered along the capillaries is negligible. Thus, if C_{pr}^P denotes the plasma concentration of proteins, we have:

$$\frac{d\left(Q^P C_{pr}^P\right)}{dx} = 0. \tag{2.14}$$

Solute Flux

To obtain plasma solute concentration profiles, we must now derive an expression for the solute flux J_S across the glomerular capillary wall. The movement of a solute is generally governed by two mechanisms, convection and diffusion. Convective transport results from the bulk motion of the fluid. Diffusion results from the random motion of molecules having thermal energy. The *Kedem-Katchalsky equation* for the flux of an uncharged solute S can be written as:

$$J_S = J_V (1 - \sigma_S) \overline{C}_S + P_S \Delta C_S, \tag{2.15}$$

where the first term represents the contribution from convection, and the second that from diffusion. P_S is the permeability of the membrane to solute S (another phenomenological coefficient), and $\overline{C}_S$ is an average membrane concentration, which in dilute solutions is given by:

$$\overline{C}_S = \frac{\Delta C_S}{\Delta \ln C_S}. \tag{2.16}$$

Models of glomerular filtration generally employ a modified form of Eq. (2.15). When applied to a portion of the membrane of infinitesimal thickness ∂y (Fig. 2.7), the Kedem-Katchalsky equation can be written as

$$J_S = J_V (1 - \sigma_S) C_S - D_S^{eff} \frac{\partial C_S}{\partial y}, \tag{2.17}$$

where the average concentration $\overline{C}_S$ is replaced by the actual concentration C_S in that infinitesimal portion, and the diffusive component of the flux is expressed using Fick's law: D_S^{eff} is the effective diffusivity of solute S in the membrane. At steady state, the volume and solute fluxes are constant and Eq. (2.17) can be rewritten as:

$$\frac{\partial C_S}{\partial y} = \frac{J_V (1 - \sigma_S) C_S}{D_S^{eff}} - \frac{J_S}{D_S^{eff}}. \tag{2.18}$$

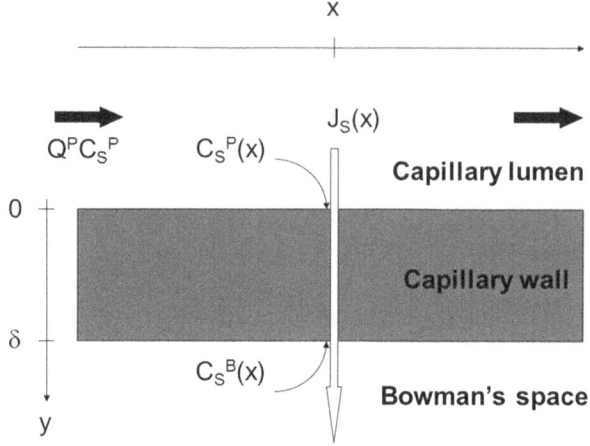

Fig. 2.7 Schematic representation of solute filtration across the capillary wall. Plasma flows in the x direction, and transversal fluxes are in the y direction

If the membrane is homogeneous, and if D_S^{eff} and σ_S are concentration-independent, integration of Eq. (2.18) between 0 and a given depth y yields:

$$C_S(y) = b_1 \exp(Pe\, y/\delta) + b_2, \tag{2.19}$$

where b_1 and b_2 are constants that will be determined below. The dimensionless Péclet number, Pe, is a measure of the importance of convection relative to diffusion:

$$Pe = \frac{J_V(1-\sigma_S)\delta}{D_S^{eff}}. \tag{2.20}$$

The permeability P_S is related to the diffusivity as $P_S = D_S^{eff}/\delta$, and the Péclet number is defined alternately as:

$$Pe = \frac{J_V(1-\sigma_S)}{P_S}. \tag{2.21}$$

A Péclet number much smaller than unity means that diffusive transport occurs much faster than convective transport. Conversely, if $Pe \gg 1$, convection predominates. The integration constants b_1 and b_2 in Eq. (2.19) can be determined knowing the boundary conditions at $y = 0$ and δ (Fig. 2.7):

$$C_S = C_S^P \quad \text{at } y = 0, \tag{2.22a}$$

$$C_S = C_S^B \quad \text{at } y = \delta. \tag{2.22b}$$

Substituting these boundary conditions into Eq. (2.19) yields:

$$b_1 = \frac{C_S^B - C_S^P}{\exp(Pe) - 1}, \quad b_2 = \frac{C_S^P \exp(Pe) - C_S^B}{\exp(Pe) - 1}. \tag{2.23}$$

2.3 Material Balance Equations

After re-arranging, we obtain:

$$C_S(y) = \left(\frac{\left(C_S^B - C_S^P\right) \exp\left(-Pe\left(1 - y/\delta\right)\right) + C_S^P - C_S^B \exp(-Pe)}{1 - \exp(-Pe)} \right). \quad (2.24)$$

Substituting Eq. (2.24) into Eq. (2.17) yields the solute flux as a function of the volume flux:

$$J_S = J_V (1 - \sigma_S) \left(\frac{C_S^P - C_S^B \exp(-Pe)}{1 - \exp(-Pe)} \right). \quad (2.25)$$

Equation (2.25) is known as the *Patlak equation* (Patlak et al. 1963). In the particular case of glomerular filtration, the Bowman's space concentration of each solute is assumed equal to the ratio of solute flux to volume flux, that is, $C_S^B = J_S/J_V$. Substituting this expression into Eq. (2.25) and rearranging yields:

$$J_S = \frac{J_V (1 - \sigma_S) C_S^P}{1 - \sigma_S \exp(-Pe)}. \quad (2.26)$$

2.3.3 Protein Plasma Concentration Profile

In 1963, Landis and Pappenheimer developed an equation that predicts the osmotic pressure of proteins as a function of total protein concentration and albumin fraction. Glomerular filtration models usually employ the following quadratic approximation of the original cubic equation:

$$\Pi_{pr}^P = a_1 C_{pr}^P + a_2 \left(C_{pr}^P\right)^2, \quad (2.27)$$

where $a_1 = 1.629$ mmHg/(g/dl) and $a_2 = 0.2935$ mmHg/(g/dl)^2. Equation (2.14) states that the molar flow rate of proteins in plasma is constant, so that $Q^P(x) = Q^A C_{pr}^A / C_{pr}^P(x)$, where the superscript "A" denotes afferent plasma values, i.e., at $x = 0$. We thus have:

$$\frac{dQ^P}{dx} = -\frac{Q^A C_{pr}^A}{\left(C_{pr}^P\right)^2} \frac{dC_{pr}^P}{dx}. \quad (2.28)$$

Substituting Eqs. (2.6, 2.9, and 2.27) into Eq. (2.28) yields:

$$\frac{dC_{pr}^P}{dx} = \frac{\left(C_{pr}^P\right)^2}{Q^A C_{pr}^A} \left(\frac{L_p S^P}{L} \right) \left[\Delta P - a_1 C_{pr}^P + a_2 \left(C_{pr}^P\right)^2 \right]. \quad (2.29)$$

If the hydraulic pressure difference is specified as a function of position, Eq. (2.29) can be integrated numerically to yield $C_{pr}^P(x)$. Changes in hydraulic pressure along the capillary wall are known to be small, so that ΔP can be approximated by a constant (ΔP_R) to which a small, linear term is added:

$$\Delta P(x) = \Delta P_R \left[1 - \varepsilon \left(x/L - 0.5\right)\right], \tag{2.30}$$

where the small parameter ε is taken to be <0.10. More often, ΔP is taken to remain constant along the capillary wall (i.e., $\varepsilon = 0$). Assuming a constant ΔP, Eq. (2.29) can be integrated analytically to yield an implicit equation for $C_{pr}^P(x)$. If we define the non-dimensional plasma protein concentration as $C^* \equiv C_{pr}^P/C_{pr}^A$, C^* satisfies (Deen et al. 1972):

$$\left(\frac{L_p S^P \Delta P_R}{L Q^A}\right) x + I = \frac{A_1}{2} \ln\left(\frac{C^{*2}}{1 - A_1 C^* - A_2 C^{*2}}\right) - \frac{1}{C^*} \\ + \left(\frac{A_1^2 + 2A_2}{2\sqrt{A_1^2 + 4A_2}}\right) \ln\left(\frac{\sqrt{A_1^2 + 4A_2} + A_1 + 2A_2 C^*}{\sqrt{A_1^2 + 4A_2} - A_1 - 2A_2 C^*}\right), \tag{2.31}$$

where I is an integration constant found by setting x to 0 and C^* to 1, and the coefficients A_1 and A_2 are given by:

$$A_1 = \frac{a_1 C_{pr}^A}{\Delta P_R}, \quad A_1 = \frac{a_2 \left(C_{pr}^A\right)^2}{\Delta P_R}.$$

2.3.4 Fundamental Equations of Glomerular Filtration

In summary, the starting point for models of glomerular filtration is the set of differential equations expressing fluid and solute conservation:

$$\frac{dQ^P}{dx} = -\frac{S^P}{L} J_V, \tag{2.32}$$

$$\frac{d\left(Q^P C_S^P\right)}{dx} = -\frac{S^P}{L} J_S, \tag{2.33}$$

$$\frac{d\left(Q^P C_{pr}^P\right)}{dx} = 0. \tag{2.34}$$

The boundary conditions are specified at the afferent end of the capillary:

$$Q^P(x=0) = Q^A, \quad C_S^P(x=0) = C_S^A, \quad C_{pr}^P(x=0) = C_{pr}^A,$$

where Q^A is the afferent plasma flow, and C_{pr}^A is the total protein concentration in afferent plasma. The volume and solute fluxes are respectively given by:

$$J_V = L_p \left(\Delta P - \Pi_{pr}^P \right), \tag{2.35}$$

$$J_S = \frac{J_V (1 - \sigma_S) C_S^P}{1 - \sigma_S \exp(-Pe)}, \tag{2.36}$$

where

$$\Pi_{pr}^P = a_1 C_{pr}^P + a_2 \left(C_{pr}^P \right)^2, \tag{2.37}$$

$$Pe = \frac{J_V (1 - \sigma_S)}{P_S}. \tag{2.38}$$

The value of ΔP is usually taken to be a constant between 30 and 50 mmHg. The ultrafiltration coefficient K_f (the product of L_p and S^P) can be estimated if measurements of GFR and/or FF are available:

$$K_f = \frac{GFR}{\left(\Delta P - <\Pi_{pr}^P> \right)} \approx \frac{GFR}{\left(\Delta P - \Pi_{pr}^A \right)}, \tag{2.39}$$

or

$$K_f \approx \frac{FF \, Q^A}{\left(\Delta P - \Pi_{pr}^A \right)}, \tag{2.40}$$

where Π_{pr}^A is the oncotic pressure evaluated at $x = 0$, knowing C_{pr}^A.

To integrate the differential equations along the x axis, solute permeabilities (P_S) and osmotic reflection coefficients (σ_S) must be specified in addition to the other inputs (Q^A, C_{pr}^A, ΔP, and possibly K_f). Once the integration is complete, solute concentrations in Bowman's space can be calculated and compared with experimental values to validate the model. The purpose of the following sections is to show how to choose appropriate and physically meaningful values for L_p, P_S, and σ_S.

2.4 Isoporous Model

2.4.1 General Assumptions

Early models of glomerular filtration represented the capillary wall as an isoporous membrane formed of parallel, cylindrical pores of uniform radius r_o. The hindered transport of uncharged, spherical solutes through uniform cylindrical pores has been extensively investigated, and the results of hydrodynamic theory can thus be employed to describe glomerular filtration across an isoporous capillary wall.

The first phenomenon to consider is partitioning, that is, the partial exclusion from the pore of a given macromolecule, by virtue of its size, shape, and charge. Consider an uncharged, spherical molecule of radius r_S. At equilibrium, its concentration within the pore depends on the volume available to the sphere. Since the distance between the center of the sphere and the pore wall must be greater than r_S, the ratio of the average solute concentration in the pore to that in the external fluid is given by (Anderson and Quinn 1974):

$$\phi_S = (1 - r_S/r_o)^2 = (1 - \lambda)^2, \tag{2.41}$$

where $\lambda = r_S/r_o$ is the ratio of the solute radius to that of the pore. The pore-to-bulk fluid solute concentration ratio at equilibrium, ϕ_S, is known as the solute *partition coefficient*. For charged or nonspherical solutes, more complex expressions of ϕ_S must be used.

In addition to steric (size-based) exclusion, the pore walls exert retarding effects on solute movement. These hydrodynamic effects are embodied in two factors, W_S and H_S, which respectively represent the hindrance to convective and diffusive solute transport. The factor W_S accounts for the fact that the solute velocity (evaluated at the particle center) differs from that of the fluid; this factor is equivalent to $(1 - \sigma_S)$. The factor H_S is the ratio of the pore-to-bulk fluid solute diffusivity, D_S^{eff}/D_S^{∞}.

Within this conceptual framework, the molar flux of solute S (per unit capillary surface area) is written as:

$$J_S = J_V W_S C_S - f H_S D_S^{\infty} \frac{\partial C_S}{\partial y}, \tag{2.42}$$

where f is the fraction of the capillary surface area that is occupied by pores. This factor is needed to distinguish J_S from the local solute flux within a pore; the volume flux J_V in Eq. (2.42) is also expressed per unit capillary surface area. By similarity with Eq. (2.26), the steady-state value of J_S is given by:

$$J_S = \frac{J_V W_S C_S^P}{1 - (1 - W_S) \exp(-Pe)}, \tag{2.43}$$

$$Pe = \frac{J_V W_S \delta}{H_S D_S^{\infty} f}. \tag{2.44}$$

The diffusivity D_S^{∞} of a spherical molecule of radius r_S is given by the Stokes-Einstein equation:

$$D_S^{\infty} = \frac{kT}{6\pi \eta r_S}, \tag{2.45}$$

where k is the Boltzmann's constant, and η is the viscosity of the fluid, usually taken as that of water (0.7 cP at 37 °C).

2.4.2 Hindrance Factors

The theory of hindered transport was first elaborated in the 1950s by Pappenheimer, Renkin and colleagues (Pappenheimer et al. 1951), who sought to describe the passage of molecules across capillary walls. Since then, many theoretical studies have focused on predicting hindered transport coefficients based upon the shape, size, and electrical charge of both solutes and pores. A comprehensive review of these theoretical developments can be found in Dechadilok and Deen (2006).

If the membrane consists of uniform cylindrical pores, W_S and H_S depend on the solute-to-pore radius, $\lambda = r_S/r_o$. In the absence of charge effects, steric and hydrodynamic hindrance becomes negligible as solute size becomes infinitely small ($\lambda \to 0$), and both factors tend towards unity. Conversely, as the radius of the solute approaches that of the pore ($\lambda \to 1$), transport is increasingly restricted, and W_S and H_S tend toward zero. For intermediate λ values, the hindrance factors are determined by solving the Navier-Stokes equations for flow past a spherical solute within a cylindrical pore, and calculating the hydrodynamic force and torque exerted on the solute. The computations are complex, and the results are often presented in tabular form. The expressions for W_S and H_S developed by Bungay and Brenner by asymptotic matching are among the very few analytical correlations found to be accurate over the entire range of λ values (Bungay and Brenner 1973). They are given here for convenience:

$$W_S = \frac{K_s \phi_S (2 - \phi_S)}{2 K_t}, \qquad (2.46)$$

$$H_S = \frac{6\pi \phi_S}{K_t}, \qquad (2.47)$$

where

$$K_t(\lambda) = \frac{9}{4}\pi^2 \sqrt{2} (1-\lambda)^{-5/2} \left[1 - \frac{73}{60}(1-\lambda) + \frac{77,293}{50,400}(1-\lambda)^2 \right] \\ - 22.5083 - 5.6117\lambda - 0.3363\lambda^2 - 1.216\lambda^3 + 1.647\lambda^4, \qquad (2.48)$$

$$K_s(\lambda) = \frac{9}{4}\pi^2 \sqrt{2} (1-\lambda)^{-5/2} \left[1 + \frac{7}{60}(1-\lambda) - \frac{2,227}{50,400}(1-\lambda)^2 \right] \\ + 4.0180 - 3.9788\lambda - 1.9215\lambda^2 + 4.392\lambda^3 + 5.006\lambda^4. \qquad (2.49)$$

2.4.3 Ultrafiltration Coefficient

The hydraulic conductivity of an isoporous capillary wall, L_P, can also be calculated explicitly under certain assumptions. For Poiseuille flow, the average velocity (U) in a pore of length δ is related to the axial pressure drop ΔP as:

$$U = \frac{r_o^2}{8\eta\delta}\Delta P. \qquad (2.50)$$

The water flux across the capillary surface area (i.e., $S^P J_V$) is also given by $f S^P U$. It can be shown that:

$$L_p = f\left(\frac{r_o^2}{8\eta\delta}\right). \qquad (2.51)$$

Hence, if K_f is known, the ratio of pore surface area-to-pore length can be calculated as:

$$\frac{fS^P}{\delta} = K_f\left(\frac{8\eta}{r_o^2}\right), \qquad (2.52)$$

which can be obtained by multiplying Eq. (2.51) by S^P and applying the relation $S^P L_p = K_f$.

As described below, it is also helpful to express the Péclet number as a function of r_o. Substituting Eqs. (2.35) and (2.51) into the expression for Pe (Eq. 2.44) yields:

$$Pe = \left(\frac{r_o^2}{8\eta}\right)\left(\frac{W_S}{H_S D_S^\infty}\right)(\Delta P - \Pi_{pr}^P). \qquad (2.53)$$

2.4.4 Fitting the Model to Experimental Data

In the isoporous model, the capillary wall is essentially characterized by one parameter, r_o. If the ultrafiltration coefficient cannot be estimated, the pore surface area-to-length ratio constitutes another unknown. This (or these) parameter(s) are chosen so as to minimize the difference between model predictions and experimental data. The following procedure is used to do so:

1. An initial guess for r_o is made. If K_f is given, then $f S^P/\delta$ is determined using Eq. (2.52), otherwise this quantity must also be guessed.
2. For each filtered solute that is being considered, W_S and H_S are calculated as described in Sect. 2.4.2.
3. The afferent values of Q^P, C_S^P and C_{pr}^P are prescribed at $x = 0$, and the corresponding differential equations are integrated along the x axis; volume and solute fluxes are updated at each step.
4. Once the integration from $x = 0$ to L is complete, filtrate-to-plasma concentration ratios are calculated as described immediately below. These predicted values are then compared to experimental data.
5. If the fit is poor, the sum of squared errors (SSE in Eq. 2.3) can be minimized by an iterative procedure so as to yield a better estimate of the parameter r_o and possibly the other unknowns.

2.5 Heteroporous Models

The filtrate-to-plasma concentration ratio of solute S is equal to its average concentration in Bowman's space divided by that in afferent plasma (C_S^A):

$$\theta_S(r_o) = \frac{1}{C_S^A} \frac{\int_0^L J_S(x)dx}{\int_0^L J_V(x)dx}. \tag{2.54}$$

As described above, this ratio is equal to the sieving coefficient of the solute if the molar flow rate of the later does not vary along renal tubules. Hence, for the purpose of validating the model, "test" solutes that are neither reabsorbed nor secreted by the tubules are administered to experimental subjects, and their sieving coefficient measured. To obtain the best fit, these test molecules should encompass a wide range of solute radii, so that predicted filtrate-to-plasma concentration ratios match experimental sieving values over a large distribution of solute size.

2.4.5 Isoporous Model Limitations

The isoporous model has the advantage of being relatively easy to formulate and implement. This model successfully predicts –and helps to interpret– clearance data in some cases, such as in normal rats and those with nephritic syndrome (a glomerular disorder characterized by the presence of red blood cells and proteins in urine). However, isoporous model predictions have been deemed incompatible with experimental results in several human diseases, such as diabetic nephropathy and glomerulonephritis. In both cases, the fractional clearances of dextrans in patients with severe injury were found to be lower for the smallest dextrans, and higher for the largest dextrans, compared with those in healthy, or less nephrotic, individuals, which is inconsistent with an isoporous representation of the capillary wall (Deen et al. 1985). Thus, more sophisticated representations of the glomerular capillary wall were subsequently developed, as described below.

2.5 Heteroporous Models

2.5.1 Model Formulation

Heteroporous models assume that the glomerular barrier can be represented by a distribution of pore sizes. As discussed below, their ability to describe clearance data in nephrotic humans was found to be significantly greater than that of isoporous models. Here, we first describe the model equations for an arbitrary distribution of pore sizes, and then focus on particular distributions that are currently being used by nephrologists for interpreting clinical data.

The pore size distribution is taken to be uniform over the capillary length, and is characterized by a function $g(r)$ such that $\int_r^{r+dr} g(s)ds$ is the fraction of pores with radii comprised between r and $(r+dr)$. Similarly, $\int_r^{r+dr} \Omega(s)ds$ is the fraction of the filtrate volume passing through pores with radii between r and $(r+dr)$. Note that by definition:

$$\int_0^\infty g(r)dr = \int_0^\infty \Omega(r)dr = 1. \tag{2.55}$$

Poiseuille flow indicates that $\Omega(r)$ should scale with $r^4 g(r)$ if the pressure drop is identical across all pores. In fact, since very large pores are permeable to proteins whereas small ones are not, the filtrate-to-plasma oncotic pressure difference decreases (and the net pressure difference increases) with increasing pore size. There is, however, a counteracting effect: filtrate viscosity increases in the presence of protein, i.e., η increases with r. Assuming that these competing effects counterbalance each other, we may assume that $\Omega(r)$ is proportional to $r^4 g(r)$. Given the normalization condition (Eq. 2.55), this means that:

$$\Omega(r) = \frac{r^4 g(r)}{\int_0^\infty r^4 g(r)dr}. \tag{2.56}$$

Next, we define $N_V(x, r)$ such that $\int_r^{r+dr} N_V(x, s)ds$ is the portion of the volume flux $J_V(x)$ that is attributable to pores with radii between r and $(r+dr)$. Given the definition of $\Omega(r)$, we have:

$$N_V(x, r) = \Omega(r) J_V(x). \tag{2.57}$$

We also define $N_S(x, r)$ such that $\int_r^{r+dr} N_S(x, s)ds$ is the portion of the solute flux $J_S(x)$ that is attributable to pores with radii between r and $(r+dr)$. There is no simple relationship between $N_S(x, r)$ and $J_S(x)$. Instead we can use Eqs. (2.43) and (2.53) to relate N_S and N_V for a given pore size:

$$N_S(x, r) = \frac{N_V(x, r) W_S(r) C_S^P(x)}{1 - [1 - W_S(r)] \exp(-Pe(x, r))}, \tag{2.58}$$

$$Pe(x, r) = \left(\frac{r^2}{8\eta}\right) \left(\frac{W_S(r)}{H_S(r) D_S^\infty}\right) (\Delta P - \Pi_{pr}^P(x)), \tag{2.59}$$

where $W_S(r)$ and $H_S(r)$ are calculated as described above, replacing r_o with r. Note that by definition,

2.5 Heteroporous Models

$$J_V(x) = \int_0^\infty N_V(x,r)\,dr, \qquad (2.60)$$

$$J_S(x) = \int_0^\infty N_S(x,r)\,dr. \qquad (2.61)$$

The filtrate-to-plasma concentration ratio for solute S is then given by:

$$\theta_S = \frac{1}{C_S^A} \frac{\int_0^L \int_0^\infty N_S(x,r)\,dr\,dx}{\int_0^L J_V(x)\,dx}. \qquad (2.62)$$

By inverting the integration order, it can be shown that θ_S may be calculated as:

$$\theta_S = \int_0^\infty \Omega(r)\theta_S(r)\,dr, \qquad (2.63)$$

where $\theta_S(r)$ is the fractional clearance determined using the isoporous model with $r_o = r$. In other words, the contribution of a given pore size to the overall fractional clearance is proportional to the fraction of volume that is filtered across that pore size. Finally, the relationship between K_f and fS/δ is similar to that obtained for the isoporous model:

$$\frac{fS}{\delta} = 8\eta K_f \frac{\int_0^\infty r^2 g(r)\,dr}{\int_0^\infty r^4 g(r)\,dr}. \qquad (2.64)$$

2.5.2 Continuous Pore Size Distributions

A commonly used distribution of pore sizes is the lognormal distribution. Its two parameters, u and ς, respectively characterize the mean and spread of the distribution:

$$g(r) = \frac{1}{\sqrt{2\pi}\, r\, \ln(\varsigma)} \exp\left[-\frac{1}{2}\left(\frac{\ln(r/u)}{\ln(\varsigma)}\right)^2\right]. \qquad (2.65)$$

The normal distribution, with parameters μ and ν, is also used sometimes:

$$g(r) = \frac{\gamma}{\nu} \exp\left[-\frac{1}{2}\left(\frac{r-\mu}{\nu}\right)^2\right]. \qquad (2.66)$$

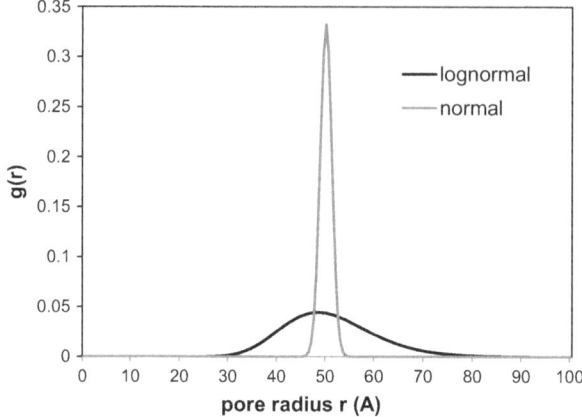

Fig. 2.8 Probability density function for the lognormal and normal distributions of pore sizes. The parameters u and μ are taken as 50 Å, and the parameters ς and ν as 1.20 Å

Note that the constant γ is not equal to $\sqrt{2\pi}$, as in standard probability theory, because the distribution is restricted to positive values of r. Instead, it depends on μ and ν, and must be evaluated so that $g(r)$ satisfies the normalization condition Eq. (2.55). Examples of lognormal and normal distributions are plotted on Fig. 2.8.

2.5.3 Discrete Pore Size Distributions

A popular alternative to these continuous distributions is the isoporous-plus-shunt model. This representation assumes two discrete populations of pores, one with a uniform radius r_o, and one with a radius so large that it is not selective and can be viewed as a shunt. This shunt pathway is characterized by ω, the fraction of the filtrate volume passing through the nonselective pores. The overall solute flux is thus written as the sum of two contributions:

$$J_S = (1-\omega)\, J_S\,(r_o) + \omega J_V C_S, \qquad (2.67)$$

where $J_S(r_o)$ is the "isoporous" solute flux evaluated using Eq. (2.43). The second term on the RHS of Eq. (2.67) reflects the hypothesis that $W_S = H_S = 1$ across the shunt pathway. The fraction ω is usually $\ll 1$, ranging from 0.001 in normal subjects to $\sim$0.02 in patients with severe nephrotic range proteinuria. Thus, Eq. (2.67) can be simplified as:

$$J_S = J_S\,(r_o) + \omega J_V C_S. \qquad (2.68)$$

2.5 Heteroporous Models

Note that ω is not an intrinsic membrane property, in that it depends on position along the capillary, even if the size and fraction of the small and nonselective pores remain constant. Indeed, the driving force for fluid flow across the small pores $(\Delta P - \Pi_{pr}^P)$ varies along the capillary length, whereas that across non-selective pores (ΔP) does not. Hence, the fraction of the filtrate volume going through the shunts also varies with x. A characteristic of the membrane per se is the fraction of the filtrate volume that would pass through the non-selective pores if plasma proteins were absent. Denoting this parameter ω_o, it can be shown that (see Problem 2.3):

$$\omega(x) = \frac{1}{1 + \left(\frac{1-\omega_o}{\omega_o}\right)\left(\frac{\Delta P - \Pi_{pr}^P(x)}{\Delta P}\right)\left(\frac{\eta^P}{\eta^S}\right)}, \tag{2.69}$$

where η^P/η^S is the plasma-to-saline viscosity ratio (taken as 1.6) and reflects the difference in filtrate properties between small and large pores. The two parameters r_o and ω_o suffice to fully determine the isoporous-plus-shunt distribution.

2.5.4 Approximate Integration of Mass Balance Equations

As with the isoporous model, the parameters of a given heteroporous model are determined by minimizing the differences between predicted and measured values of θ_S for solutes that are neither secreted nor reabsorbed.

There are several ways to numerically integrate the mass balance equations and determine fractional clearances using heteroporous models:

- The first one consists in evaluating $\theta_S(r)$ for the range of pore radii considered, using the isoporous model for each value of r and following the procedure described in Sect. 2.4.4. The overall sieving coefficient can then be evaluated using Eq. (2.63).
- The second method consists in considering the pore size distribution at each step of the integration process. At a given position x, the volume flux $J_V(x)$ is calculated using Eq. (2.35).
    - Assuming a continuous distribution $g(r)$, $N_V(x,r)$ and $N_S(x,r)$ are then determined for each value of r with Eqs. (2.57) and (2.58). The solute flux $J_S(x)$ is subsequently obtained by integrating $N_S(x,r)$ over all the r values (Eq. 2.61).
    - Assuming an isoporous-plus-shunt representation, the solute flux is calculated based upon Eq. (2.68) instead. Knowing J_V and J_S, the plasma and solute flows at the next step can be determined.

  Once the mass balance equations are integrated along the entire x axis, the overall sieving coefficient is determined using Eq. (2.62).
- The third method consists in approximating the volume and solute fluxes with analytical expressions, to avoid the numerical integration of the mass balance

equations. Since plasma proteins are not filtered by the glomerulus, their concentration increases along the capillary, thereby reducing the driving force for fluid reabsorption. The J_V decrease can be approximated by an exponential decay such that:

$$J_V(x) = J_V^A \exp(-bx/L), \tag{2.70}$$

where J_V^A is the volume flux at the afferent end of the capillary, which can be calculated based on the boundary conditions at $x = 0$. The constant b is obtained by integrating the plasma flow equation (Eq. 2.32) from 0 to L:

$$\int_0^L \frac{dQ^P}{dx} dx = -\frac{S^P}{L} \int_0^L J_V dx, \tag{2.71}$$

$$Q^P(L) - Q^A = S^P J_V^A \left(\frac{\exp(-b) - 1}{b} \right). \tag{2.72}$$

By definition, the filtration fraction FF equals $1 - Q^P(L)/Q^A$, and Eq. (2.72) can be expressed as:

$$\frac{b}{1 - \exp(-b)} = \left(\frac{S^P J_V^A}{FF \, Q^A} \right). \tag{2.73}$$

The constant b can thus be determined based on known parameters. Similarly, the rate at which solute concentration increases along the capillary length is assumed to be exponential:

$$C_S^P(x) = C_S^A \left[1 + a_S \left(1 - \exp(-bx/L) \right) \right]. \tag{2.74}$$

The constant a_S is obtained by noting that the molar flow of solute at the capillary outlet must equal that at the inlet minus that in Bowman space, which after rearrangement yields (see Problem 2.2):

$$a_S = \frac{FF (1 - \theta_S)}{(1 - FF)(1 - \exp(-b))}. \tag{2.75}$$

The ultimate objective here is to calculate sieving coefficients more easily, without numerical integration of the differential equations. To do so, we must derive an analytical expression for solute fluxes too. Replacing the analytical expression for J_V into Eq. (2.43) yields:

$$J_S = \frac{J_V^A W_S C_S^A \left[1 + a_S \left(1 - \exp(-bx/L) \right) \right]}{1 - (1 - W_S) \exp(-Pe)}, \tag{2.76}$$

where the Péclet number equals, for a given pore radius:

2.5 Heteroporous Models

Table 2.1 Sum of squared errors (SSE) for different pore-size distributions

Distribution	Normal	Grade I	Grade III
Isoporous	1.75	3.40	2.34
Isoporous with shunt	0.473	0.205	0.095
Lognormal	0.653	0.399	0.251
Normal	0.711	0.517	0.359

Adapted from Deen et al. (1985)
For each pore size distribution, the characteristic parameters (e.g., u and ς for the lognormal distribution) were chosen so as to minimize the difference between measured and predicted sieving coefficients. The lowest SSE values of the different distributions were then compared. The lower SSE, the better the ability of the model to simulate the dextran fractional data shown in Fig. 2.3. Note that a 10 % difference between measured and predicted sieving coefficients for each of the 17 dextran sizes examined would yield SSE = 0.17

$$Pe = \left(\frac{r^2}{8\eta}\right) \left(\frac{W_S}{H_S D_S^\infty}\right) \left(\Delta P - \Pi_{pr}^A\right) \exp\left(-bx/L\right). \tag{2.77}$$

The sieving coefficient corresponding to a given pore radius is then given by:

$$\theta_S(r) = \frac{W_S b/L}{1 - \exp(-b)} \int_0^L \frac{[1 + a_S (1 - \exp(-bx/L))]}{1 - (1 - W_S) \exp(-Pe)} dx. \tag{2.78}$$

The overall sieving coefficient is then determined by integrating over all pore sizes (Eq. 2.63). How big are the errors using this approximate method? Deen et al. (1985) examined 36 cases in which they varied Q^A, ΔP, and solute radius, and found that the absolute value of the relative error (i.e., the relative difference between the exact and approximate values of θ_S) averaged 1.7 %.

Once mass balance equations are integrated following either of these three approaches, model parameters are adjusted by minimizing the sum of squared errors (SSE in Eq. 2.3) as described above.

2.5.5 Heteroporous Model Performance

What can these pore models tell us about changes in the properties of the capillary wall in disease states? The nephrotic syndrome is a group of symptoms which include the leak of proteins into urine. Deen et al. (1985) used the sieving curves of healthy and nephrotic patients (shown in Fig. 2.3) to determine the parameters of several hypothetical pore distributions under these different conditions. The model with the best ability to predict all sieving curves was then chosen to interpret in physical terms the effects of proteinuria on the filtration barrier.

Shown in Table 2.1 are the SSE values for four different distributions (isoporous, isoporous with shunt, lognormal, and normal) and three different conditions

Table 2.2 Optimal parameter values for the isoporous-plus-shunt model

	Normal	Grade I	Grade III
r_o (Å)	57.5	54.1	55.9
ω_o	0.0018	0.0072	0.0202

Adapted from Deen et al. (1985)
The model is characterized by two parameters: r_o is the radius of the small pores, and ω_o is the fraction of the filtrate that would pass through the large non-selective pores (i.e., the shunts) in the absence of plasma proteins

(normal, nephrotic grade I, and nephrotic grade III) each. It can be seen that the isoporous-plus-shunt model consistently outperforms the other models in terms of its ability to fit experimental sieving curves.

The optimal parameter values for this model are given in Table 2.2. The most probable radius of the small pores varies little amongst the three patient populations. In contrast, the contribution of the shunt pathway increases very significantly going from normal controls to grade I and then grade III nephrotics: ω_o is respectively four- and tenfold higher in grade I and grade III patients, relative to controls. These results suggest overall that the more severe the degree of proteinuria (as assessed by the fractional clearance of IgG), the greater the amount of filtrate volume that passes through the non-selective shunt pathway, and the less size-selective the filtration barrier. In grade III nephrotics, as much as 2 % of GFR is predicted to flow through the shunt pathway.

2.5.6 Heteroporous Model Limitations

Even though the isoporous-plus-shunt model adequately simulated dextran sieving curves in the cases examined just above, it was not able to reproduce experimental measurements of albumin and IgG fractional clearances. There may have been at least two reasons for this discrepancy: variations in molecular charge and molecular configuration. The pore models described above apply to the transport of non-charged solutes, whereas albumin is highly anionic at physiological pH values. In addition, dextran does not behave as a neutral, rigid sphere, which is why it was replaced as a test molecule by Ficoll in the 1990s. Another important limitation of the pore models is that they do not take into account the sophisticated ultrastructure of the capillary wall, the three layers of which greatly differ in their size- and charge-selectivity properties (see below).

Nonetheless, due to the ease with which pore models can be used and their results interpreted, they are still today preferentially used by biophysicists and nephrologists to interpret disease- or agent-mediated changes in the selectivity of the glomerular barrier; as an example, see the study of Sangalli et al. (2011).

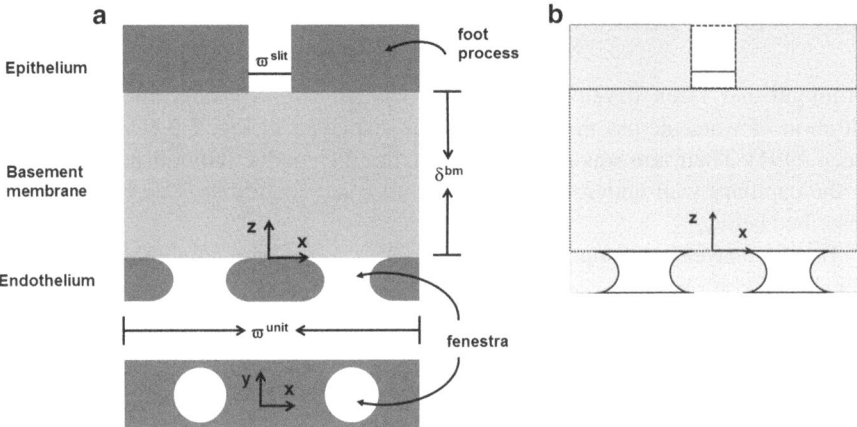

Fig. 2.9 (a) Structural unit of the glomerular capillary wall. *Top*: cross-sectional view, with the three layers of the barrier. *Bottom*: endothelial layer with fenestrated openings. The ultrastructural model represents the wall as a series of such identical units, and assumes a zipper configuration for the filtration slit (Fig. 2.2). The filtrate flows along the z-axis. (**b**) Representation of computational domains: upper rectangle with dashed contour, epithelial slit; middle rectangle with dotted contour, glomerular basement membrane; lower domains with solid contours, endothelial fenestrae (Adapted from Drumond and Deen (1994))

2.6 Ultrastructural Model of Glomerular Filtration

Starting in the early 1990s, Deen and collaborators began to develop new models of glomerular filtration based on the specific ultrastructure of the capillary wall. The goal of such models is to relate the permeability properties of the wall to its unique cellular, and even molecular, characteristics. In this perspective, the "effective pore" approach is replaced by a meticulous analysis of the contribution of each layer.

Since ultrastructural models of water and solute filtration are both very detailed and complex, we merely summarize the main underlying concepts below. A more thorough description can be found in several publications (Drumond and Deen 1994; Edwards et al. 1999; Deen et al. 2001).

The capillary wall is represented as a series of identical, 3-dimensional, repeating basic structural units (shown in Fig. 2.9). Important geometrical parameters include the width of the filtration slit (ϖ^{slit} ~40 nm in both rats and humans), the thickness of the glomerular basement membrane (δ^{bm} ~200 nm in rats, 400 nm in humans), the dimensions of each fenestra and the number of fenestrae per filtration slit, and the width of the filtration unit (ϖ^{unit}). The latter, which is determined based on the fraction of surface area occupied by slits, is estimated as 360 nm in rats and 500 nm in humans.

2.6.1 Water Filtration

Drumond and Deen developed a highly detailed hydrodynamic model for the filtration of water across the structural unit displayed in Fig. 2.9 (Drumond and Deen 1994). Their aim was to predict the hydraulic conductivity (or permeability) of the capillary wall under normal and pathological conditions. Key concepts are described below.

The three layers constitute resistances in series. Since permeability is the inverse of resistance, we have:

$$\frac{1}{L_p^{gcw}} = \frac{1}{L_p^{en}} + \frac{1}{L_p^{bm}} + \frac{1}{L_p^{ep}}, \qquad (2.79)$$

where the subscripts "gcw", "en", "bm" and "ep" respectively denote the glomerular capillary wall, the endothelium, the basement membrane, and the epithelium. In turn, the hydraulic conductivity of a layer j is calculated as:

$$L_p^j = \frac{\bar{v}_z^j}{\overline{\Delta P}_j}, \qquad (2.80)$$

where z is the direction of filtration (perpendicular to the glomerular barrier), $\bar{v}_z^j$ is the average of the z-component of the velocity (determined over the entire layer width), and $\overline{\Delta P}_j$ is the average pressure drop across the layer.

Epithelium

Across the filtration slits, the velocity profile and hydraulic conductivity are determined by solving the *Stokes and continuity equations*:

$$\nabla P = \eta \nabla^2 \underline{v}, \qquad (2.81)$$

$$\nabla \cdot \underline{v} = 0, \qquad (2.82)$$

where $\underline{v}$ is the 3-dimensional velocity vector. Note that the Stokes equation is used instead of Navier-Stokes because the Reynolds number is close to zero (Re $\sim 10^{-6}$). The continuity equation expresses local conservation of mass (i.e., incompressibility). The corresponding computational domain is shown in Fig. 2.9. The boundary conditions specify the velocity at the interface with the foot processes and the basement membrane, as well as downstream from the filtration slits, that is, at the interface with Bowman's space. Given the complex 3-dimensional geometry of the slit diaphragm, a numerical solution must be sought. Using a finite-element

2.6 Ultrastructural Model of Glomerular Filtration

approach, L_p^{ep} is estimated as 8.6×10^{-9} m·s^{-1}·Pa^{-1} for normal rats (Drumond and Deen 1994).

Glomerular Basement Membrane

In fibrous media such as the glomerular basement membrane, fluid flow may be described by *Darcy's law*, provided that the dimensions of the entire layer are much larger than those of the fibers. In this approach, the velocity and pressure are averaged over a length scale that is large compared to the size of each fiber, but small relative to that of the overall barrier. That is, micro-structural details are not explicitly considered, but embedded in a microscale parameter, the Darcy permeability (κ) of the medium. Darcy's law is given by:

$$\underline{v} = -\frac{\kappa}{\eta}\nabla P. \tag{2.83}$$

This equation is solved together with the continuity equation (2.82), with prescribed velocity boundary conditions at all boundaries of the basement membrane (see Fig. 2.9). Assuming that κ equals 2.7 nm^2, L_p^{bm} is calculated as 8.3×10^{-9} m·s^{-1}·Pa^{-1} for normal rats (Drumond and Deen 1994).

Endothelium

Assuming that the endothelial fenestrae are filled with water, the pressure and velocity profiles in each fenestra are obtained by solving the Stokes and continuity equations (Eqs. 2.81 and 2.82) in the computational domains shown in Fig. 2.9. The no-slip boundary condition must be satisfied at the fenestra walls (at the interface with the endothelial cells), and the pressure at the entrance of the fenestra is set to the luminal pressure. At the interface between the fenestrae and the basement membrane, the pressure, velocities and viscous stress must match. However, because Darcy's law does not involve velocity derivatives, it can give rise to discontinuities in shear stress or velocity at boundaries. For this reason, the *Brinkman equation* is used in a small region of the basement membrane next to the fenestrae:

$$\nabla P = \eta \nabla^2 \underline{v} - \frac{\eta}{\kappa}\underline{v}. \tag{2.84}$$

This equation is a semi-empirical combination of the Stokes equation and Darcy's law. Because it includes derivatives of $\underline{v}$, it makes it possible to equate the viscous stresses on either side of the basement membrane-fenestra interface:

$$(\tau_{zr})_f = (\tau_{zr})_{bm}, \tag{2.85a}$$

Table 2.3 Hydraulic conductivity calculations

	Case 1: glycocalyx-filled fenestrae	Case 2: water-filled fenestrae
L_p^{en}	1.3×10^{-8} (24 %)	2.0×10^{-7} (2 %)
L_p^{bm}	8.3×10^{-9} (39 %)	8.3×10^{-9} (50 %)
L_p^{ep}	8.6×10^{-9} (37 %)	8.6×10^{-9} (48 %)
L_p^{gcw}	3.2×10^{-9}	4.1×10^{-9}

Hydraulic conductivity units are $m \cdot s^{-1} \cdot Pa^{-1}$. Numbers in parenthesis indicate the fractional resistance, relative to that of the overall barrier

$$(\tau_{zz})_f = (\tau_{zz})_{bm}, \quad (2.85b)$$

where the subscript "f" denotes fenestrae, and the viscous stress for a Newtonian fluid with constant density is given by:

$$\underline{\underline{\tau}} = \mu \left(\nabla \underline{v} + \left(\nabla \underline{v} \right)^t \right). \quad (2.86)$$

Whether the fenestrae are filled with fluid or with glycocalyx remains uncertain. Assuming that they contain a sparse fiber matrix instead of water, the pressure and velocity profiles in the fenestrae are determined using Brinkman's equation, with the same boundary conditions as described above. If the Darcy permeability of the glycocalyx equals that of the basement membrane, L_p^{en} is estimated as 1.3×10^{-8} $m \cdot s^{-1} \cdot Pa^{-1}$ for normal rats. However, since the value of the glycocalyx κ is unknown, that estimate is very uncertain. When, alternatively, the Stokes equation is used to determine the hydraulic resistance of water-filled fenestrae, L_p^{en} is computed instead as 2.0×10^{-7} $m \cdot s^{-1} \cdot Pa^{-1}$ (Drumond and Deen 1994).

Overall Barrier

Lastly, the hydraulic conductivity of the entire wall (L_p^{gcw}) is then computed using Eq. (2.79). The predicted values of L_p^{gcw}, on the order of 4×10^{-9} $m \cdot s^{-1} \cdot Pa^{-1}$ as summarized in Table 2.3, are in good agreement with experimental measurements, which range from 3×10^{-9} to 5×10^{-9} $m \cdot s^{-1} \cdot Pa^{-1}$ (Drumond and Deen 1994).

It has been noted that the zipper configuration is likely too tight in view of sieving measurements, and the contribution of the epithelial layer to L_p^{gcw} may have been overestimated. However, that of the endothelial layer may have been underestimated. Altogether, these results suggest that the resistance of the glomerular basement membrane to water flow accounts for approximately half that of the capillary wall (Deen et al. 2001).

2.6 Ultrastructural Model of Glomerular Filtration

Pathophysiological Applications

The hydrodynamic model described above has been successfully applied to a number of pathophysiological conditions. To give one illustration, in a group of patients with membranous nephropathy, kidney biopsies showed a significant reduction in filtration slit frequency accompanied by a thickening of the glomerular basement membrane (Squarer et al. 1998). The corresponding parameters ϖ^{unit} and δ^{bm} were found to be approximately four- and twofold higher than in controls. The model therefore predicted a 66 % reduction in L_p^{gcw} in those patients. This reduction was partly counterbalanced by a 37 % increase in the filtration surface area, caused by glomerular hypertrophy. Overall, K_f was predicted to decrease by 52 % in membranous nephropathy, which would explain by itself the observed 45 % decrease in GFR, from 102 to 56 ml/min/1.73 m² (Squarer et al. 1998).

2.6.2 Filtration of Macromolecules

Theoretical efforts to relate the solute permeability of the capillary wall to its 3-layer structure have also begun, but mathematical models have yet to incorporate a number of complex phenomena, as discussed further below.

Whereas the overall resistance to water flow is equal to the *sum* of the individual resistances of each layer (Eq. 2.79), the overall sieving coefficient can be determined as the *product* of the individual sieving coefficients:

$$\theta_S = \theta_S^{en} \theta_S^{bm} \theta_S^{ep}, \qquad (2.87)$$

where θ_S^j is the concentration of solute S at the downstream edge of layer j divided by that at the upstream edge. Equation (2.87) is obtained by matching concentrations at the interface between the endothelium and the basement membrane, and at that between the basement membrane and the epithelium. Note that this can only be done at the level of each structural unit, since concentrations vary along the length of the capillary. In other words, Eq. (2.87) is valid locally. To compute sieving coefficients for the entire capillary, average solute concentrations in Bowman's space must be determined.

One consequence of this relationship is that relative changes in either θ_S^{en}, θ_S^{bm}, or θ_S^{ep} impact θ_S to similar degrees: whether the individual sieving coefficient is ~ 1 (low perm-selectivity) or $\ll 1$ (high perm-selectivity), a 10 % variation will affect the overall θ_S by 10 % approximately (since individual sieving coefficients are interdependent, as described below, θ_S does not vary by exactly 10 %).

Individual sieving coefficients are obtained by solving for concentration profiles in each layer, wherein the three-dimensional flux of solute S ($\underline{N}_S$) is expressed as:

$$\underline{N}_S = \underline{v} \, W_S C_S - H_S D_S^\infty \nabla C_S. \qquad (2.88)$$

Equation (2.88) is the 3-dimensional form of Eq. (2.42). At steady state, conservation of mass yields:

$$\nabla \cdot \underline{N}_S = 0. \quad (2.89)$$

This conservation equation is coupled with appropriate boundary conditions at solid surfaces and at the interfaces between adjacent layers (where fluxes and concentrations must match). It is solved numerically to determine local concentrations in all three layers, from which an overall sieving coefficient can then be computed.

A one-dimensional approximation of the glomerular basement membrane (GBM) model can yield some insight into the structural determinants of permselectivity. Assuming that the GBM extends from $y = 0$ to δ^{bm}, and that the fluid velocity v_y is constant, it can be shown that (Problem 2.4):

$$\theta_S^{bm} = \frac{\phi_S W_S}{\theta_S^{ep}(1-\exp(-Pe)) + \phi_S W_S \exp(-Pe)}, \quad (2.90)$$

where ϕ_S is the equilibrium partition coefficient of solute S, which taken to be equal on both sides of the GBM. The Péclet number is given by:

$$Pe = \frac{v_y W_S \delta^{bm}}{H_S D_S^\infty}. \quad (2.91)$$

This simplified analysis serves to illustrate several points. Firstly, individual sieving coefficients are not independent: θ_S^{bm} is a function of θ_S^{ep}. Not only that, but if θ_S^{ep} is sufficiently small, θ_S^{bm} can become greater than unity, as illustrated in Fig. 2.10. In other words, when $\theta_S^{ep} \ll 1$, solute concentration within the GBM may increase in the direction of flow. This phenomenon, known as concentration polarization, stems from the fact that in the presence of very restrictive slit diaphragms, the GBM must also limit solute flux: the GBM concentration increase serves to drive solute diffusion in the opposite direction, thereby reducing transport towards the slits.

Figure 2.10 also illustrates the dependence of θ_S^{bm} on Pe. For very small values of Pe, θ_S^{bm} is close to unity, independently of other parameter values; i.e., as convection becomes negligible, the concentration field in the GBM becomes uniform. As Pe rises, θ_S^{bm} either increases above 1 if $\theta_S^{ep} < \phi_S W_S$ — which is when concentration polarization occurs — or decreases below 1 if $\theta_S^{ep} > \phi_S W_S$.

2.6.3 Current Limitations

The models presented thus far do not account for charge selectivity. A number of experiments have suggested that the filtration of negatively charged macromolecules

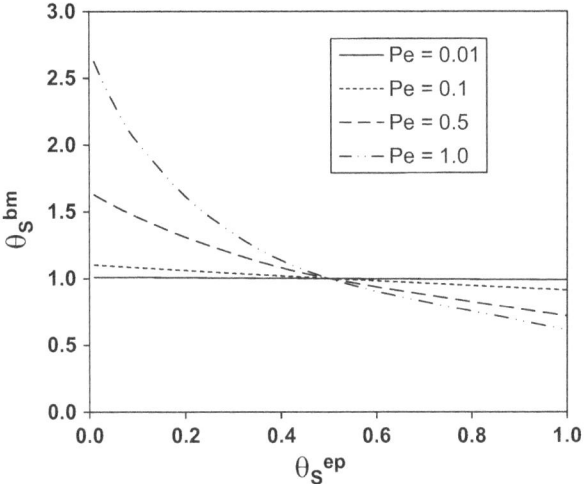

Fig. 2.10 Glomerular basement membrane (GBM) sieving coefficient (θ_S^{bm}) as a function of epithelial slit sieving coefficient (θ_S^{ep}) and Péclet number (*Pe*). In this simplified 1D model of the GBM, θ_S^{bm} is given by Eq. (2.90). The value of $\phi_S W_S$ is taken as 0.5, within the estimated range for a macromolecule with a 3–5 nM radius

across the glomerular capillary wall is more restricted than that of neutral molecules of similar size and configuration (Guasch et al. 1993; Lindstrom et al. 1998). However, others have disputed these findings. In particular, the selectivity of the barrier to albumin and the origin of proteinuria remain highly controversial (Russo et al. 2007; Comper et al. 2008; Jarad and Miner 2009; Peti-Peterdi 2009). None of the structure-based models built so far considers charge effects.

The sieving coefficients of test macromolecules such as Ficoll have been shown to vary with protein concentration (Ohlson et al. 2001). This results from the fact that steric interactions between tracers and proteins are enhanced in a concentrated solution, thereby lowering the energy barrier for tracer entry into adjacent fibrous or porous material (Deen et al. 2001). In other words, the presence of proteins such as albumin affects the partitioning of other solutes into the capillary wall. There have been some attempts to incorporate the effect of proteins on sieving coefficients (Edwards et al. 1999), but a rigorous theoretical approach has yet to be implemented.

2.7 Problems

Problem 2.1. Calculate the ultrafiltration coefficient for two groups of Munich Wistar rats with extensive kidney ablation.

After removal of the right kidney and segmental infarction of 2/3rds of the left kidney, Group I received no therapy, whereas Group 2 was given the Angiotensin I-

Table 2.4 Parameters for Problem 2.1

	Q^A (nl/min)	FF	P^{GC} (mmHg)	P^T (mmHg)	C_{pr}^A (g/100 ml)	C_{pr}^E (g/100 ml)
Group 1	234	0.31	68	18	5.5	8.0
Group 2	242	0.28	53	17	5.5	7.6

Data taken from Anderson et al. (1986)
P^{GC} and P^T denote the hydraulic pressure in the capillary and in the proximal tubule. C_{pr}^A and C_{pr}^E denote the afferent and efferent arteriolar plasma protein concentration

converting enzyme inhibitor, enalapril. Based on the parameters given in Table 2.4, determine K_f (in nl/s/mmHg) for each group. Comment on the results.

Problem 2.2. Show that when using an approximate integration of the mass balance equations (Eq. 2.74), the constant a_S is given by (Eq. 2.75):

$$a_S = \frac{FF(1-\theta_S)}{(1-FF)(1-\exp(-b))}.$$

Problem 2.3. Demonstrate that the fraction of the filtrate volume passing through the nonselective pores at a given position along the glomerular capillary is given by Eq. (2.69), that is:

$$\omega = \frac{1}{1+\left(\frac{1-\omega_0}{\omega_0}\right)\left(\frac{\Delta P - \Pi_{pr}^P}{\Delta P}\right)\left(\frac{\eta^P}{\eta^S}\right)}.$$

Problem 2.4. Show that, using a one-dimensional approximation of the GBM, the basement membrane sieving coefficient can be calculated as (Eq. 2.90):

$$\theta_S^{bm} = \frac{\phi_S W_S}{\theta_S^{ep}(1-\exp(-Pe)) + \phi_S W_S \exp(-Pe)}.$$

References

Anderson, J.L., Quinn, J.A.: Restricted transport in small pores: a model for steric exclusion and hindered particle motion. Biophys. J. **14**(2), 130–150 (1974)

Anderson, S., Rennke, H.G., et al.: Therapeutic advantage of converting enzyme inhibitors in arresting progressive renal disease associated with systemic hypertension in the rat. J. Clin. Invest. **77**(6), 1993–2000 (1986)

Brenner, B.M., Troy, J.L., et al.: The dynamics of glomerular ultrafiltration in the rat. J. Clin. Invest. **50**, 1776–1780 (1971)

Bungay, P.M., Brenner, H.: The motion of a closely-fitting sphere in a fluid-filled tube. Int. J. Multiphase Flow. **1**, 25–56 (1973)

Chang, R.L.S., Robertson, C.R., et al.: Permselectivity of the glomerular capillary wall to macromolecules. I. Theoretical considerations. Biophys. J. **15**, 861–886 (1975)

Comper, W.D., Haraldsson, B., et al.: Resolved: normal glomeruli filter nephrotic levels of albumin. J. Am. Soc. Nephrol. **19**(3), 427–432 (2008)

References

Dechadilok, P., Deen, W.M.: Hindrance factors for diffusion and convection in pores. Ind. Eng. Chem. Res. **45**, 6953–6959 (2006)

Deen, W.M., Bridges, C.R., et al.: Heteroporous model of glomerular size selectivity: application to normal and nephrotic humans. Am. J. Physiol. Renal Physiol. **249**(3), F374–F389 (1985)

Deen, W.M., Robertson, C.R., et al.: A model of glomerular ultrafiltration in the rat. Am. J. Physiol. **223**(5), 1178–1183 (1972)

Deen, W.M., Lazzara, M.J., et al.: Structural determinants of glomerular permeability. Am. J. Physiol. Renal Physiol. **281**(4), F579–F596 (2001)

Drumond, M.C., Deen, W.M.: Structural determinants of glomerular hydraulic permeability. Am. J. Physiol. Renal Physiol. **266**(1), F1–F12 (1994)

Edwards, A., Daniels, B.S., et al.: Ultrastructural model for size selectivity in glomerular filtration. Am. J. Physiol. Renal Physiol. **276**, F892–F902 (1999)

Guasch, A., Deen, W.M., et al.: Charge selectivity of the glomerular filtration barrier in healthy and nephrotic humans. J. Clin. Invest. **92**, 2274–2282 (1993)

Hora, K., Ohno, S., et al.: Three-dimensional study of glomerular slit diaphragm by the quick-freezing and deep-etching replica method. Eur. J. Cell Biol. **53**, 402–406 (1990)

Jarad, G., Miner, J.H.: Albuminuria, wherefore art thou? J. Am. Soc. Nephrol. **20**(3), 455–457 (2009)

Kedem, O., Katchalsky, A.: Thermodynamic analysis of the permeability of biological membranes to non-electrolytes. Biochim. Biophys. Acta **27**, 229–246 (1958)

Lindstrom, K.E., Johnson, E., et al.: Glomerular charge selectivity for proteins larger than serum albumin as revealed by lactate dehydrogenase isoforms. Acta Physiol. Scand. **162**, 481–488 (1998)

Ohlson, M., Sorensson, J., et al.: A gel-membrane model of glomerular charge and size selectivity in series. Am. J. Physiol. Renal Physiol. **280**(3), F396–F405 (2001)

Pappenheimer, J.R., Renkin, E.M., et al.: Filtration, diffusion and molecular sieving through peripheral capillary membranes: a contribution to the pore theory of capillary permeability. Am. J. Physiol. **167**(1), 13–46 (1951)

Patlak, C.S., Goldstein, D.A., et al.: The flow of solute and solvent across a two-membrane system. J. Theor. Biol. **5**(3), 426–442 (1963)

Pavenstadt, H., Kriz, W., et al.: Cell biology of the glomerular podocyte. Physiol. Rev. **83**(1), 253–307 (2003)

Peti-Peterdi, J.: Independent two-photon measurements of albumin GSC give low values. Am. J. Physiol. Renal Physiol. **296**(6), F1255–F1257 (2009)

Rodewald, R., Karnovsky, M.J.: Porous substructure of the glomerular slit diaphragm in the rat and mouse. J. Cell Biol. **60**(2), 423–433 (1974)

Russo, L.M., Sandoval, R.M., et al.: The normal kidney filters nephrotic levels of albumin retrieved by proximal tubule cells: retrieval is disrupted in nephrotic states. Kidney Int. **71**(6), 504–513 (2007)

Sangalli, F., Carrara, F., et al.: Effect of ACE inhibition on glomerular permselectivity and tubular albumin concentration in the renal ablation model. Am. J. Physiol. Renal Physiol. **300**(6), F1291–F1300 (2011)

Squarer, A., Lemley, K.V., et al.: Mechanisms of progressive glomerular injury in membranous nephropathy. J. Am. Soc. Nephrol. **9**(8), 1389–1398 (1998)

Starling, E.H.: The glomerular functions of the kidney. J. Physiol. **24**, 317–330 (1899)

Chapter 3
Urine Concentration

Abstract During water deprivation, the kidney of a mammal can conserve water by producing a urine that is more concentrated than blood plasma. That hypertonic urine is produced when water is reabsorbed, in excess of solutes, from the collecting ducts and into the renal vasculature, thereby concentrating the collecting duct fluid, which eventually emerges as urine. In this chapter, we introduce mathematical models that simulate the urine concentrating process. To learn how to build those models, we first derive equations that represent tubular flow, transmural water flux, and transmural solute fluxes along a renal tubule. We then develop models that simulate countercurrent multiplication in a loop, and we study factors that affect the efficiency of the concentrating mechanism.

3.1 Biological Background: How Does an Animal Produce a Concentrated Urine?

When a mammal is deprived of water, its kidney can conserve water by increasing solute concentration (or, osmolality) in urine to a level well above that of blood, so that solutes are excreted in excess of water. This process of urine concentration occurs in the renal medulla, and has the effect of stabilizing blood plasma osmolality. Some animals can concentrate urine better than others. Maximum reported urine osmolalities in several animals are shown in Table 3.1. For comparison, blood plasma osmolality is $\sim$300 mOsm/kg H_2O. The values in Table 3.1 indicate that the human kidney can produce a urine that is $\sim$4.8 times more concentrated than that of plasma. Note that is the *maximum* value ever measured, so it is fair to say that most of us don't do that well. That human maximum urine osmolality value is also the reason that one should refrain from drinking sea water to quench thirst, given that sea water osmolality ranges from 2,000 to 2,400 mOsm/kg H_2O. The kidney of an Australian hopping mouse, which lives in the desert, can produce an amazingly concentrated urine that has an osmolality >30 times above that of blood plasma.

Table 3.1 Maximum measured urine osmolalities in selected animals. For comparison, blood plasma osmolality is about 300 mOsm/kg H_2O

Animal	Urine osmolality mOsm/kg H_2O
Domestic pig	1,075
Human	1,430
Rat	2,849
Mouse	2,950
Chinchilla	7,599
Australian hopping mouse	9,374

A urine that has an osmolality higher than blood plasma is said to be hypertonic. A hypertonic urine is concentrated in the final stages of urine production: water is absorbed, in excess of solutes, from the collecting ducts and into the vasculature of the medulla, thus increasing the osmolality of the collecting duct fluid—fluid that is called urine after it emerges from the collecting ducts. In the outer medulla, water absorption from the collecting ducts is driven by the active transepithelial transport of NaCl from the water-impermeable thick ascending limbs into the surrounding interstitium, where the NaCl promotes, via osmosis, water absorption from collecting ducts, descending limbs, and some blood vessels. The countercurrent configuration of renal tubules and blood vessels in the outer medulla augments this concentrating effect, as a function of depth, along the cortico-medullary axis, so that an osmolality gradient is generated along all the structures of the outer medulla, from the cortico-medullary boundary to the outer-inner medullary boundary. Although this concentrating mechanism is well-established in the outer medulla—by both physiological experiments and theoretical investigation—the nature of the concentrating mechanism in the inner medulla remains to be elucidated.

3.2 Modeling Flow Along a Renal Tubule

In this section, we will derive equations that model tubular flow and transmural fluxes along a renal tubule. The system is assumed to be at steady state.

3.2.1 Mass Conservation Equations

We will derive the differential equations that describe the conservation of water and solutes along a renal tubule. We will first consider water transport along the tubule, which extends from $x = 0$ to $x = L$, as shown in Fig. 3.1. For simplicity, we assume that the tubule is rigid. Of course, technically speaking, tubular walls are comprised of cells that are, to some extent, flexible. However, the structures surrounding the tubules in vivo likely reduce that degree of compliance, which makes the rigid-wall

3.2 Modeling Flow Along a Renal Tubule

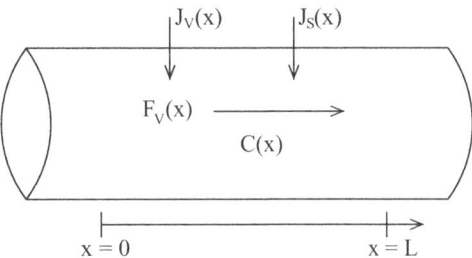

Fig. 3.1 Schematic drawing for model renal tubule, illustrating water flow (F_V), water flux (J_V), and solute flux (J_S)

assumption reasonable. It is also reasonable to describe the flow in the tubules as plug flow (i.e., flow with no radial component and constant velocity across any cross-section).

To derive a differential equation that describes water conservation along the tubule, consider the tubular segment in Fig. 3.1. The change in water flow rate must equal the sum of the water flux out of (or into) the tubule through its walls between $x = 0$ and $x = L$. This reasoning can be written as

$$F_V(L) = F_V(0) + 2\pi r \int_0^L J_V(x)\, dx, \quad (3.1)$$

where r denotes tubular radius, assumed constant. $F_V(x)$ denotes the volume flow rate along the tubule, the units of which are typically nl/min for renal tubules. $J_V(x)$ denotes water flux through the tubular walls, taken positive into the tubule. J_V is computed at a point along the circumference of the tubule, hence the multiplication by the factor $2\pi r$. Rewriting Eq. (3.1) in differential form, we get

$$\frac{\partial}{\partial x} F_V(x) = 2\pi r J_V(x). \quad (3.2)$$

Next we consider solute conservation along the tubule. Such a solute can be NaCl or urea or protein. The rate of flow of a given solute at position x is given by the product of its concentration $C(x)$ and the rate of flow of water $F_V(x)$, i.e., $F_V(x)C(x)$. Let the amount of solute transported inward through the tubule walls at x per unit area per unit time be denoted by $J_S(x)$. Then, through a procedure similar to the one we used to derive the water conservation equation (3.2), we can describe the solute conservation along the renal tubule by

$$\frac{\partial}{\partial x}(F_V(x)C(x)) = 2\pi r J_S(x). \quad (3.3)$$

The conservation equations (3.2) and (3.3) are general and apply to all types of renal tubules. Of course, tubules in the kidney differ widely in their transport properties, and those differences are reflected in the flux terms J_V and J_S.

3.2.2 Water Fluxes

Water can be driven through a cell membrane by hydrostatic pressure, oncotic pressure, and osmotic pressure. Oncotic pressure, discussed in Chap. 4, is exerted by proteins in blood plasma. Because in a healthy kidney, virtually no proteins are filtered by the glomerulus, oncotic pressure can be assumed to be zero along the loops of Henle and collecting ducts.

Osmotic pressure is the pressure that must be applied to a solution to stop the inflow of water across a water-permeable membrane. Water tends to move through a water-permeable membrane when the solutions on the two sides of the membrane have different *osmolalities*. Osmolality is given by a weighted sum of the concentrations of all the solutes in the solution:

$$\text{osmolality} = \sum_k \sigma_k C_k, \tag{3.4}$$

where C_k is the concentration of the kth solute, and σ_k is the osmotic coefficient of that solute.

Consider a membrane that is permeable to water but impermeable to a given solute. Suppose the difference in the concentration of that solute between the two sides of the membrane is ΔC. Then, for a small solute, the osmotic pressure exerted by that solute can be approximated by

$$\text{osmotic pressure} = RT\sigma\Delta C, \tag{3.5}$$

where R is the universal gas constant (62.36×10^{-3} mmHg·K^{-1}·mM^{-1}), and T is the absolute temperature. Even a small concentration gradient can exert a substantial osmotic pressure. Let $\Delta C = 1$ mM, $\sigma = 1$, and $T = 310.15$ K (human body temperature, ≈ 37 C). The osmotic pressure is about 19.3 mmHg.

Hydrostatic pressure is frequently assumed negligible, because the transmembrane hydrostatic pressure difference, which is likely on the order of 1 mmHg, is much smaller than the osmotic pressure exerted by a concentration gradient of 1 mM (which is ~ 19.3 mmHg).

To derive the equation that describes water flux across a renal tubule, we make another simplifying assumption, which is that water transport across tubular walls can be represented as single-barrier transport. We make the same assumption in our description of solute fluxes below as well. Renal tubular and vascular walls are made up of a single layer of cells (epithelial cells for loops of Henle and collecting ducts, and endothelial cells for vasa recta). A fluid or solute particle can be transported through the cells, or paracellularly through the junctions between cells. To move from the tubular lumen through the cells into the surrounding interstitium, the particle must first move through the apical cell membrane into the cytoplasm of the cell, diffuse through the cytoplasm, and then move through

3.2 Modeling Flow Along a Renal Tubule

a second cell membrane, the basolateral membrane. The transport properties of the two cell membranes (apical and basolateral) are often different. However, because the transport properties of individual membranes are frequently not well known, and because transcellular transport can be complicated, we assume that the transport between luminal and interstitial compartments can be represented as a single-barrier flux.

Given the above discussion, water flux into a renal tubule in Fig. 3.1 can be described by

$$J_V(x) = L_p(x) RT\sigma \left(C(x) - C^e(x) \right), \tag{3.6}$$

where $L_p(x)$ is the water permeability of the tubule, and $C^e(x)$ denotes the interstitial (i.e., external) solute concentration at position x. As discussed above, oncotic and hydrostatic pressures are assumed negligible. For this simple model, only one solute is represented. If multiple solutes are represented, the osmotic pressure is given by a summation as in Eq. (3.4).

3.2.3 Solute Fluxes

Transepithelial solute fluxes may be driven by electrochemical potential gradients, by pumps (i.e., active transport), or via coupled transport systems. In Chap. 8 we discuss how to model these fluxes in details. Here we take a simpler approach and make the same single-barrier transport assumption that we have made for water fluxes. A typical simple model considers two pathways by which a solute may be transported across renal tubular walls, passive and active:

$$J_S(x) = -\frac{V_{\max}(x) C(x)}{K_M + C(x)} + P_S(x) \left(C^e(x) - C(x) \right). \tag{3.7}$$

For simplicity, the solute is assumed to be uncharged (e.g., urea or NaCl). The first term on the right represents active solute transport, characterized by Michaelis-Menten kinetics, which is one of the simplest and best-known models of enzyme kinetics in biochemistry, named after German biochemist Leonor Michaelis and Canadian physicist Maud Menten. Here, $V_{\max}$ represents the maximum transport rate achieved by the system at solute concentration C, and the Michaelis constant K_M is the solute concentration at which the reaction rate is half of $V_{\max}$. Thus, the transport rate increases as C increases from 0, but it levels off and approaches $V_{\max}$ as C approaches infinity. The negative sign implies that the active transport flux is outward-directed. The second term in the equation represents transmural diffusion, with solute permeability P_S.

3.3 Countercurrent Multiplication in a Loop

We will develop a model of the loop of Henle that illustrates the principle of countercurrent multiplication. The paradigm of countercurrent multiplication was proposed by Werner Kuhn, a brilliant Swiss physical chemist who had studied with giants such as Niels Bohr and Ernest Rutherford. With his colleague Kaspar Ryffel, Kuhn published a 34-page treatise describing and actually testing several arrangements by which an osmolality gradient could be generated along parallel but opposing flows in adjacent tubes that were made contiguous by a hair-pin turn. By the principle of *countercurrent multiplication*, a transfer of solute from one tubule to another (a "single" effect) augments ("multiplies," or reinforces) the axial osmolality gradient in the parallel flow ("Vervielfältigung des Einzeleffektes"). Thus, a small transverse osmolality difference (a small single effect) is multiplied into a much larger osmolality difference along the axis of tubular flow.

To exemplify the principle of countercurrent multiplication, we will construct a model that represents a loop, with a descending limb and an ascending limb. The two limbs are assumed to be in direct contact with each other. A schematic diagram of the model configuration is shown in Fig. 3.2a. The model represents only one solute, say, NaCl. In addition, we make the following simplifying assumptions:

1. We assume that the descending limb is water impermeable but infinitely permeable to solute. This is of course a simplification, because a large portion of the descending limb is known to be highly water permeable. Nonetheless, we make this assumption to make things easy. The conservation equations become

$$\frac{\partial}{\partial x} F_{DL,V}(x) = 0, \tag{3.8}$$

$$\frac{\partial}{\partial x} (F_{DL,V}(x) C_{DL}(x)) = 2\pi r_{DL} J_{DL,S}(x), \tag{3.9}$$

   where the subscript 'DL' denotes the descending limb.

2. We assume that the ascending limb is water impermeable. And we assume that the solute is pumped out of the ascending limb at a fixed rate of A. A fixed pump rate is assumed instead of the (nonlinear) Michaelis-Menten kinetics in Eq. (3.7) so that we can derive an analytical solution. Additionally, we assume that all of that solute goes into the descending limb. Thus, $2\pi r_{DL} J_{DL,S} = A$ and $2\pi r_{AL} J_{AL,S} = -A$, where the subscript 'AL' denotes the ascending limb. The conservation equations for the ascending limb are

$$\frac{\partial}{\partial x} F_{AL,V}(x) = 0, \tag{3.10}$$

$$\frac{\partial}{\partial x} (F_{AL,V}(x) C_{AL}(x)) = -A. \tag{3.11}$$

3. Because the descending and ascending limbs are assumed to be contiguous, at the loop bend ($x = L$) we have

3.3 Counter current Multiplication in a Loop

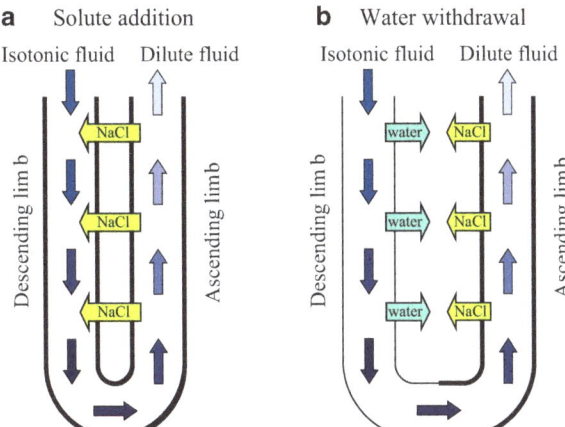

Fig. 3.2 Two paradigms for countercurrent multiplication. (**a**) Countercurrent multiplication by NaCl transfer from an ascending flow to a descending flow: the concentration of the descending flow is progressively concentrated by NaCl addition. (**b**) Countercurrent multiplication by water withdrawal from a descending flow: NaCl transport from the ascending flow into the interstitium raises interstitial osmolality; this results in passive water transport from the descending flow, which has lower osmolality than the interstitium. In both paradigms, a steady state is achieved in which NaCl concentration is raised in the descending limb so that tubular fluid achieves a maximum concentration at the loop bend. In both figure panels, tubular fluid flow direction is indicated by *blue arrows*; increasing osmolality is indicated by *darkening shades of blue*. Thick black lines indicate that a tubule is water impermeable; *thin lines* indicate high permeability to water (Figure modified from Layton and Layton 2011)

$$F_{\text{DL},V}(L) = -F_{\text{AL},V}(L), \tag{3.12}$$

$$C_{\text{DL}}(L) = C_{\text{AL}}(L). \tag{3.13}$$

In Eq. (3.12) we assume that flow is positive in the x direction; thus, flow rate along the ascending limb is negative.

4. Finally, to complete the system, we must specify the boundary conditions at the entrance of the descending limb:

$$F_{\text{DL},V}(0) = F_{V,0}, \tag{3.14}$$

$$C_{\text{DL}}(0) = C_0. \tag{3.15}$$

We now have enough information to determine $C_{\text{DL}}(x)$ and $C_{\text{AL}}(x)$. Since the entire loop is assumed to be water impermeable, $F_{\text{DL},V}(x) = F_{V,0}$ and $F_{\text{AL},V}(x) = -F_{V,0}$. Plugging this into Eq. (3.9), we have

$$F_{V,0}\frac{\partial}{\partial x}C_{\text{DL}}(x) = A, \tag{3.16}$$

which can be integrated, and combined with the boundary condition (3.15), to yield

$$C_{DL}(x) = C_0 + \left(\frac{A}{F_{V,0}}\right) x. \quad (3.17)$$

Now to compute solute concentration along the ascending limb, we evaluate C_{DL} at $x = L$, use that as the initial condition for the ODE (3.11) to get

$$C_{AL}(x) = C_{DL}(L) - \left(\frac{A}{F_{V,0}}\right)(L - x)$$

$$= C_0 + \left(\frac{A}{F_{V,0}}\right) x = C_{DL}(x). \quad (3.18)$$

This simple model predicts that (1) the concentrations along the descending and ascending limbs are the same at any given position x; (2) solute concentration increases linearly along the x direction; and thus (3) the longer the loop, the higher the loop-bend concentration.

3.4 Countercurrent Multiplication in a Loop, Revisited

The preceding example assumes that solute is directly secreted from the ascending limb into the descending limb. While experimental studies support active NaCl transport from thick ascending limbs, experiments also indicate that descending limbs are not highly permeable to NaCl. Instead, those segments of the descending limbs are highly permeable to water. These observations suggest that the accumulation of NaCl from thick limbs may concentrate descending limb tubular fluid principally by means of osmotic water absorption from descending limbs rather than by NaCl secretion into descending limbs. We will modify our model to capture this mechanism.

A schematic diagram of the model is shown in Fig. 3.2b. We assume that the descending and ascending limbs of the loop interact through a common, external compartment, which represents extratubular structures, such as the interstitium, interstitial cells and vasculature. Both the NaCl that is actively pumped out of the ascending limb and the water that is reabsorbed from the descending limb are taken up by the external compartment.

3.4.1 Model Assumptions

Here are the new model assumptions:

1. We assume that the descending limb is impermeable to solute, but is highly permeable to water. In fact, we assume the descending limb is so permeable

3.4 Countercurrent Multiplication in a Loop, Revisited

to water that its concentration equilibrates with the external solute concentration C^e, i.e.,

$$C_{\mathrm{DL}}(x) = C^e(x). \tag{3.19}$$

The solute conservation equation is

$$\frac{\partial}{\partial x}\left(F_{\mathrm{DL},V}(x)C_{\mathrm{DL}}(x)\right) = 0, \tag{3.20}$$

since there is no solute flux, i.e., $J_{\mathrm{DL},S}(x) = 0$. The water conservation equation is

$$\frac{\partial}{\partial x}F_{\mathrm{DL},V}(x) = 2\pi r_{\mathrm{DL}} J_{\mathrm{DL},V}(x). \tag{3.21}$$

2. The conservation equations for the ascending limb are the same as before: Eqs. (3.10) and (3.11).
3. For the external compartment, we assume that the reabsorbate (i.e., NaCl from the ascending limb and water from the descending limb) is picked up locally. That is, we assume no axial flow in this compartment. Thus, by mass conservation, the external compartment concentration $C^e(x)$ can be related to the solute and water fluxes by

$$C^e(x) = \frac{2\pi r_{\mathrm{AL}} J_{\mathrm{AL},S}(x)}{2\pi r_{\mathrm{DL}} J_{\mathrm{DL},V}(x)} = -\frac{A}{2\pi r_{\mathrm{DL}} J_{\mathrm{DL},V}(x)}. \tag{3.22}$$

3.4.2 Model Solution

We will first compute water flow and solute concentration along the descending limb. Equation (3.20) implies that, because the descending limb is solute-impermeable, solute flow is constant along the limb. That is, we can write

$$F_{\mathrm{DL},V}(x)C_{\mathrm{DL}}(x) = F_{\mathrm{DL},V}(0)C_{\mathrm{DL}}(0), \tag{3.23}$$

$$\Rightarrow F_{\mathrm{DL},V}(x) = F_{\mathrm{DL},V}(0)\frac{C^e(0)}{C^e(x)}. \tag{3.24}$$

since we assume that the descending limb concentration equilibrates with the external concentration. To get $C^e(x)$, we eliminate $J_{\mathrm{DL},V}(x)$ from Eq. (3.21) using Eq. (3.22) to get

$$\frac{\partial}{\partial x}F_{\mathrm{DL},V}(x) = -\frac{A}{C^e(x)}. \tag{3.25}$$

We then rewrite Eq. (3.20) as

$$C^e(x)\frac{\partial}{\partial x}F_{\text{DL},V}(x) + F_{\text{DL},V}(x)\frac{\partial}{\partial x}C^e(x) = 0, \qquad (3.26)$$

with $C_{\text{DL}}(x)$ replaced by $C^e(x)$. Next, we eliminate $F_{\text{DL},V}$ and its spatial derivative from the above equation, using Eqs. (3.24) and (3.25):

$$A = F_{\text{DL},V}(0)\frac{C^e(0)}{C^e(x)}\frac{\partial}{\partial x}C^e(x), \qquad (3.27)$$

which can be written as

$$\frac{\partial}{\partial x}C^e(x) = \frac{A}{F_{\text{DL},V}(0)C^e(0)}C^e(x). \qquad (3.28)$$

The ODE can be integrated to give the solute concentrations along the external compartment as well as the descending limb:

$$C^e(x) = C_{\text{DL}}(x) = C^e(0)\exp\left(\frac{Ax}{F_{\text{DL},V}(0)C^e(0)}\right). \qquad (3.29)$$

The above solution indicates that the descending limb and external solute concentrations increase exponentially along the model medulla.

Now let's consider the ascending limb. To compute its flow rate and concentration, we need its boundary conditions, i.e., flow rate and concentration at the loop bend. By evaluating Eqs. (3.24) and (3.29) at $x = L$, we have

$$F_{\text{AL},V}(L) = -F_{\text{DL},V}(L) = -F_{\text{DL},V}(0)\frac{C_{\text{DL}}(0)}{C^e(L)}, \qquad (3.30)$$

$$C_{\text{AL}}(L) = C^e(L) = C^e(0)\exp\left(\frac{AL}{F_{\text{DL},V}(0)C^e(0)}\right). \qquad (3.31)$$

Because the ascending limb is assumed to be water impermeable, its water flow rate doesn't change, i.e., $F_{\text{AL},V}(x) = F_{\text{AL},V}(L)$. Its solute concentration does change, though. In fact, we expect it to progressively decrease towards $x = 0$ as NaCl is actively pumped out. Using Eq. (3.31) as the initial condition for the solute conservation equation (3.11), we obtain

$$C_{\text{AL}}(x) = C^e(0)\exp\left(\frac{AL}{F_{\text{DL},V}(0)C^e(0)}\right) - \frac{Ax}{F_{V,DL}(L)}. \qquad (3.32)$$

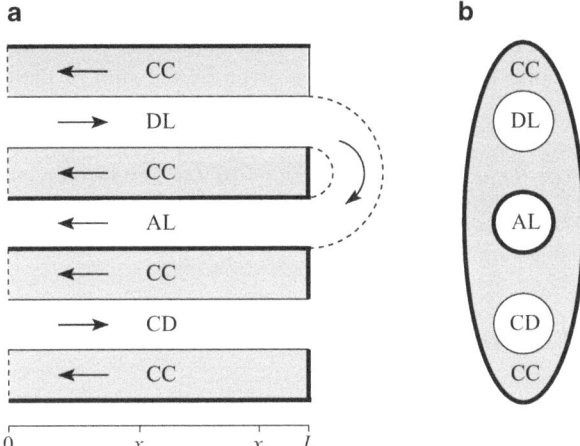

Fig. 3.3 Schematic diagram of the central core model. Panel (**a**), tubules along spatial axis. *DL* descending limb, *AL* ascending limb, *CD* collecting duct, *CC* central core. *Arrows*, steady-state flow directions. *Heavy lines*, water-impermeable boundaries. Panel (**b**), cross-section showing connectivity between CC and other tubules (Reprinted from Layton and Layton 2002)

3.5 The Central Core Model

In the model we have just considered, water and solute absorbed from tubules into the interstitium are assumed to enter the peritubular capillaries directly, at each medullary level, and afterwards, that absorbate is assumed to have no further interaction with the medulla, because we assume that there is no axial flow outside of the loop. Consequently, relatively concentrated ascending fluid does not equilibrate with progressively less concentrated surrounding interstitium. And as a result, that model may be unrealistically dissipative of the axial osmolality gradient.

We now consider an alternative model formulation, the *central core assumption*. A schematic diagram of the central core model is shown in Fig. 3.3. The central core was developed by John Stephenson (1955–2010), a former faculty member at the Weill Cornell Medical College in New York City. In the central core formulation, blood vessels, interstitial cells, and interstitial spaces are merged into a single compartment, with which the loops of Henle and collecting ducts interact. Axial flow is allowed within the central core. The central core formulation assumes maximum countercurrent exchange by the vasculature, and, compared to the model in Sect. 3.4, is much less dissipative of the axial osmolality gradient. The effects of the vasculature on the concentrating mechanism are considered in Chap. 4.

We augment the previous model (Sect. 3.4) in two ways. First, we use the central core assumption to represent the interactions among the tubules and the vasculature. Second, we also represent the collecting duct, which, together with the loops of Henle, are surrounded by, and interact through, a central core. The solute that is pumped out of the ascending limb, or the water and solute that are reabsorbed from the descending limb and collecting duct, are picked up by the capillaries that are represented by the central core. Thus, by water and solute conservation, the water and solute fluxes into the central core are given by the sum of the corresponding tubular fluxes:

$$2\pi r_{CC} J_{CC,V} = 2\pi \left(-r_{DL} J_{DL,V} - r_{AL} J_{AL,V} - r_{CD} J_{CD,V}\right), \quad (3.33)$$

$$2\pi r_{CC} J_{CC,S} = 2\pi \left(-r_{DL} J_{DL,S} - r_{AL} J_{AL,S} - r_{CD} J_{CD,S}\right). \quad (3.34)$$

3.5.1 Model Assumptions

We make the following assumptions in this model:

1. We assume that the descending limb and collecting duct are infinitely water permeable. As a result, the intratubular concentrations of the descending limb and collecting duct nearly equilibrate with the central core, and, to a good approximation,

$$C_{DL}(x) = C_{CD}(x) = C_{CC}(x) \equiv C(x). \quad (3.35)$$

   We denote the common concentration by $C(x)$.
2. The descending and ascending limbs are contiguous, and the boundary conditions Eqs. (3.12) and (3.13) hold.
3. We assume that the ascending limb is water impermeable. Thus, $J_{AL,V} = 0$, and it follows that $F_{AL,V}(x) = -F_{DL,V}(L)$ for all x.
4. We assume that the descending limb and collecting duct are solute permeable. Thus, from Eq. (3.34), we have

$$r_{DL} J_{DL,S}(x) + r_{CD} J_{CD,S}(x) + r_{CC} J_{CC,S}(x) = -r_{AL} J_{AL,S}(x). \quad (3.36)$$

5. We further assume that the central core is closed at $x = L$, which corresponds to the papillary tip. This assumption implies that there is no convective entry of solute or fluid at $x = L$. Thus, $F_{CC,V}(L) = 0$.

3.5.2 Model Solution

If we add up the solute conservation equations for the descending limb, collecting duct, and central core, we get

$$\frac{\partial}{\partial x} \left(F_{DL,V} C_{DL} + F_{CD,V} C_{CD} + F_{CC,V} C_{CC}\right) = 2\pi \left(r_{DL} J_{DL,S} + r_{CD} J_{CD,S} + r_{CC} J_{CC,S}\right), \quad (3.37)$$

3.5 The Central Core Model

or,

$$2\pi (r_{DL} J_{DL,V} + r_{CD} J_{CD,V} + r_{CC} J_{CC,V}) C + (F_{DL,V} + F_{CD,V} + F_{CC,V}) \frac{\partial}{\partial x} C$$
$$= -2\pi r_{AL} J_{AL,S}. \tag{3.38}$$

Because, by water conservation, $r_{DL} J_{DL,S} + r_{CD} J_{CD,S} + r_{CC} J_{CC,S} = 0$, the above equation simplifies to an ODE for $C(x)$:

$$\frac{\partial}{\partial x} C(x) = \frac{-2\pi r_{AL} J_{AL,S}}{F_{DL,V} + F_{CD,V} + F_{CC,V}}, \tag{3.39}$$

which says that the rate of increase of the concentration in the descending limb, collecting duct, and central core is the ratio of the solute reabsorption from the ascending limb to the net water flow rate in the other three tubules. Now we will rewrite the above equation in terms of the solute flow, given by $F_{i,S} = F_{i,V} C$ for tubule i. Dividing Eq. (3.39) by $C(x)$, we have

$$\frac{C'(x)}{C(x)} = \frac{-2\pi r_{AL} J_{AL,S}}{F_{DL,S} + F_{CD,S} + F_{CC,S}}. \tag{3.40}$$

By solute conservation, we have for the collecting duct and central core

$$F_{CD,S}(x) = F_{CD,S}(0) + 2\pi r_{CD} \int_0^x J_{CD,S}(s)\, ds, \tag{3.41}$$

$$F_{CC,S}(x) = -2\pi \int_L^x \left(r_{DL} J_{DL,S}(s) + r_{CD} J_{CD,S}(s) + r_{AL} J_{AL,S}(s) \right) ds, \tag{3.42}$$

which together give

$$F_{CD,S}(x) + F_{CC,S}(x) = F_{CD,S}(L) - 2\pi \int_x^L \left(r_{DL} J_{DL,S}(s) + r_{AL} J_{AL,S}(s) \right) ds. \tag{3.43}$$

Upon substituting into Eq. (3.40), we get

$$\frac{C'(x)}{C(x)} = \frac{-2\pi r_{AL} J_{AL,S}(x)}{F_{DL,S}(x) + F_{CD,S}(L) - 2\pi \int_x^L \left(r_{DL} J_{DL,S}(s) + r_{AL} J_{AL,S}(s) \right) ds}. \tag{3.44}$$

After integrating this ODE, we obtain the following expression

$$\frac{C(x)}{C(0)} = \exp\left(\int_0^x \frac{-2\pi r_{AL} J_{AL,S}(y)}{F_{DL,S}(y) + F_{CD,S}(L) - 2\pi \int_y^L \left(r_{DL} J_{DL,S}(s) + r_{AL} J_{AL,S}(s) \right) ds}\, dy \right). \tag{3.45}$$

Fig. 3.4 A comparison of interstitial concentration profile $C(x)$ obtained using Eq. (3.29) for the countercurrent multiplication model in Sect. 3.4 with the profile obtained using Eq. (3.46) for the central core model in Sect. 3.5

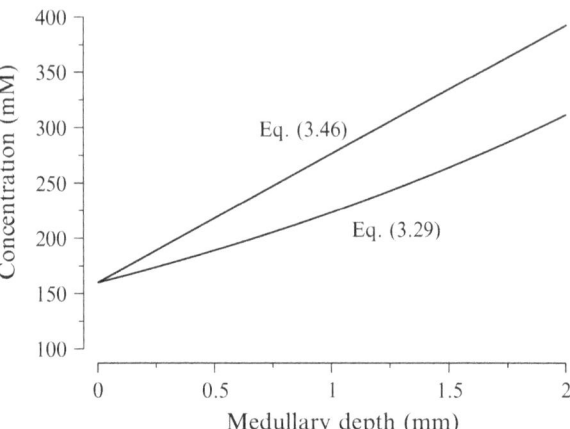

The above expression, which is very general, gives the concentration ratio attained along the medulla as a function only of solute flow along the descending limb, flow exiting the end of the collecting duct, and the solute fluxes from the loop.

Now in the mammalian kidney, the descending limbs have a low permeability to NaCl. So let's assume $J_{\mathrm{DL},S} = 0$. As a result, $F_{\mathrm{DL},S}(x) = F_{\mathrm{DL},S}(0)$. We further assume that the solute is pumped out of the ascending limb at a fixed rate of A. With these assumptions, the integral (3.45) can be evaluated:

$$C(x) = C(0) \left(\frac{F_{\mathrm{DL},S}(0) + F_{\mathrm{CD},S}(L) - (L-x)A}{F_{\mathrm{DL},S}(0) + F_{\mathrm{CD},S}(L) - LA} \right). \tag{3.46}$$

Let's plug in some numbers and plot the above expression. Let's suppose $F_{\mathrm{DL},S}(0) = 1.6\,\mathrm{nmol/min}$, $F_{\mathrm{CD},S}(L) = 0.2\,\mathrm{nmol/min}$, $C(0) = 160\,\mathrm{mM}$, and $L = 2\,\mathrm{mm}$. We assume that 2/3 of the salt is pumped out of the ascending limb, consistent with what happens in the rat outer medulla; so $A = (2/3 \times 1.6)/2 = 0.533\,\mathrm{nmol/(min \cdot mm)}$. With these numbers, the fluid osmolality in the descending limb, collecting duct, and central core increases from 160 at $x = 0$ to 393 mOsm/kg H_2O at $x = L$, i.e., by a factor of 2.45.

What can we learn from the formula (3.46)? First, the higher the active transport rate of the ascending limb (A), the larger the concentrating effect. Second, the smaller the "load" on the concentrating mechanism, the larger the axial osmolality gradient. By "load" we mean the water flow rate of the descending limb and collecting duct. For example, if there is no urine "load" on the system, i.e., $F_{\mathrm{CD},S}(L) = 0$, then the descending limb and central core fluid will be concentrated to 480 mOsm/(kg H_2O), a factor of about 3.

To understand how the central core model solution compares with the earlier model in Sect. 3.4, which assumes that there is no axial flow outside of the loop, we calculate interstitial concentration profiles $C(x)$ for both models, using Eqs. (3.29) and (3.46). Those concentration profiles are shown in Fig. 3.4. As you can see, the central core model produces a significantly higher concentrating effect. That is because axial flow within the central core allows absorbate from the deep medulla (i.e., closer to $x = L$), which has a high concentration, to interact with and concentrate the tubular fluid in the upper medulla (i.e., closer to $x = 0$), thereby augmenting the overall concentrating effect of the system.

3.6 The Distributed-Loop Model

Early models of the urine concentrating mechanism typically represent one loop of Henle and one collecting duct. These single-loop models may be sufficient to illustrate certain simple principles, e.g., countercurrent multiplication. But it has long been recognized that the loops of Henle differ from one another greatly. In the rat kidney, there are two populations of loops: the *short* loops of Henle, which turn near the boundary between the outer and inner medullas; and the *long* loops of Henle, which reach into the inner medulla. And not all long loops are alike either! Those long loops of Henle turn at differing depths of the inner medulla, some turn near the outer-inner medullary boundary, some reach deeper, and a small fraction reach all the way to the papillary tip.

Based on this observation, some models used the *discrete-loop representation*. Typically, such models represent a finite, usually small, number of loops. Say, two loops, one short loop and one long loop that reaches to the papillary tip. Some models represent a few more loops. But a rat kidney typically has approximately 30,000–40,000 loops, and it is simply not practical to represent each loop individually.

In his doctoral thesis, Harold Layton (now professor at Duke University) developed a model representation using *continuously distributed loops of Henle*. The reasoning is that because there are tens of thousands of loops of Henle in a kidney, we might as well assume a continuous distribution of those loops. We consider only one spatial direction that corresponds to the fluid flow direction, with the assumption that fluid flow and composition are homogeneous in the radial direction. However, we allow the tubular fluid flow rate and composition, as well as transmural fluxes, to differ among loops of different lengths. So each variable, e.g., solute concentration, is a function of two spatial variables x and y, i.e., $C(x, y)$. Here x denotes the location at which we are evaluating C, and y denotes the medullary depth at which the loop turns. With this notation, $C(x, y_1)$ and $C(x, y_2)$ denote the concentration values at location x of two different loops, one turning at depth y_1 and the other at y_2. $C(x_1, y)$ and $C(x_2, y)$ denote the concentration values of the same loop at two different locations, x_1 and x_2. We use the same notation for water flow $F_V(x, y)$, and fluxes $J_V(x, y)$ and $J_S(x, y)$ (Fig. 3.5).

A kidney likely behaves very differently if most of its loops are short and only a fraction are long (like in a rat), than if most of its loops are long ones (like in chinchilla). So we need a way to describe the population distribution of the loops. This can be done using a function $w(x)$ that specifies the fraction of loops that

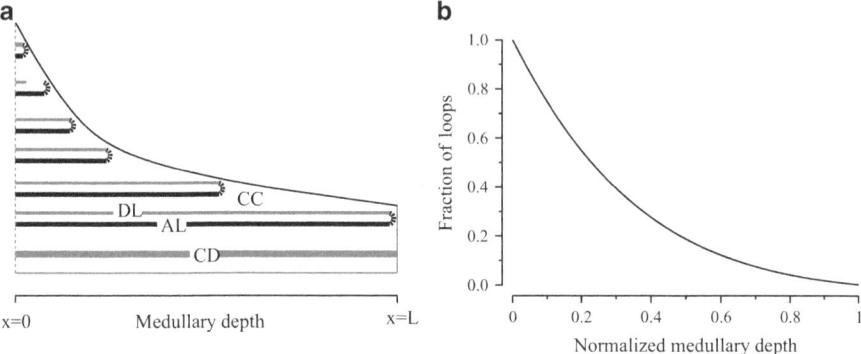

Fig. 3.5 Panel (**a**), schematic diagram of the distributed-loop model, showing loops of Henle (descending limb, *DL* and ascending limb, *AL*), collecting duct (*CD*), and central core (*CC*). Only six representative loops are drawn, but the model represents a continuously decreasing population. Panel (**b**), fraction of loops of Henle remaining ($w(x)$) as a function of medullary depth

remain at location x. So $w(x)$ is a monotonically decreasing function of x, starting at $w(0) = 1$ and decreasing to $w(L) = 0$ at the papillary tip.

As an example, we will revisit the central core model. This time, we replace the single loop in the previous example with a continuously distributed loop with population $w(x)$. Consider the sum of water fluxes into the central core at spatial location x. We must take into account water fluxes from the collecting duct, as well as from all loops that turn at a medullary level at or below x (i.e., at $x \le y$). Loops with length shorter than x have already turned and thus make no contribution. The total water flux from all descending limbs that are present at x is given by

$$2\pi r_{\text{DL}} \int_x^L J_{\text{DL}}(x, y) \left(-\frac{dw(y)}{dy}\right) dy. \tag{3.47}$$

Since $w(y)$ is the fraction of loops remaining at level y, $-dw(y)/dy$ gives the rate at which loops turn at y. (Since w is monotonically decreasing, the negative sign gives us a positive rate.) Hence, Eq. (3.47) is the integral of water fluxes from all loops that turn beyond x, weighted by the population density of loops at each length. A similar integral is applied to the ascending limbs (but not the collecting duct). Together, the total water and solute fluxes into the central core are given by

$$2\pi r_{\text{CC}} J_{\text{CC},V}(x) = -2\pi r_{\text{DL}} \int_x^L J_{\text{DL},V}(x, y) \left(-\frac{dw(y)}{dy}\right) dy$$
$$- 2\pi r_{\text{AL}} \int_x^L J_{\text{AL},V}(x, y) \left(-\frac{dw(y)}{dy}\right) dy - 2\pi r_{\text{CD}} J_{\text{CD},V}(x). \tag{3.48}$$

$$2\pi r_{CC} J_{CC,S}(x) = -2\pi r_{DL} \int_x^L J_{DL,S}(x, y) \left(-\frac{dw(y)}{dy}\right) dy$$

$$-2\pi r_{AL} \int_x^L J_{AL,S}(x, y) \left(-\frac{dw(y)}{dy}\right) dy - 2\pi r_{CD} J_{CD,S}(x). \tag{3.49}$$

Making the same assumptions as we did in Sect. 3.5 and following the derivation there, we obtain an expression for $C(x)$, which is the solute concentration for the central core, as well as the infinitely water-permeable descending limb and collecting duct:

$$\frac{C(x)}{C(0)} = \exp\left(\int_0^x \frac{2\pi r_{AL} \int_z^L -J_{AL,S}(z, y)(-w'(y)) \, dy}{F_{DL,S}^{tot}(z) + F_{CD,S}(L) - J_{loop,S}^{tot}(z)} \, dz\right), \tag{3.50}$$

where $F_{DL,S}^{tot}(z) \equiv \int_z^L F_{DL,S}(z, y)(-w'(y)) \, dy$ and

$$J_{loop,S}^{tot}(z) \equiv 2\pi \int_z^L \int_s^L r_{DL}(-w'(y)) J_{DL,S}(s, y) + r_{AL}(-w'(y)) J_{AL,S}(s, y) \, dy \, ds.$$

3.7 Current State of Affairs

The concentrating mechanism in the outer medulla of the mammalian kidney is believed to be well understood. That mechanism involves processes similar to those represented in the central core model in Sect. 3.5: the thick ascending limbs of the loop of Henle actively transport NaCl into the surrounding interstitium to generate an increasing osmolality gradient along all tubules and vessels.

However, the epithelial cells in the inner-medullary portion of the ascending limbs are very different from those in the outer medulla. In the inner medulla, those cells look "thinner" and have different transport properties. In particular, the thin ascending limbs found in the inner medulla have no significant active transepithelial transport of NaCl or of any other solute. As a result, active solute transport coupled with countercurrent flow does not explain the concentrating process in this region. This is particularly puzzling because the inner medulla is believed to be where the steepest osmotic gradient is generated.

Decades of efforts, both theoretical and experimental, have been dedicated to elucidating the urine concentrating mechanism of the inner medulla, which has remained one of the longest-standing mysteries in traditional physiology. Even though the inner medullary urine concentrating mechanism is still controversial, progress has been made. Anatomical studies have revealed that, perhaps unsurprisingly, the kidney is more complicated than we thought. New transporters continue to be discovered. As a result, our knowledge of the transport properties of the tubules, as well as their interactions, is constantly revised. Mathematical models have been built to shed light into the roles of these new findings in the mammalian urine concentrating mechanism. For more details, you may refer to reviews by Layton (2002), Layton et al. (2009), and Pannabecker et al. (2008).

3.8 Problems

Problem 3.1. To a good approximation, the descending limbs of the loops of Henle in the Japanese quail kidney are water impermeable.

(a) Using the central core model described in Sect. 3.5, compute an expression for $R \equiv C(L)/C(0)$.
(b) Let

$$A = 2\pi \int_0^L (r_{\mathrm{DL}} J_{\mathrm{DL},S} + r_{\mathrm{AL}} J_{\mathrm{AL},S})\, dx. \tag{3.51}$$

Show that

$$\lim_{A \to F_{\mathrm{CD},S}(L)} R = \infty.$$

(c) Why is the relation $A > F_{\mathrm{CD},S}(L)$ prohibited in the model? Explain in terms of flows and concentrations.
(d) In the Japanese quail kidney, the descending limb is slightly water permeable, and, of course, there is a vasculature with counter-current exchange rather than a "central core." Also, $C_{\mathrm{CD}}(0) = C_{\mathrm{CC}}(0)$ will not be enforced. Explain why $A > F_{\mathrm{CD},S}(L)$ is a condition that will not be prohibited in a bird renal medulla. (Actual maximum avian concentration ratio R is about 2.)

Problem 3.2. In the outer medulla of the rat kidney, the lower half of about 2/3 of the descending limb is now thought to be water impermeable; the remaining descending limbs appear to be highly water permeable throughout the outer medulla. Assume that all descending limbs are solute impermeable.

(a) Assume that the collecting duct and the water-permeable population of the descending limbs are infinitely water permeable. Assume also that the ascending limbs are water impermeable, and have active solute transport that is independent of luminal solute concentration (but may depend on space). Using the central core framework, derive an expression for $R = C(L)/C(0)$.
(b) Let M be the total amount of solute entering all descending limbs. Assume that $J_{\mathrm{AL},S}$ is constant, that $2\pi r_{\mathrm{AL}} \int_0^L J_{\mathrm{AL},S}\, ds = M/2$, and that $F_{\mathrm{CD},S}(L) = M/10$. Evaluate R.

References

Layton, H.E.: Mathematical models of the mammalian urine concentrating mechanism. In: Layton, H.E., Weinstein, A.M. (eds.) Membrane Transport and Renal Physiology. The IMA Volumes in Mathematics and Its Applications, vol. 129, pp. 233–272. Springer, New York (2002)

Layton, A.T., Layton, H.E.: A semi-Lagrangian semi-implicit numerical method for models of the urine concentrating mechanism. SIAM J. Sci. Comput. **23**(5), 1526–1548 (2002)

Layton, A.T., Layton, H.E.: Countercurrent multiplication may not explain the axial osmolality gradient in the outer medulla of the rat kidney. Am. J. Physiol. Ren. Physiol. **301**, F1047–F1056 (2011)

Layton, A.T., Layton, H.E., Pannabecker, T.L., Dantzler, W.H.: The mammalian urine concentrating mechanism: hypotheses and uncertainties. Physiology **24**, 250–256 (2009)

Pannabecker, T.L., Dantzler, W.H., Layton, H.E., Layton, A.T.: Role of three-dimensional architecture in the urine concentrating mechanism of the rat renal inner medulla. Am. J. Physiol. Ren. Physiol. **295**, F1217–F1285 (2008)

Chapter 4
Counter-Current Exchange Across Vasa Recta

Abstract The microvessels of the renal medulla, known as vasa recta, form a counter-current arrangement. They play an essential role in the delivery of oxygen and other nutrients to renal tissue, and the removal of water and solutes reabsorbed by renal tubules. The first part of this chapter describes the principles of counter-current exchange. In the following sections we formulate the equations that represent the transport of water and solutes across the plasma and red blood cell compartments of vasa recta. Lastly, we examine the specific case of oxygen, which is supplied by vasa recta and provides the energy needed for active reabsorption across renal tubules.

4.1 The Renal Medullary Microcirculation

4.1.1 Background

The renal microcirculation plays an essential role in the delivery of oxygen and other nutrients to renal tissue, the removal of water and solutes reabsorbed by renal tubules, and the preservation of the cortico-medullary osmolality gradient.

The renal cortex contains a dense web of peritubular, fenestrated capillaries. Their high permeability to water, combined with their large surface area, makes it possible to remove the great amounts of water that are reabsorbed from proximal tubules. To date, there have been few quantitative descriptions of the cortical microcirculation. Mathematical models that account for transport across cortical tubules do not explicitly represent peritubular capillaries; instead, they assume that the composition of the cortical interstitium is similar to that of plasma.

This chapter focuses on the microcirculation of the renal medulla. Until recently, models of the urinary concentrating mechanism neglected its contribution to renal fluid and solute handling, but this has begun to change in light of evidence that the microcirculation modulates fluid and electrolyte excretion, and thereby affects extracellular fluid homeostasis and arterial blood pressure. Many studies, reviewed in Pallone et al. (2012), have shown that variations in renal medullary perfusion alter sodium and water excretion; nevertheless, the underlying mechanisms remain to be fully elucidated. Thus, the medullary microcirculation remains an active area of study, both experimental and theoretical.

4.1.2 Anatomy of the Medullary Microcirculation

The microvessels of the renal medulla, known as vasa recta, form a counter-current arrangement, and their number decreases in the direction of the papillary tip. As shown in Fig. 4.1, descending vasa recta (DVR) originate from the efferent arterioles of juxtamedullary glomeruli and supply all blood flow to the renal medulla. In the inner stripe of the outer medulla, the DVR coalesce into vascular bundles, where they lie in close proximity to ascending vasa recta (AVR) returning from the inner medulla. DVR in the center of vascular bundles pursue their "downward" trajectory to the inner medulla, whereas those on the bundle periphery peel off to supply blood flow to the outer medullary capillary plexus. The blood that runs through the interbundle capillary network returns to the cortex without passing through vascular bundles. In contrast, AVR originating from the inner medulla ascend through the bundles. The first mathematical models of vasa recta neglected the capillary plexus and considered instead that DVR were directly converted to AVR. More recent models explicitly represent the capillaries in between, assuming that capillary plasma equilibrates with the interstitial fluid. These models can thus account for diffusion across capillary red blood cells, which is significant for solutes such as oxygen.

The diameter of DVR ranges between 12 and 18 μm. The DVR endothelium is continuous, with tight junctions, throughout most of the vessel length; in rats, it is fenestrated along the last 1.5–2.0 mm of the papilla. DVR are surrounded by pericytes, vascular smooth muscle-like cells that impart contractile properties to the vessels. AVR are larger and more numerous than DVR (the AVR-to-DVR number ratio lies between 2 and 3), and they are highly fenestrated.

The renal medullary microcirculation is also characterized by a low hematocrit (i.e., the red blood cell-to-blood volume ratio). The hematocrit in systemic vessels is the 40–50 % range, versus 25 % in papillary DVR and AVR. These low values are thought to arise from red blood cell (RBC) shrinkage as blood encounters increasingly hypertonic regions and water is shifted out of RBCs, and from Fahraeus effects. As described by Fahraeus (1929), RBC migrate towards the center in small vessels, where the velocity is highest. As a consequence of this, it is thought that a relatively cell-free blood is "skimmed" from the periphery of interlobular arteries to enter the afferent arterioles of deep glomeruli, from which DVR subsequently arise. A detailed description of these phenomena can be found in the review of Pallone et al. (1990).

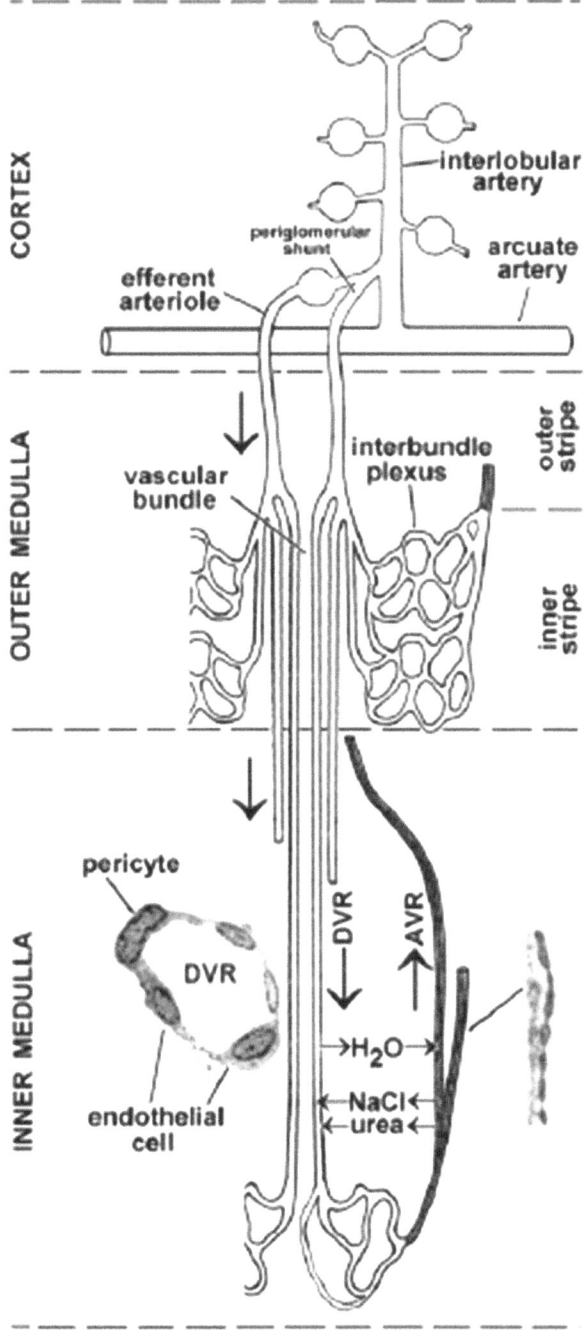

Fig. 4.1 Anatomy of the renal medullary microcirculation. In the outer medulla, juxtamedullary efferent arterioles give rise to descending vasa recta (*DVR*). The latter coalesce into vascular bundles in the inner stripe, where they lie in parallel with ascending vasa recta (*AVR*) returning from the inner medulla. DVR at the periphery of the bundles peel off to form the interbundle capillary plexus that perfuses outer medullary tubules (not shown). DVR in the center of the bundles penetrate into the inner medulla, where the bundles vanish, and where DVR and AVR are scattered among renal tubules (not shown). The endothelium is continuous in DVR and highly fenestrated in AVR (*insets*) (Reproduced from Pallone et al. (2003))

4.2 Counter-Current Exchange

4.2.1 Purpose

The vasa recta fulfill two essential functions. They bring nutrients to, and remove metabolic end products from the renal medulla. In addition, vasa recta must carry back to the general circulation the significant amounts of water and solutes that are reabsorbed from the descending loops of Henle and the collecting ducts. This second task must be performed without abolishing the cortico-medullary concentration gradient that allows water (and sodium) reabsorption to occur. If DVR and AVR were not arranged in a counter-flow manner, they would act to dissipate the osmolality gradient. The principle of counter-current transfer is to maximize radial exchanges of solute (or heat) while minimizing solute (or heat) loss from the extremities. The importance of the counter-current arrangement in the kidney was first recognized by Kuhn and his colleagues in the 1950s; the relevant references are in German, but a translation of one of their seminal articles appeared recently (Hargitay and Kuhn 2001). The need for efficient counter-exchange specifically across vasa recta was subsequently highlighted by Berliner et al. (1958), with an elegant analogy between heat and solute transfer. They showed that just as the maximum temperature attained in a heat exchanger with counter-current fluid flow is significantly greater than with straight flow, blood solute concentrations increase considerably more in a counter-current capillary loop than in a co-current arrangement.

4.2.2 Determinants of Counter-Current Exchange Efficiency

In order to examine the factors that affect the efficiency of counter-current exchange, we analyze a simplified model with an analytical solution, illustrated in Fig. 4.2. We regard blood as a homogeneous compartment (i.e., plasma and RBCs are not considered separately), and we assume that the vessels are impermeable to water, so that blood flow rate is constant; this unrealistic assumption is used here to illustrate basic principles, and will be abandoned further below. Another assumption of this simplified model is that the interstitial solute concentration profile is known a priori and linear, i.e.:

$$C_S^I(x) = C_0 + (C_L - C_0)\frac{x}{L}, \tag{4.1}$$

where C_S^I denotes the interstitial concentration of a given solute S, and C_0 and C_L are the values of C_S^I at $x = 0$ and L respectively.

4.2 Counter-Current Exchange

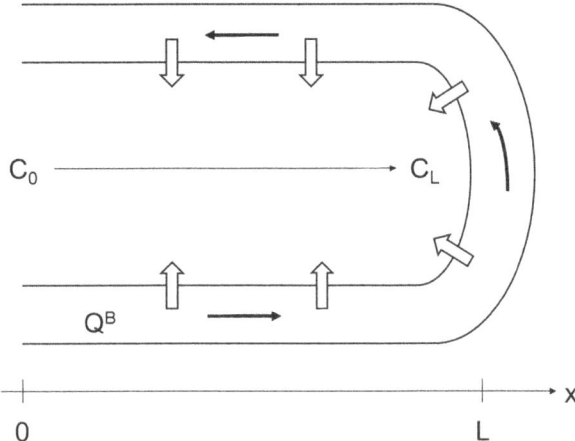

Fig. 4.2 Counter-current flow in a capillary loop, where solute (but not water) is exchanged via a common interstitium. The *black arrows* represent blood flow, and the *white arrows* transversal solute fluxes

The blood flow rate is taken to be positive in DVR, and negative in AVR; its absolute value is denoted Q^B. As derived earlier (see Eq. 2.33) the solute concentration in DVR (superscript "D") satisfies:

$$Q^B \frac{dC_S^D}{dx} = -\frac{S^P}{L} J_S^D(x), \tag{4.2}$$

where S^P is the surface area of the vessel and L its length. In the absence of water reabsorption, the outward solute flux J_S^D is given by (see Eq. 2.15):

$$J_S^D(x) = P_S \left[C_S^D(x) - C_S^I(x) \right], \tag{4.3}$$

where the solute permeability P_S is taken to be identical for DVR and AVR, so as to simplify calculations. The corresponding equations in AVR (superscript "A") are written as:

$$-Q^B \frac{dC_S^A}{dx} = -\frac{S^P}{L} J_S^A(x), \tag{4.4}$$

$$J_S^A(x) = P_S \left[C_S^A(x) - C_S^I(x) \right]. \tag{4.5}$$

Note that the "−" sign on the LHS of Eq. (4.4) arises because AVR flow is in the opposite direction. At the cortico-medullary junction ($x = 0$), the solute concentration in DVR plasma is taken to be equal to that in the interstitium:

$$C_S^D(0) = C_0. \tag{4.6}$$

Concentrations at the AVR inlet are not known. Instead, continuity implies:

$$C_S^A(L) = C_S^D(L). \tag{4.7}$$

The differential equations can be integrated to obtain solute concentration profiles along DVR and AVR. It can be shown that (see Problem 4.1):

$$C_S^D(x) = C_S^I(x) - \frac{(C_L - C_0)}{\Omega}\left[1 - \exp(-\Omega x/L)\right], \tag{4.8}$$

$$C_S^A(x) = C_S^I(x) + \frac{(C_L - C_0)}{\Omega}\left[1 + \exp(-\Omega(2 - x/L)) - 2\exp(-\Omega(1 - x/L))\right], \tag{4.9}$$

where the dimensionless parameter Ω is given by:

$$\Omega = \frac{P_S S^P}{Q^B}. \tag{4.10}$$

These last equations indicate that DVR concentrations consistently lag behind those in the interstitium, whereas, for sufficiently large Ω values, AVR concentrations remain slightly above interstitial values, except near the papilla (x ~ L). This lag in equilibration is due to the finite value of the permeability, and is amplified by high blood flow. The higher P_S (or S^P), or the lower Q^B, the larger Ω and the smaller the lag. This can also be view on Fig. 4.3, which displays concentration profiles for different values of Ω.

An ideal counter-current exchanger would maximize radial mass (or heat) transfers between adjacent limbs without removing solute (or heat) from the system. In that sense, the efficiency of our exchanger is inversely correlated with the amount of solute that is carried away from the renal medulla by the microcirculation, which is given by:

$$M_S = Q^B\left[C_S^A(0) - C_S^D(0)\right]. \tag{4.11}$$

Substituting Eqs. (4.8 and 4.9) into Eq. (4.11) yields:

$$M_S = Q^B \frac{(C_L - C_0)}{\Omega}\left[1 + \exp(-2\Omega) - 2\exp(-\Omega)\right]. \tag{4.12}$$

That is,

$$M_S = (C_L - C_0)\frac{(Q^B)^2}{P_S S^P}\left[1 + \exp(-2P_S S^P/Q^B) - 2\exp(-P_S S^P/Q^B)\right]. \tag{4.13}$$

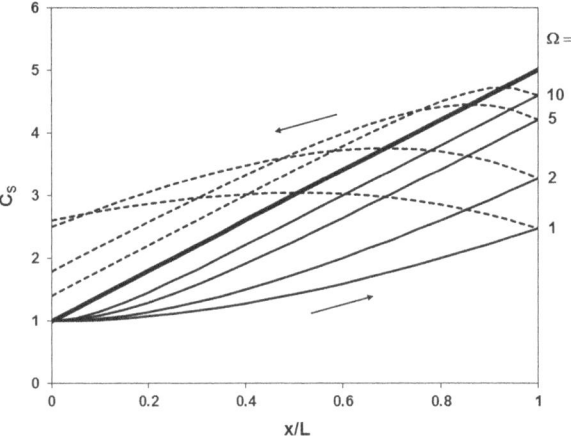

Fig. 4.3 DVR (*solid curves*) and AVR (*dashed curves*) concentration profiles in an idealized counter-current exchanger, for different values of the parameter $\Omega = P_S S^P/Q^B$ (see text). *Arrows* indicate the direction of flow. The *thick line* denotes the concentration in the surrounding medium (i.e., interstitium), taken to increase linearly along the exchanger axis, from 1 at $x = 0$ to 5 at $x = L$. Concentrations in DVR lag behind those in the interstitium. The lag in equilibration and the rate of solute removal are both reduced as Ω increases

Thus, the same factors that reduce the lag in equilibration also decrease the rate of solute removal and increase counter-current efficiency. Equation (4.13) also makes clear that blood flow exerts an especially strong dissipative, "wash-out" effect, since the rate of solute removal is proportional to the square of Q^B.

4.3 Conservation Equations in Vasa Recta

The counter-exchange model described above is an elegant way to illustrate how blood flow and effective permeability govern the rate of solute removal by the microcirculation, but it is too simple a representation of the vasa recta. In this section and the next, we develop more realistic transport equations.

We distinguish between the plasma compartment (superscript "P") and the red blood cells (superscript "R"). The net volume flux out of the plasma compartment equals the volume flux from plasma to interstitium (J_V^P) minus that from RBCs to plasma (J_V^R). Hence, conservation of volume in plasma and RBCs can be written as:

$$\frac{dQ^P}{dx} = -2\pi\, r \left(J_V^P - \psi J_V^R \right), \tag{4.14}$$

$$\frac{dQ^R}{dx} = -2\pi\, r\, \psi\, J_V^R, \tag{4.15}$$

where Q^P and Q^R are the plasma and RBC volume flows, r is the vessel radius ($2\pi r$ being equivalent to S^P/L), and ψ is the ratio of RBC-to-vessel surface area. We consider henceforth that Q^P and Q^R are negative in AVR, because of the flow direction – this eliminates the need for varying signs in the conservation equations.

The RBC-to-vessel surface area ratio varies with position and is computed as follows. The surface area and volume of a single RBC are denoted s^R and v^R, respectively. Whereas s^R is assumed constant (129 µm²), v^R varies as RBC shrink or swell; its value at $x=0$ is taken as 61 µm³. Consider a volume element within a vessel of length Δx and cross-sectional area $A = \pi r^2$. By definition of Ψ, we have:

$$\Psi = \frac{s^R N}{S^P (\Delta x/L)}, \qquad (4.16)$$

where N is the average number of RBCs within the volume element $A\Delta x$. This number is equal to the total volume occupied by RBCs within $A\Delta x$ divided by the volume of a single RBC:

$$N = \frac{A\Delta x}{v^R} \left(\frac{Q^R}{Q^P + Q^R} \right). \qquad (4.17)$$

The combination of these two equations yields:

$$\Psi = \frac{AL\, s^R}{S^P v^R} \left(\frac{Q^R}{Q^P + Q^R} \right) = \frac{r\, s^R}{2v^R} \left(\frac{Q^R}{Q^P + Q^R} \right). \qquad (4.18)$$

This expression can be further simplified by considering the conservation of RBCs: the number of RBCs flowing at a given location per unit time does not vary. In other words:

$$\frac{Q^R}{v^R} = \frac{Q_0^R}{v_0^R}, \qquad (4.19)$$

where the subscript "0" refers to values in DVR at $x=0$. Substituting Eq. (4.19) into Eq. (4.18), we finally obtain:

$$\Psi = \frac{r\, s^R}{2v_0^R} \left(\frac{Q_0^R}{Q^P + Q^R} \right). \qquad (4.20)$$

The conservation equations for a given solute S in plasma and RBC are written as:

$$\frac{d\left(Q^P C_S^P\right)}{dx} = -2\pi r \left(J_S^P - \Psi J_S^R\right), \qquad (4.21)$$

$$\frac{d\left(Q^R C_S^R\right)}{dx} = -2\pi \, r \, \psi \, J_S^R, \qquad (4.22)$$

where C_S^P and C_S^R denote the plasma and RBC concentration of solute S, and J_S^P and J_S^R the corresponding outward fluxes. Exchanges of sodium, albumin, hemoglobin and other non-urea solutes between plasma and RBCs are generally assumed to be negligible, so that $J_S^R = 0$ for these solutes. The last two equations implicitly assume that the solute is non-reactive. How to handle reactive solutes such as oxygen is described further below.

4.4 Water Transport Across Vas Rectum Walls

Prior to solving the system of differential equations representing mass conservation, we must specify how volume and solute fluxes are calculated. The vasa recta wall is viewed as a homogeneous membrane, and we use the generalized form of the Kedem-Katchalsky equation to determine the volume flux (see Eq. 2.7):

$$J_V^P = L_p^P \left(\Delta P - \sum_j \sigma_j \Delta \Pi_j \right), \qquad (4.23)$$

where L_p^P is the hydraulic conductivity of the vessel wall, ΔP is the transmembrane (plasma-to-interstitium) difference in hydraulic pressure, $\Delta \Pi_j$ is the transmembrane difference in osmotic pressure due to solute j, and σ_j is the osmotic reflection coefficient of the wall to solute j. Small solutes ("ss") and plasma proteins ("pr") may follow different transport pathways, so it is helpful to distinguish their contribution to the driving force and to rewrite the outward volume flux as:

$$J_V^P = L_p^P \left[\left(P^P - P^I\right) - \sigma_{pr}\left(\Pi_{pr}^P - \Pi_{pr}^I\right) - \sum_{ss} \sigma_{ss} \Delta \Pi_{ss} \right], \qquad (4.24)$$

where the superscript "I" denotes the interstitium. The small solutes that are exchanged between plasma and interstitium are essentially sodium (which is meant to represent NaCl) and urea. The oncotic pressure due to plasma proteins can be calculated using the Landis and Pappenheimer (1963) equation:

$$\Pi_{pr} = 2.1 \, C_{pr} + 0.16 \, \left(C_{pr}\right)^2 + 0.009 \, \left(C_{pr}\right)^3, \qquad (4.25)$$

where C_{pr} is the plasma protein concentration (in g/dl) in the compartment (plasma or interstitium) being considered. Water transport pathways differ between DVR and AVR, so we must now examine them separately.

4.4.1 Descending Vasa Recta

The following description applies only to the non-fenestrated portion of DVR. In rats, the DVR lumen oncotic pressure ($\Pi_{pr}^P \sim 20\text{--}25$ mmHg) is higher than the hydraulic pressure ($P^P \sim 6\text{--}10$ mmHg) both at the base and the tip of the papilla. The interstitial hydraulic pressure (P^I) is about 5 mmHg. The net driving force should therefore favor water influx into DVR, unless (a) the interstitial oncotic pressure is very high, or (b) small solutes exert a significant counteracting effect. In fact, micropuncture measurements have shown that the concentration of plasma protein increases along DVR, implying fluid loss (i.e., water efflux) along descending vasa recta. The first hypothesis, namely, a very high interstitial oncotic pressure, is incompatible with volume uptake by adjacent AVR, which is necessary to preserve the medullary water balance. Hence, fluid loss from descending vessels must result from transcapillary osmotic forces (i.e., $\Delta \Pi_{ss}$).

Due to the lag in equilibration between the vessels and their surroundings, small solute concentrations are higher in the interstitium than in DVR plasma at a given depth. Thus, if σ_{ss} is non-zero, the transcapillary osmotic pressure difference can in principle explain fluid loss from DVR. This hypothesis was experimentally confirmed in rats treated with furosemide (a loop diuretic that abolishes NaCl reabsorption in the thick ascending limb): elimination of the corticomedullary concentration gradient led to virtual abolition of water efflux from DVR. Prior to the discovery of water channels, σ_{ss} was calculated to be ≥ 0.05 based on Eq. (4.24) and water flux estimates.

The finding that DVR express aquaporin-1 (AQP-1) water channels modified the understanding of the underlying mechanisms. The DVR wall transports water via two routes: (1) a high conductance ("large pore"), presumably paracellular, shared pathway, which is permeable to both water and solutes, and (2) a transcellular pathway consisting of AQP-1 water channels, which exclude solutes. The experimental data can be reconciled by expressing the DVR plasma flux as the sum of two contributions:

$$J_V^{DVR} = J_{V,p}^{DVR} + J_{V,t}^{DVR}, \qquad (4.26)$$

$$J_{V,p}^{DVR} = L_{p,p}^{DVR} \left(\Delta P - \sigma_{pr} \Delta \Pi_{pr} \right), \qquad (4.27)$$

$$J_{V,t}^{DVR} = L_{p,t}^{DVR} \left(\Delta P - \Delta \Pi_{pr} - \sum_{ss} \Delta \Pi_{ss} \right), \qquad (4.28)$$

where $L_{p,p}^{DVR}$ and $L_{p,t}^{DVR}$ are respectively the DVR paracellular and transcellular hydraulic conductivity. It is thought that the high conductance pathway is not restrictive for small solutes, hence $\sigma_{ss} = 0$ in Eq. (4.27). Conversely, since AQP-1 is impermeable to solutes, all osmotic reflection coefficients for the transcellular pathway are taken to be 1. The osmotic pressure exerted by a small solute ss is

4.4 Water Transport Across Vas Rectum Walls

approximated as $\Pi_{ss} \approx \gamma_{ss} RTC_{ss}$, where γ_{ss} is the activity coefficient of the solute, and Eq. (4.28) is rewritten as:

$$J_{V,t}^{DVR} = L_{p,t}^{DVR} \left(\Delta P - \Delta \Pi_{pr} - RT \sum_{ss} \gamma_{ss} \Delta C_{ss} \right). \quad (4.29)$$

What is the order of magnitude of DVR transport parameters? Experimentally, hydraulic conductivity values are determined by imposing concentration gradients across vasa recta walls. When NaCl concentration gradients were employed to drive water flux across DVR walls in rats, the osmotic water permeability P_f was measured as 1,100 μm/s. Note that $P_f = L_p RT/\bar{v}_w$, where $\bar{v}_w$ is the partial molar volume of water (at 37 °C, $RT/\bar{v}_w = 1.074 \times 10^6$ mmHg); thus $L_{p,t}^{DVR}$ was estimated as 1.02×10^{-7} cm·s^{-1}·mmHg^{-1}. When albumin gradients were employed instead, the measured conductivity was insensitive to pCMBS (a blocker of AQP-1), suggesting that the paracellular pathway predominated under these conditions; $L_{p,p}^{DVR}$ was then estimated as 1.56×10^{-6} or 1.75×10^{-6} cm·s^{-1}·mmHg^{-1} (i.e., P_f ~16,700 μm/s), assuming an osmotic reflection coefficient to albumin of 1 or 0.89, respectively.

Physiologically, both small solutes and plasma proteins exert osmotic forces across the DVR wall, and paracellular and transcellular fluxes should be considered simultaneously. Models of the medullary microcirculation that account for both transport routes have confirmed that under normal conditions, the transcapillary concentration gradients of sodium and urea induce water efflux from DVR via AQP1, whereas classic Starling (i.e., hydraulic and oncotic) forces induce water uptake via the shared pathway.

It should be noted that recent studies in the AQP1 null mice suggest the existence of a third pathway for water transport across the DVR wall. In these AQP1 knock-out mice, urea (MW 60), glucose (MW 180), and raffinose (MW 594) were found to drive water movement across an AQP1-independent route. This additional pathway may consist of UTB urea carriers, but this hypothesis has not yet been confirmed.

4.4.2 Ascending Vasa Recta

Since there is net fluid loss from DVR, all the water that is reabsorbed from descending limbs and collecting ducts must be removed by the AVR. Water is thought to be carried exclusively across AVR fenestrations; AVR do not express AQP1, and small solute concentration gradients do not induce water flow across the AVR wall. The fenestrations impart a high permeability to AVR, which favors a rapid rate of water uptake. The volume flux through this pathway is given by:

$$J_V^{AVR} = L_p^{AVR} \left(\Delta P - \sigma_{pr} \Delta \Pi_{pr} \right). \quad (4.30)$$

Measurements of AVR properties are limited since these vessels cannot be isolated for ex vivo studies. Instead, experimenters have performed micropuncture and microperfusion of rat AVR on the surface of the exposed papilla (after removing the pelvis of the ureter). The hydraulic conductivity of AVR has thus been estimated as 12.5×10^{-6} cm $\cdot$ s^{-1} $\cdot$ mmHg^{-1}, with a reflection coefficient to albumin around 0.70. Note that the AVR-to-DVR water conductivity ratio is on the order of 10.

4.5 Solute Transport Across Vas Rectum Walls

We now consider explicitly the flux of a given solute S from DVR or AVR plasma into the interstitium. If the solute is carried through a pathway that is shared with water, the solute flux across this route can be expressed as (see Eq. 2.25):

$$J_S^P = J_{V,p}^P \left(1 - \sigma_S^P\right) \left(\frac{C_S^P - C_S^I \exp(-Pe)}{1 - \exp(-Pe)}\right), \quad (4.31)$$

where $J_{V,p}^P$ denotes the volume flux via the shared (presumably paracellular) pathway, and σ_S^P is the reflection coefficient of the vessel wall to solute S; for small solutes such as sodium and urea, $\sigma_S^P = 0$, as described above. The Péclet number, which measures the importance of convection relative to diffusion, is given by:

$$Pe = \frac{J_{V,p}^P \left(1 - \sigma_S^P\right)}{P_S^P}, \quad (4.32)$$

where P_S^P is the permeability of the shared pathway to solute S. Since sodium and urea have very similar diffusivities in dilute solution, they should have similar permeabilities across non-restrictive, large conductance pathways. The urea-to-sodium permeability ratio of inner medullary DVR and AVR was measured as $\sim$1 in rats, as expected. However, that ratio was found to be >4 in outer medullary DVR, suggesting the existence of an additional, separate pathway for urea transport. Indeed, it was later found that DVR express the urea endothelial carrier UTB, as do RBCs. The urea flux via the UTB (transcellular) pathway across the DVR wall is calculated as:

$$J_u^P = P_{UTB}^P \left(C_u^P - C_u^I\right), \quad (4.33)$$

where P_{UTB}^P denotes the permeability of DVR UTB to urea ($\sim 300 \times 10^{-5}$ cm/s in the outer medulla). Urea concentration increases steeply from the cortico-medullary junction to the papillary tip (by a factor >100 in the antidiuretic rat), whereas sodium concentration increases significantly less (by a factor of $\sim$5). UTB carriers provide a way for the DVR lumen (and the RBC cytosol) to rapidly equilibrate with the surrounding interstitium.

4.6 Transport Across Red Blood Cells

The non-homogeneous nature of blood, in which plasma and cells form distinct layers, is important when considering the transport of nutrients such as oxygen. In this section, we first describe the RBC fluxes of water and non-reactive solutes, and then focus on oxygen transport.

4.6.1 Water and Non-reactive Solutes

The RBC flux equations are similar to those of plasma. The RBC-to-plasma water flux is calculated assuming that there is no hydraulic pressure difference across the membrane:

$$J_V^R = L_p^R \left[\Pi_{pr}^P - \Pi_{hem}^R - RT \sum_{ss} \gamma_{ss} \left(C_{ss}^R - C_{ss}^P \right) \right]. \tag{4.34}$$

The first term within the brackets represents the oncotic pressure due to plasma proteins, and the second that due to hemoglobin. The latter is calculated using an equation fitted to experimental data:

$$\Pi_{hem}^R = RT \left[C_{hem}^m + 0.106 \left(C_{hem}^m \right)^2 + 0.020 \left(C_{hem}^m \right)^3 \right], \tag{4.35}$$

$$C_{hem}^m = \left(\frac{5.1}{34.4} \right) \frac{C_{hem}}{1 - \bar{v}_{hem} C_{hem}}, \tag{4.36}$$

where C_{hem}^m is the solvent-based molar (or molal) concentration of hemoglobin in RBC (in mmol/l solvent), C_{hem} is the hemoglobin concentration expressed in units of g/dl, and $\bar{v}_{hem} = 0.0075$ dl/g is the partial specific volume of hemoglobin. Note that here, small solutes include not only sodium and urea, but also RBC ions such as potassium and magnesium.

As mentioned above, RBC-to-plasma fluxes of sodium, hemoglobin, and plasma proteins are deemed negligible. Urea is carried across the RBC membrane via UTB carriers (characterized by a permeability P_{UTB}^R), so that:

$$J_u^R = P_{UTB}^R \left(C_u^R - C_u^P \right). \tag{4.37}$$

4.6.2 Oxygen Transport

A key role of the microcirculation is to bring oxygen (O_2) to the medulla. Renal oxygen tension (P_{O2}) in the rat kidney ranges from 40 to 50 mmHg in the cortex to

10–20 mmHg in the medulla. The low medullary P_{O2} stems from the high metabolic requirements of medullary thick ascending limbs (mTALs). As described in Chap. 3, the production of concentrated urine is contingent upon the active reabsorption of NaCl in mTALs, a process that is highly energy-dependent: the O_2 consumption-to-supply ratio is estimated as 80 % in the outer medulla.

Oxygen is carried by blood in free form (O_2) but predominantly as oxyhemoglobin (HbO_2). It is estimated that >95 % of O_2 is delivered to the medulla in the form of HbO_2. As it flows down DVR, a fraction of O_2 unbinds from hemoglobin, diffuses from RBC to adjacent layers, and is either consumed for metabolic purposes or flows back up along AVR. Conservation equations for O_2 must account for all these processes.

Oxygen Conservation Equations

Oxygen is a reactive solute, and its mass balance must therefore include a net generation term that accounts for the formation or disappearance of O_2 by chemical reaction (including binding). In plasma and RBCs, the O_2 conservation equations can be written as:

$$\frac{d\left(Q^P C^P_{O2}\right)}{dx} = -2\pi\, r \left(J^P_{O2} - \psi J^R_{O2}\right) + A^P \Phi^P_{O2}, \qquad (4.38)$$

$$\frac{d\left(Q^R C^R_{O2}\right)}{dx} = -2\pi\, r\, \psi J^R_{O2} + A^R \Phi^R_{O2}, \qquad (4.39)$$

where Φ^k_{O2} denotes the net rate of O_2 generation (i.e., production minus consumption) per unit volume in compartment k (k = P and R), and A^k is the cross-sectional area of compartment k. In RBCs, the O_2 generation rate accounts for O_2 dissociation from hemoglobin. In plasma, it accounts for the metabolic O_2 consumption that occurs in the adjacent endothelial layer (which is not explicitly considered); hence the parameter A^P reflects the cross-sectional area of the endothelium rather than that of plasma.

Oxygen Binding

Hemoglobin (Hb) has four O_2 binding sites, and its affinity for O_2 varies according to the number of occupied sites. A complex mathematical model of the O_2 dissociation curve was developed by Gilbert Adair in 1925 and others have been formulated since. These models generally involve many parameters and are cumbersome to implement in renal medullary transport models. Thus, we use instead the simpler, empirical equation formulated by Archibald Hill in 1910, which provides a satisfactory fit of the HbO_2 dissociation curve over physiological saturation ranges. The dissociation of HbO_2 into O_2 and hemoglobin is expressed as a one-step reaction:

4.6 Transport Across Red Blood Cells

$$HbO_2 \underset{}{\overset{k_1/k_{-1}}{\longleftrightarrow}} Hb + O_2$$

Thus, the net volumetric rate of O_2 formation in RBCs is given by:

$$\Phi_{O2}^R = k_1 C_{HbO2}^R - k_{-1} C_{Hb}^R C_{O2}^R. \tag{4.40}$$

Given that the kinetics of HbO_2 dissociation is significantly faster than the diffusion of O_2, it is generally assumed that the reaction is at equilibrium even during O_2 unloading. As shown by Hill, HbO_2 saturation (S_{HbO2}) can be described by the following equation:

$$S_{HbO2} \equiv \frac{C_{HbO2}^R}{C_{HbO2}^R + C_{Hb}^R} = \frac{\left(C_{O2}^R/C_{50}\right)^n}{1 + \left(C_{O2}^R/C_{50}\right)^n}, \tag{4.41}$$

where C_{50} is the O_2 concentration at half-saturation (equivalent to 26.4 mmHg) and n (= 2.6) characterizes the degree of binding cooperativity. Note that the solubility coefficient for oxygen (i.e., the C_{O2}/P_{O2} conversion factor) is 1.34 μM/mmHg in plasma and tubular fluid, and 1.56 in RBCs. The dissociation constant k_1 is fixed (49 s^{-1}), and the association constant is calculated at each level as a function of the local O_2 concentration, so as to yield compatibility with the Hill equilibrium curve:

$$k_{-1} = k_1 \frac{\left(C_{O2}^R\right)^{n-1}}{(C_{50})^n}. \tag{4.42}$$

The HbO_2 saturation curve predicted by the Hill equation is depicted in Fig. 4.4. Its sigmoidal shape accounts for the fact the affinity of hemoglobin for O_2 first increases, then decreases, as four successive O_2 bind to one Hb. The binding of the first O_2 molecule facilitates the binding of the second and third, but steric crowding then makes binding of the forth O_2 molecule more difficult. As described above, P_{O2} in the renal medulla hovers between 10 and 20 mmHg: in this range (i.e., the steeper portion of the curve), a small decrease in P_{O2} leads to significant dissociation of HbO_2, so as to release large amounts of O_2 to oxygen-poor tissues.

Metabolic Oxygen Consumption

The rate of O_2 consumption for basal metabolic purposes (i.e., to maintain vital functions, such as respiration and circulation, at rest) is usually described using an O_2-dependent Michaelis-Menten relationship, reflecting the fact that O_2 consumption decreases with decreasing O_2 availability:

$$\Phi_{O2} = \frac{\Phi_{O2}^{max} C_{O2}}{K_{M,O2} + C_{O2}}. \tag{4.43}$$

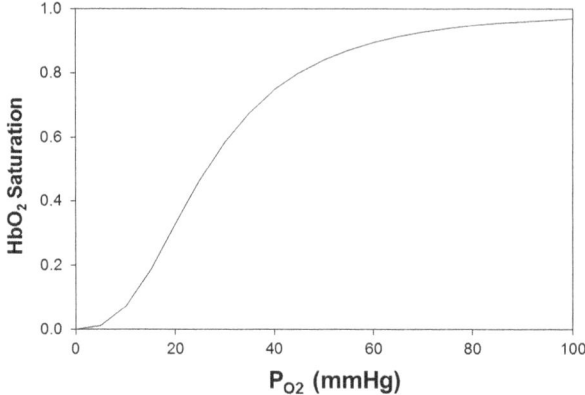

Fig. 4.4 Oxygen-hemoglobin equilibrium curve as predicted by the Hill model (Eq. 4.41). HbO_2 saturation (the fraction of hemoglobin that is oxygenated) is plotted as a function of oxygen tension. The partial pressure of O_2 at which HbO_2 is half saturated (P_{50}) is about 26.4 mmHg under normal conditions. An increase in P_{50} (i.e., a decrease in O_2 binding affinity) shifts the curve to the right, and facilitates HbO_2 dissociation and O_2 release. Conversely, a decrease in P_{50} shifts the curve to the left, so that hemoglobin binds O_2 more easily and unloads it more slowly. Factors that shift the curve to the right include an increase in temperature and in CO_2, and a decrease in pH (Bohr effect)

The maximal consumption rate $\left(\Phi_{O2}^{\max}\right)$ varies with the tissue being considered, and the parameter $K_{M,O2}$ may depend on factors known to affect O_2 conversion, such as nitric oxide availability.

It should be noted that active transport processes, such as those involving ATPase pumps, also consume significant amounts of O_2. As noted above, the active reabsorption of NaCl across mTALs, in particular, requires significant energy. Under optimal conditions, the number of Na^+ moles actively reabsorbed per mole of O_2 consumed (also known as the T_{Na^+}/Q_{O_2} ratio) is 18; the high mTAL Na^+ transport rate therefore significantly depletes O_2 in surrounding tissue. A full description of O_2 transport across renal tubules is beyond the scope of this book, but can be found elsewhere (Chen et al. 2009).

4.7 Full Model Specification

Flow rates and concentrations in vasa recta are obtained by solving the system of conservation equations in plasma and RBCs (Eqs. 4.14, 4.15, 4.21, and 4.22), using the water and solute flux expressions given above. Since plasma fluxes depend on interstitial pressures and concentrations, the latter must be specified or simultaneously determined. In addition, the number of vasa recta fluctuates along the cortico-medullary axis, since the depth at which DVR turn back to form AVR varies. We now describe possible ways to handle these complications.

4.7 Full Model Specification

4.7.1 Interstitial Values

If the vasa recta are included into a larger model of the renal medulla (such as the models described in Chap. 3), one that incorporates renal tubules, then mass balances can be written for the interstitium. In this case, the conservation equations for vasa recta, tubules, and interstitium are solved simultaneously, yielding flow rates and concentrations in all compartments.

Otherwise, some assumptions must be made. One possibility is to stipulate interstitial concentration profiles, by extrapolating experimental data. Some models for example specify the interstitial osmolarity, as well as the fraction of that osmolarity that is due to sodium, along the cortico-medullary axis. Another approach consists in specifying interstitial "generation" rates, i.e., the rates at which water and solutes are reabsorbed from renal tubules. The significant drawback of these two approaches is that they cannot easily account for the coupling between medullary vessels and tubules.

4.7.2 Varying Number of Vasa Recta

Let $N(x)$ denote the number of DVR (or AVR) at level x, and $q^P(x)$ the plasma flow rate in a single DVR (or AVR) at x. Given the large number of vessels (and nephrons) in mammalian kidneys, we assume that $N(x)$ is a continuous, decreasing function of x. The rate at which the vasa recta end at x is equal to $-dN(x)/dx$. $N(x)$ is analogous to the loop of Henle distribution function $w(x)$ discussed in Sect. 3.6. Note that we assume that at a given medullary depth, all vasa recta share the same physical and transport properties, whereas those of the loops of different lengths may differ.

The total plasma flow in DVR varies along the cortico-medullary axis because (a) plasma exchanges water with its surrounding compartments, and (b) the number of vasa recta varies as DVR are converted to AVR. Hence, the difference in total DVR plasma flow between depths x_1 and x_2, which is written as $N(x_2) q^P(x_2) - N(x_1) q^P(x_1)$, equals the amount of plasma entering the DVR lumen across vessel walls and RBC membranes between x_1 and x_2, minus the amount of plasma that is shunted to AVR in each of the DVR that ends between x_1 and x_2. In other words:

$$N(x_2) q^P(x_2) - N(x_1) q^P(x_1) = \\ -\int_{x_1}^{x_2} 2\pi r \left[J_V^P(x) - \psi J_V^R(x) \right] N(x) \, dx - \int_{x_1}^{x_2} \left(-\frac{dN(x)}{dx} \right) q^P(x) \, dx. \quad (4.44)$$

Note that the transmural fluxes J_V^P and J_V^R are based on a single capillary, as defined above. The differential form of Eq. (4.44) is:

$$\frac{d\left(Nq^P\right)}{dx} = -2\pi\, r\left(J_V^P - \psi J_V^R\right) N + \frac{dN}{dx} q^P. \tag{4.45}$$

Equation (4.45) can be re-written in terms of the total plasma flow rate, $Q^P = Nq^P$, yielding:

$$\frac{dQ^P}{dx} = -2\pi\, r\left(J_V^P - \psi J_V^R\right) N + \frac{dN}{dx}\left(\frac{Q^P}{N}\right). \tag{4.46}$$

Similarly, variations in the total RBC flow rate are given by:

$$\frac{dQ^R}{dx} = -2\pi\, r\, \psi\, J_V^R N + \frac{dN}{dx}\left(\frac{Q^R}{N}\right). \tag{4.47}$$

The conservation equations for solute S in DVR (or AVR) plasma and RBC are derived using the same approach:

$$\frac{d\left(Q^P C_S^P\right)}{dx} = -2\pi\, r\left(J_S^P - \psi J_S^R\right) N + \frac{dN}{dx}\left(\frac{Q^P C_S^P}{N}\right), \tag{4.48}$$

$$\frac{d\left(Q^R C_S^R\right)}{dx} = -2\pi\, r\, \psi\, J_S^R N + \frac{dN}{dx}\left(\frac{Q^R C_S^R}{N}\right). \tag{4.49}$$

4.7.3 Boundary Conditions

Boundary conditions for DVR and AVR flow rates and concentrations must be prescribed. The DVR flow rate and composition at the cortico-medullary junction (at $x = 0$) are estimated based on those of efferent arterioles, from which they arise. Typical DVR inlet values are given in Table 4.1. The boundary conditions for AVR are obtained by continuity with DVR, assuming that they are directly connected. That is, at the level at which an AVR is formed, its plasma and RBC volume and molar flow rates are equal to those of the DVR from which it arises.

The system of differential equations representing mass balance is coupled and non-linear, and is usually solved using an iterative procedure. Typically, an initial guess is made for flow and concentration profiles in both DVR and AVR, and the equations are integrated iteratively, until the normalized difference between the current and previous estimates of each variable at any given depth is less than a specified tolerance.

4.8 Problems

Table 4.1 Boundary values for DVR at $x = 0$

Single vessel blood flow rate	9.0 nl/min
Hematocrit	0.25
Plasma protein concentration	6.8 g/dl
Plasma concentration of sodium	150 mM
Plasma concentration of urea	5 mM
RBC concentration of urea	5 mM
RBC concentration of hemoglobin	5.1 mM (or 34.4 g/dl)
RBC concentration of other small solutes	292 mOsm/l

The activity coefficient of urea is taken as 0.9, and that of sodium (which implicitly represents NaCl) as 1.86

4.8 Problems

Problem 4.1. Derive equations (4.8) and (4.9), that is, show that for the idealized counter-current exchanger described in Sect. 4.2, the concentrations in DVR and AVR are given by:

$$C_S^D(x) = C_S^I(x) - \frac{(C_L - C_0)}{\Omega}[1 - \exp(-\Omega \, x/L)],$$

$$C_S^A(x) = C_S^A(x) + \frac{(C_L - C_0)}{\Omega}[1 + \exp(-\Omega \, (2 - x/L)) - 2\exp(-\Omega \, (1 - x/L))].$$

Problem 4.2. Estimate the paracellular and transcellular volume fluxes across the DVR endothelial wall (in cm/s). Examine two limiting cases: (a) the oncotic pressure due to proteins in the interstitium is negligible, or (b) it is equal to that in DVR plasma. Assume that the transcapillary concentration gradient is 10 mM each for sodium and urea. State any other assumption you might make.

Problem 4.3. Calculate the amount (in mol/s) of O_2 supplied by a single DVR using the parameters given in Table 4.1, assuming that $P_{O2} = 50$ mmHg at the cortico-medullary junction.

Problem 4.4. Compare the rate of oxygen uptake in counter-current and co-current flows. As illustrated in Fig. 4.5, O_2 is transferred from a fluid F (e.g., air or water) to blood (B); the two compartments are separated by a membrane of permeability γ. The volume flow rates in F (Q^F) and B (Q^B) are taken to be constant. Assume for simplicity that the O_2 solubility coefficient is the same in F and B.

(a) Show the conservation equations for oxygen tension (denoted P) can be written as:

$$\frac{dP^F(x)}{dx} = -a\left[P^F(x) - P^B(x)\right],$$

$$\frac{dP^B(x)}{dx} = -\sigma b\left[P^F(x) - P^B(x)\right],$$

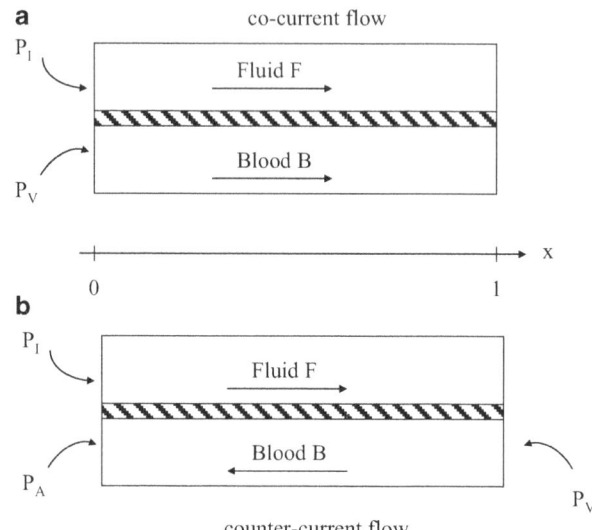

Fig. 4.5 Model representation of the co-current (**a**) and counter-current (**b**) exchange of oxygen between F and B. P_I and P_V are the O_2 tension values at the inlet of F and B, respectively

where $\sigma = -1$ for counter-current flow, and $\sigma = +1$ for co-current flow, and we have introduced the parameters $a = \gamma/Q^F$ and $b = \gamma/Q^B$.

(b) Determine P^F and P^B for each flow configuration (assume $a = b$). Express the results in terms of the inlet values, P_I and P_V.

(c) Determine the rate of oxygen removal (R_{O2}) from fluid F between $x = 0$ and $x = 1$ for both configurations.

(d) Plot the counter-current to co-current R_{O2} ratio for values of a ranging from 0.01 to 10. Comment on the efficiency of counter-current exchange.

References

Berliner, R.W., Levinski, N.G., et al.: Dilution and concentration of the urine and the action of the antidiuretic hormone. Am. J. Med. **24**, 730–744 (1958)

Chen, J., Layton, A.T., et al.: A mathematical model of O2 transport in the rat outer medulla. I. Model formulation and baseline results. Am. J. Physiol. Renal Physiol. **297**(2), F517–F536 (2009)

Fahraeus, R.: The suspension stability of the blood. Physiol. Rev. **9**, 241–274 (1929)

Hargitay, B., Kuhn, W.: The multiplication principle as the basis for concentrating urine in the kidney: [Chemie 55(6): 539-558, 1951 (with comments by Bart Hargitay and S. Randall Thomas)]. J. Am. Soc. Nephrol. **12**(7), 1566–1586 (2001)

Landis, EM., Pappenheimer, JR.: Exchange of substances through the capillary walls. In: Hamilton, WF. (ed.) Handbook of Physiology, Section 2. Circulation. **2**, 961–1034. American Physiological Society, Washington, DC (1963)

Pallone, T., Robertson, C., et al.: Renal medullay microcirculation. Physiol. Rev. **70**, 885–920 (1990)
Pallone, T.L., Turner, M.R., et al.: Countercurrent exchange in the renal medulla. Am. J. Physiol. Regul. Integr. Comp. Physiol. **284**(5), R1153–R1175 (2003)
Pallone, T.L., Edwards, A., et al.: Renal medullary circulation. Compr. Physiol. **2**, 97–140 (2012)

Chapter 5
Tubuloglomerular Feedback

Abstract Tubuloglomerular feedback (TGF) contributes to hemodynamics control by adjusting the single nephron glomerular filtration rate according to the chloride concentration sensed downstream. To analyze the TGF system, which is a negative feedback loop, we first formulate model equations consisting of a partial differential equation that describes solute conservation along the thick ascending limb, and a delay equation that describes the feedback response. Depending on model parameters, in particular the feedback delay and gain, the model may predict limit-cycle oscillations or a time-independent steady state, following a transient perturbation. We analyze the dynamic behaviors of the TGF model by linearizing the model equations and deriving a characteristic equation. Numerical simulations can also be conducted to assist in the interpretation of the analysis.

5.1 A Negative Feedback Loop

Normal renal function requires that the fluid flow through the nephron be kept within a narrow range. When tubular flow rate falls outside of that range, the ability of the nephron to maintain salt and water balance may be compromised. Tubular flow rate depends, in large part, on glomerular filtration rate (GFR), which is regulated by several mechanisms. One of these is the tubuloglomerular feedback (TGF): TGF provides a mechanism by which changes in GFR can be detected and rapidly corrected for on a minute-to-minute basis as well as over sustained periods. When changes in nephron flow rate are detected, feedback signals are initiated that give rise to a cascade of events that aim to return GFR to an appropriate level.

The TGF system is a negative feedback loop in which the chloride ion concentration is sensed downstream in the nephron tubule by a specialized cluster of cells, the macula densa, that are located in the tubular wall of the thick ascending limb in the region where it comes into close contact with the glomerulus; see Fig. 5.1. The thick ascending limb is an important tubular segment for TGF function. The epithelial cells of the thick ascending limb vigorously pump NaCl from the tubular

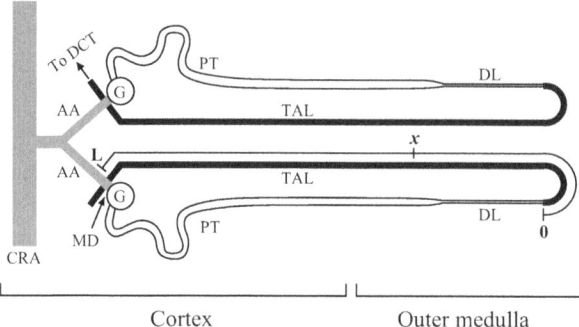

Fig. 5.1 A schematic drawing of two short-looped nephrons and their afferent arterioles (*AA*). The arterioles branch from a small connecting artery (unlabeled), which arises from a cortical radial artery (*CRA*). The nephron consists of the glomerulus (*G*) and a tubule having several segments, including: the proximal tubule (*PT*), the descending limb (*DL*), the thick ascending limb (*TAL*), and the distal convoluted tubule (*DCT*). Each nephron has its glomerulus in the renal cortex, and each short-looped rat nephron has a loop that extends into the outer medulla of the kidney. The macula densa (MD), a localized plaque of specialized cells, forms a portion of the TAL wall that is separated from the AA by a few layers of extraglomerular mesangial cells; in this figure, the macula densa is part of the short TAL segment that passes behind the AA. Fluid from the DCT enters the collecting duct system (not shown), from which urine ultimately emerges. Structures labeled on one nephron apply to both nephrons (Figure and legend adapted from Pitman et al. 2004)

fluid into the surrounding interstitium by means of active transport. Because the thick ascending limb walls are water impermeable, no water follows. As a result, the active reabsorption of NaCl dilutes the tubular fluid.

If the GFR increases above its normal, base-line rate, then tubular fluid flow in the thick ascending limb increases. The resulting shorter transit time of a given fluid packet along the thick ascending limb implies that a smaller fraction of filtered NaCl is reabsorbed. As a result, the chloride concentration in thick ascending limb tubular fluid alongside the macula densa is increased above its target value. This concentration increase, through a sequence of signaling events, which occur in the juxtaglomerular apparatus, results in a constriction of the afferent arteriole and a corresponding reduction in glomerular blood pressure and thus a reduction in GFR. Conversely, if GFR decreases below its base-line rate, the chloride concentration in tubular fluid alongside the macula densa is decreased below its target value, and TGF acts to increase GFR by signaling the afferent arteriole to relax. The resulting higher flow rate reduces transit time along the thick ascending limb, and raises tubular fluid chloride concentration. This TGF relation is depicted in Fig. 5.2.

Physically, the TGF system serves multiple physiological functions: TGF participates in balancing GFR with the transport capacities of the cells that form the tubular portion of the nephron; TGF plays a fundamental role in stabilizing water and electrolyte delivery to the distal nephron and to the collecting duct system; and TGF helps protect the glomerulus from damage that might arise from sufficiently large or sufficiently abrupt excursions in blood pressure. Mathematically, TGF provides a platform for learning how to model a complex biological feedback system.

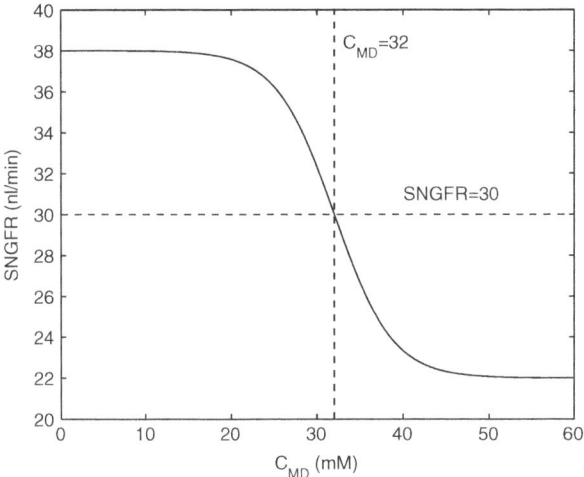

Fig. 5.2 TGF response, which gives SNGFR as a function of macula densa [Cl$^-$] (C_{MD})

5.2 Brief Introduction to Delay-Differential Equations

Delay-differential equations often arise in biological or technological control problems; the TGF system is one example. In these systems, a controller senses variations in the state of the system, and makes adjustments to return the system to its equilibrium state. Because these adjustments frequently cannot be made instantaneously, a delay arises between the observation and the control action. And as we will see later, different delay values can lead to qualitatively different system behaviors.

5.2.1 A Simple Example

Consider a simple feedback system, where the rate-of-change of a variable x at time t depends on its state a little while ago, at $t - \tau$:

$$\frac{dx}{dt} = -x(t - \tau), \tag{5.1}$$

with initial history

$$x(t) = 1, \quad t \leq 0. \tag{5.2}$$

To compute the solution to Eq. (5.1), we consider consecutive time intervals of size τ, i.e., $(0, \tau]$, $(\tau, 2\tau]$, $(2\tau, 3\tau]$, ... As an example, take $\tau = 1$. Then over the

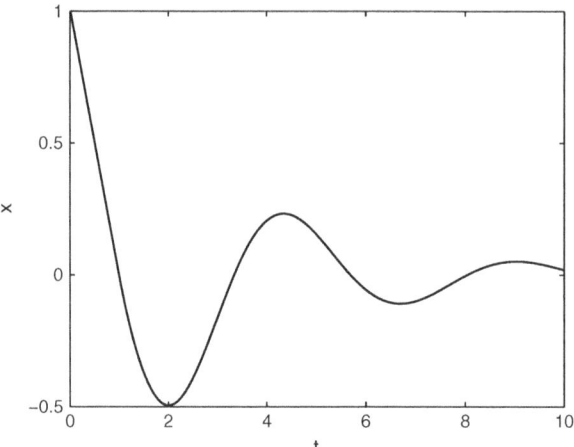

Fig. 5.3 A damped oscillatory solution for delayed ODE (5.1)

interval $t \in (0, \tau] = (0, 1]$, $x(t-1) = 1$ as given by the initial history. Thus, we have

$$\frac{dx}{dt} = -1, \quad t \in (0, 1], \tag{5.3}$$

with initial condition $x(0) = 1$. Hence,

$$x(t) = 1 - \int_0^t 1 \, ds = 1 - t. \tag{5.4}$$

Over the next interval $(1, 2]$, with initial condition $x(1) = 0$, we have

$$x(t) = 0 - \int_1^t (1 - (s-1)) \, ds = -\left(2s - \frac{1}{2}t^2\right)\Big|_1^t = \frac{3}{2} - 2t + \frac{1}{2}t^2. \tag{5.5}$$

At $t = 2$, $x(2) = -\frac{1}{2}$. In the interval $(2, 3]$,

$$x(t) = -\frac{1}{2} - \int_2^t \left(\frac{3}{2} - 2(s-1) + \frac{1}{2}(s-1)^2\right) ds \tag{5.6}$$

$$= \frac{5}{3} - \frac{3}{2}t + (t-1)^2 - \frac{1}{6}(t-1)^3. \tag{5.7}$$

The solution $x(t)$, which is a damped oscillation, is shown in Fig. 5.3 for $0 \leq t \leq 10$.

5.2.2 Stability Analysis

Much can be learned about the general behaviors of the system if we conduct a stability analysis of its equilibrium point or steady state. The procedures are similar to a stability analysis for an ODE (without delay). For Eq. (5.1), $x(t) = 0 \equiv x^*$ is a steady state for all t. To analyze the stability of x^*, we assume a time-dependent solution $x(t)$ that deviates somewhat from steady state:

$$x(t) = x^* + \tilde{x}(t). \tag{5.8}$$

Our goal is to find out if the deviation $\tilde{x}(t)$ grows in time or not. To accomplish that, we substitute the solution (5.8) into the delay-differential equation (5.1):

$$\frac{d}{dt}\left(x^* + \tilde{x}(t)\right) = -\left(x^* + \tilde{x}(t - \tau)\right). \tag{5.9}$$

Since $x^* = 0$, the above equation simplifies to

$$\frac{d\tilde{x}(t)}{dt} = -\tilde{x}(t - \tau). \tag{5.10}$$

We then assume that the above equation has an exponential solution, i.e.,

$$\tilde{x}(t) = Ae^{\lambda t}, \tag{5.11}$$

where λ is a complex number. Substituting the exponential solution (5.11) into Eq. (5.10), we get

$$\lambda Ae^{\lambda t} = -Ae^{\lambda(t-\tau)}, \tag{5.12}$$

which simplifies to the *characteristic equation*

$$\lambda + e^{-\lambda \tau} = 0. \tag{5.13}$$

Given a delay τ, we can analyze the stability of x^* by computing the solution λ to the characteristic equation (5.13). Alternatively, we can ask what values of τ yield a stable x^* and what values yield an unstable one.

For a given τ, the solution λ of Eq. (5.13) is

$$\lambda = \frac{LW(-\tau)}{\tau}, \tag{5.14}$$

where $LW(x)$ denotes the Lambert W function. The deviation $\tilde{x}(t)$ grows in time if Re $(\lambda) > 0$, and decays if Re $(\lambda) < 0$. As an example, for $\tau = 1$, a solution is $\lambda = -0.3181 + i1.337$, which decays. On the other hand, for a longer delay of $\tau = 5$, a solution is $\lambda = 0.1691 + i0.3750$; and the system is unstable.

In one important way Eq. (5.13) differs from the characteristic equation that we get in the stability analysis of an ODE (with no delay). The characteristic equation in an ODE stability analysis is a polynomial, which has a finite number of roots. If any of the solutions have positive real parts, then the equilibrium point in unstable. If all the solutions have negative real parts, then the equilibrium point is stable. In contrast, because of the exponential term $e^{-\lambda \tau}$, Eq. (5.13) has an infinite number of roots in the complex plane. We can't compute all the roots. Instead, for the TGF system, we consider only roots that have physiological relevance.

5.3 A Partial Differential Equation Model with Delayed Feedback

Now that we are comfortable with delay-differential equations, we will proceed to build a model of the TGF system in a short-looped rat nephron. The first step in building such a model, or any model, is to decide what components to represent, and at what level of details. Because the chloride ion is believed to be the principal signaling agent for TGF activation along the macula densa, it makes sense to represent in detail the portion of the loop of Henle where tubular fluid chloride concentration varies the most. (Tubular fluid contains other solutes too, e.g., calcium, urea, etc., but they are not believed to play a significant role in TGF.) That segment is the thick ascending limb, which actively pumps NaCl out of the lumen. (Actually, it is only sodium that is being pumped; the chloride ion follows down an electrochemical gradient.) Besides the thick ascending limb, other segments involved in the TGF system include the afferent arteriole, the glomerulus, the proximal tubule, and the descending limb. In a highly detailed model of the TGF, all these segments can be represented in detail. However, for now we aim for a "minimal model," i.e., one that captures the essential features of the TGF system while representing as few components in detail as possible. Thus, the actions of the afferent arteriole, glomerulus, proximal tubule, and descending limb are represented by phenomenological relations. The thick ascending limb is represented by a rigid tube. The only solute represented in the model thick ascending limb is chloride. A schematic diagram for the model is shown in Fig. 5.4.

5.3.1 Solute Conservation Along the Thick Ascending Limb

In Chap. 3, we derived a solute conservation equation along a renal tubule, Eq. (3.3), which we will use to describe solute conservation along the thick ascending limb. Now Eq. (3.3) is given for steady state, but here we will formulate a dynamic

5.3 A Partial Differential Equation Model with Delayed Feedback

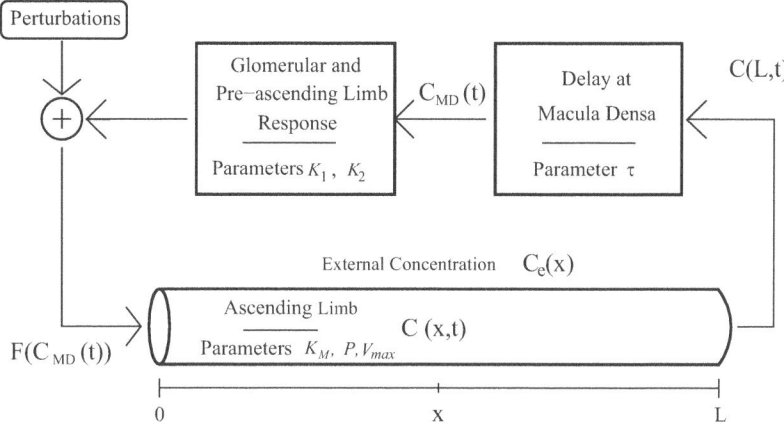

Fig. 5.4 Schematic representation of model configuration. Model represents three essential elements of the TGF pathway: thick ascending limb (cylinder), delay at the macula densa (*box at right*), and TGF response function (*box at left*). Perturbations and coupling enter as adjustments to thick ascending limb flow rate

(or, time-dependent) equation. The thick ascending limb is water impermeable, so water flux is zero and water flow rate is constant along that segment. It is natural in this model to take x to be positive in the flow direction of the thick ascending limb (which, unfortunately, is the opposite of the convention used in Chap. 3). Solute fluxes along the thick ascending limb have two components. One is passive diffusion; the other is active solute transport, characterized by Michaelis-Mention kinetics. Taken together, NaCl concentration along the thick ascending limb, denoted by $C(x,t)$ is given by

$$A(x)\frac{\partial}{\partial t}C(x,t) = -F(t)\frac{\partial}{\partial x}C(x,t) - 2\pi r(x)$$
$$\times \left(\frac{V_{\max}C(x,t)}{K_M + C(x,t)} + P\Big(C(x,t) - C^e(x)\Big)\right), \quad (5.15)$$

where A and R denote the cross-sectional area and radius of the thick ascending limb lumen, and $C^e(x)$ denotes the external (interstitial) NaCl concentration. The first term on the right corresponds to axial intratubular solute advection. As previously noted, because the thick ascending limb is water impermeable, F is constant along space, but may vary in time because of the TGF response. The two terms inside the large pair of parentheses correspond to active solute transport characterized by Michaelis-Menten kinetics, with maximum active transport rate $V_{\max}$ and Michaelis constant K_m, and transepithelial diffusion characterized by permeability P.

5.3.2 Tubuloglomerular Feedback Response

In the model, the fluid flow rate along the thick ascending limb is controlled by the TGF response. At time t, the flow rate $F(t)$ is a function of the macula densa chloride concentration some time τ ago. The delay τ arises because, as revealed in biological experiments, a change in macula densa concentration does not fully affect afferent arteriole muscle tension until after a time delay, which is approximately 3.5 s in rat. Based on empirical measurements of GFR and chloride concentration, we describe the TGF response as

$$F(t) = F_0 \bigg(1 + K_1 \tanh \Big(K_2 \big(C_{\text{op}} - C_{\text{MD}}(t - \tau) \big) \Big) \bigg), \qquad (5.16)$$

where $C_{\text{MD}}(t)$ denotes NaCl concentration at the macula densa, i.e., $C_{\text{MD}}(t) = C(L, t)$. The constant C_{op} is the time-independent steady-state thick ascending limb tubular fluid chloride concentration at the macula densa when $F(t)$ assumes a steady-state value of F_0. The dependence of $F(t)$ on C_{MD}, which gives the TGF response, is described by a hyperbolic tangent function, to approximate empirical data (see Fig. 5.2). The magnitude of the TGF response is given by, in part, K_1, and the sensitivity of $F(t)$ to deviations of C_{MD} from C_{op} is given by the product of $K_1 K_2$ (which you can confirm by taking the derivative of $F(t)$ with respect to C_{MD}).

5.4 Numerical Solution and Limit-Cycle Oscillatory Behaviors

Given the model equations (5.15) and (5.16), one can ask a number of questions: What is the steady-state chloride concentration profile? If the system is transiently perturbed, will it return to a time-independent steady-state solution, or will it evolve into regular, sustained, stable oscillations, i.e., limit-cycle oscillations? How do the dynamic behaviors of the system depend on TGF parameters such as gain and delay?

5.4.1 Time-Independent Steady-State Solution

Let's first find the steady-state solution of the system. We will call the steady-state concentration profile along the thick ascending limb $S(x)$. To find that solution, we set the tubular flow rate to the steady-state TGF operating point flow F_0, and obtain the time-independent form of Eq. (5.15) by setting the time-derivative to zero. This results in an ODE for $S(x)$:

5.4 Numerical Solution and Limit-Cycle Oscillatory Behaviors

Table 5.1 Base-case parameter values

Parameter	Description	Dimensional value
C_o	Loop-bend [Cl$^-$]	275 mM
F_o	Steady-state flow rate	6.00 nl/min
K_1, K_2	TGF response parameters	
K_M	Michaelis-Menten constant	70.0 mM
L	Thick ascending limb length	0.500 cm
P	[Cl$^-$] permeability	1.50×10^{-5} cm/s
r	Thick ascending limb luminal radius	10.0 μm
V_{max}	Maximum active NaCl transport rate	14.5 nmole·cm^{-2}·s^{-1}
τ	TGF delay	3.50 s

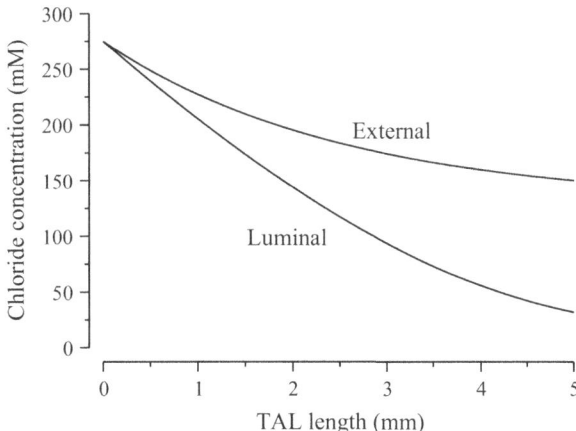

Fig. 5.5 Steady-state thick ascending limb luminal chloride concentration ($S(x)$) and external chloride concentration profiles

$$\frac{d}{dx}S(x) = -\frac{2\pi r(x)}{F_o}\left(\frac{V_{max}S(x)}{K_M + S(x)} + P\Big(S(x) - C^e(x)\Big)\right). \quad (5.17)$$

The initial condition is $S(0) = C_o$, which is the chloride concentration entering the thick ascending limb at the loop bend.

To find a solution of the initial value problem Eq. (5.17), we need a few parameters: F_o, V_{max}, K_M, $C^e(x)$, etc. Values for these parameters are given in Table 5.1. Extratubular concentration is specified by $C^e(x) = C_o(A_1 \exp(-A_3 x/L) + A_2)$, where $A_1 = (1 - 150 \text{ mM}/C_o)/(1 - \exp(-A_3))$, $A_2 = 1 - A_1$, and $A_3 = 2$. This condition yields a cortical interstitial concentration $C^e(L)$ of 150 mM.

Because an analytical solution for Eq. (5.17) does not exist, we numerically integrate Eq. (5.17). The solution is the steady-state profile $S(x)$, which is shown in Fig. 5.5, together with the external concentration profile $C^e(x)$. A few things worth pointing out about these profiles:

1. The steady-state operating concentration C_{op} corresponds to $S(L)$.
2. $S(x)$ decreases monotonically from the thick ascending limb entrance ($x = 0$) to the macula densa ($x = L$). That decrease is attributable to the outward-directed active transport of NaCl, without any accompanying water reabsorption.
3. $C^e(x)$ also decreases monotonically towards the cortex, based on the assumption that in the deeper outer medulla the NaCl reabsorption rate is higher and the water reabsorption rate is lower.
4. At each level x, $C^e(x) > S(x)$. That implies that chloride diffuses passively back into the thick ascending limb lumen. Nonetheless, $S(x)$ continues to decrease as a function of x because the rate of active NaCl chloride transport exceeds that of inward-directed passive diffusion.
5. Near the macula densa ($x = L$), $S(x)$ approaches what is called the "static head," as its slope is much reduced. This happens because as $S(x)$ becomes small, the active transport rate decreases. A "static head" is reached when the active transport is balanced by passive diffusion, i.e., when

$$\frac{V_{\max} S(x)}{K_M + S(x)} = -P\Big(S(x) - C^e(x)\Big), \tag{5.18}$$

and when $\frac{dS(x)}{dx}\big|_{x=L} = 0$.

Because the goal of the TGF system is to control chloride delivery by varying fluid flow rate, a static head is undesirable as far as the TGF system is concerned. That is because the degree to which macula densa chloride concentration can be controlled by varying flow rate is dependent on $S'(L)$. To understand that, consider the dynamic model and imagine that $F(t)$ is raised by an infinitesimal amount (perhaps in response to a macula densa chloride concentration that falls below C_{op}). Because the thick ascending limb is a water-impermeable rigid tube, that has the effect of pushing the whole column of fluid forward by a small amount. Now if $C'(L) = 0$, that would not change $C(L)$ at all! In contrast, if $C'(L) < 0$ (as in normally the case, see Fig. 5.5), $C(L)$ would increase, which is what we want.

5.4.2 Limit-Cycle Oscillations

Renal blood pressure is almost constantly perturbed, as the animal breathes or moves about, and as its heart beats, etc. Following a transient perturbation, nephron fluid pressure (or flow) may return to a time-independent steady state, or it may evolve into a limit-cycle oscillation. The asymptotic behavior depends on, among many things, model parameters such as TGF gain and delay. Given a set of model parameter values, one may predict the asymptotic behavior of the in vivo tubular fluid dynamics that occurs in response to a perturbation by means of direct computations of the numerical solution to the model equations (5.15) and (5.16).

5.4 Numerical Solution and Limit-Cycle Oscillatory Behaviors

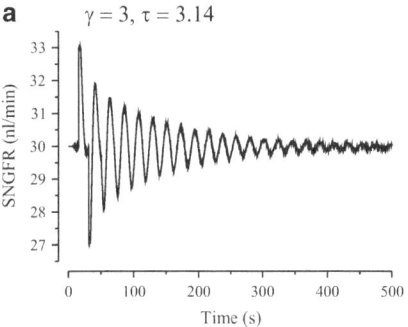
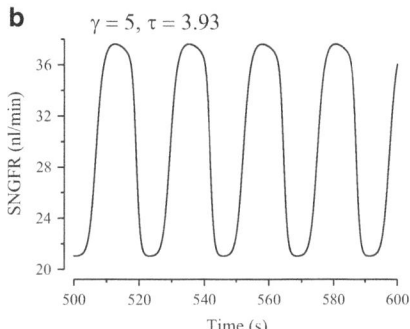

Fig. 5.6 Model equations (5.15) and (5.16) predict (a) damped oscillations for $(\gamma, \tau) = (3, 3.14\,\text{s})$, and (b) sustained oscillations for $(\gamma, \tau) = (5, 3.93\,\text{s})$. We assume that 5/6 of the fluid is reabsorbed along the proximal tubule and descending limb, so SNGFR $= 6\,F(t)$

We perform two simulations using the tubular dimensions and transport parameters in Table 5.1. The two simulations use different TGF delay τ and gain γ. τ is the delay that appears in TGF response Eq. (5.16). γ is a new parameter, defined by the product of $F'(C_{\text{op}})$ (the derivative is taken with respect to C_{MD}) and $S'(L)$ (spatial derivative), non-dimensionalized by L/F_0; i.e., $\gamma = (L/F_0)F'(C_{\text{op}})S'(L)$. To interpret γ, we note that $F'(C_{\text{op}})$ determines the degree to which F is adjusted given a small perturbation in C_{MD}. As previously noted, because tubular fluid is incompressible, a small increase (or decrease) in F would result in an instantaneous forward (or backward) translation in the $[\text{Cl}^-]$ profile, so $S'(L)$ describes the instantaneous response of C_{MD} to a small perturbation in F. Taken together, γ characterizes the strength of the TGF response, a.k.a. TGF gain.

To determine the system's response to a transient perturbation, we perform the following steps:

1. We first initialize the system to steady state. That is, we set $C(x, 0) = S(x)$ and $F(0) = F_0$.
2. Next, we apply a transient perturbation to the flow rate. That is, for $0 \leq t \leq 1\,\text{s}$, $F(t) = F_0 + 0.1F_0$. Here we ignore the TGF response Eq. (5.16).
3. We then advance the PDE Eqs. (5.15) and (5.16) in time. That is, for $t > 1\,\text{s}$, the transient perturbation stops and tubular flow rate is given by the TGF response. The goal is to see whether the system returns to a steady state, or develops sustained tubular flow rate oscillations.

As you might expect, the behavior of the system depends on the parameters. In the first simulation, we set TGF delay τ to 3.14 s and γ to 3. With these parameters, GFR gradually returns to a time-independent steady state following a transient perturbation. See Fig. 5.6a. In another simulation, we set $\tau = 3.93\,\text{s}$ and $\gamma = 5$. With these larger delay and gain values, the TGF system develops sustained limit-cycle oscillations after a transient perturbation in flow rate. See Fig. 5.6b. It is noteworthy that even when the system is unstable, the oscillations are bounded because the TGF response (Eq. 5.16) is bounded.

5.5 Characteristic Equation

We have seen that the asymptotic behaviors of the system can be studied by computing numerical solutions to the model equations (5.15) and (5.16). However, because such computations involve long-time integration of a system of coupled PDEs, they can be time-consuming and may not be feasible if one wishes to attain a thorough understanding of the systemic dependence of model behavior on all the parameter values that fall within the physiological ranges.

As an alternative, we will derive a characteristic equation from a linearization of the model equations. By analyzing the characteristic equation, we can gain some understanding of how model behavior depends on system parameters. To derive the characteristic equation, we first make the additional assumption that the tubular radius is constant, so $r(x) = r_o$ and $A(x) = A_o$. Next we introduce normalized variables by dividing dimensional variables by corresponding dimensional reference values: let $\tilde{x} = x/L$, $\tilde{t} = t/T_o$, where T_o is the reference transit time, given by $T_o = A_o L / F_{\text{op}}$, $\tilde{\tau} = \tau/T_o$, $\tilde{C}(\tilde{x}, \tilde{t}) = C(x,t)/C_o$, $\tilde{C}^e(\tilde{x}) = C^e(x)/C_o$, $\tilde{F}(\tilde{C}(1,\tilde{t})) = F(C(L,t))/F_{\text{op}}$, $\tilde{V}_{\max} = V_{\max}/(C_o F_{\text{op}}/(2\pi r_o L))$, $\tilde{K}_M = K_M/C_o$, and $\tilde{P} = P/(F_o/(2\pi r_o L))$. Then in non-dimensional form, Eq. (5.15) is given by

$$\frac{\partial}{\partial t}C(x,t) = -F(t)\frac{\partial}{\partial x}C(x,t) - \left(\frac{V_{\max}C(x,t)}{K_M + C(x,t)} + P\Big(C(x,t) - C^e(x)\Big)\right), \quad (5.19)$$

where we have dropped the tilde's to simplify the notations.

To proceed with the bifurcation analysis, we linearize $C(x,t)$ around the (non-dimensionalized) steady-state concentration profile $S(x)$, and write C as the sum of S and a deviation ϵc_ϵ:

$$C(x,t) = S(x) + \epsilon c_\epsilon(x,t), \quad (5.20)$$

where $\epsilon \ll 1$. We then substitute Eq. (5.20) into (5.15) to get

$$\frac{\partial}{\partial t}(S(x) + \epsilon c_\epsilon(x,t)) + F(S(L) + \epsilon c_\epsilon(L, t-\tau))\frac{\partial}{\partial x}(S(x) + \epsilon c_\epsilon(x,t))$$
$$= -K(S(x) + \epsilon c_\epsilon(x,t)) - P(S(x) + c_\epsilon(x,t) - C^e(x)), \quad (5.21)$$

where K denotes the Michaelis-Menten kinetics term

$$K(C) = \frac{V_{\max}C}{K_m + C}. \quad (5.22)$$

We then expand expressions in Eq. (5.21) in ϵ, allow the terms from the steady-state equation (5.17) to drop out, and keep only the remaining $\mathcal{O}(\epsilon)$ terms. After cancelling ϵ and simplifying further, we arrive at the following linear PDE (Problem 5.3):

5.5 Characteristic Equation

$$\frac{\partial}{\partial t}c_\epsilon(x,t)+\frac{\partial}{\partial x}c_\epsilon(x,t)=-K'(S(x))c_\epsilon(x,t)-F'(C_{\text{op}})S'(x)c_\epsilon(L,t-\tau)-Pc_\epsilon(x,t),\tag{5.23}$$

where the derivatives $K'(S(x))$ and $F'(C_{\text{op}})$ are taken with respective to S.

We will solve Eq. (5.23) using separation of variables. Let

$$c_\epsilon(x,t) = f(x)e^{\lambda t},\tag{5.24}$$

where $\lambda \in \mathbb{C}$. Recall that our goal is to understand the asymptotic behaviors of the system. That is, we want to know whether the deviation $c_\epsilon(x,t)$ will grow in time or not; in other words, we want to know if $\text{Re}(\lambda) > 0$.

To find λ, we substitute Eq. (5.24) into Eq. (5.23) and cancel the common factor $e^{\lambda t}$. This results in an ODE for $f(x)$:

$$f'(x) + f(x)\left(\lambda + P + K'(S(x))\right) = -F'(C_{\text{op}})S'(x)f(1)e^{-\lambda \tau},\tag{5.25}$$

with the boundary condition $f(0) = 0$, because we assume that $C(0,t)$ is fixed and thus $c_\epsilon(0,t) = 0$. The solution to the ODE (5.25) is

$$f(x) = -\exp\left(-\int_0^x \left(\lambda + P + K'(S(y))\right) dy\right) \times$$
$$\int_0^x F'(C_{\text{op}})S'(s)f(1)e^{-\lambda \tau} \exp\left(\int_0^s \left(\lambda + P + K'(S(y))\right) dy\right) ds.\tag{5.26}$$

Now take $x = 1$. After rearranging, the common factor $f(1)$ drops out and yields

$$1 = -F'(C_{op})e^{-\lambda \tau} \int_0^1 S'(x) \exp\left(-\int_x^1 \left(\lambda + P + K'(S(y))\right) dy\right) dx.\tag{5.27}$$

To simplify the above equation, we differentiate the non-dimensionalized steady-state equation

$$\frac{d}{dx}S(x) = -\left(K(S(x)) + P\left(S(x) - C^e(x)\right)\right),\tag{5.28}$$

with respect to x to get

$$K'(S) + P = \frac{PC^{e\prime}}{S'} - \frac{S''}{S'}.\tag{5.29}$$

Substituting the above expression into Eq. (5.27) we get

$$1 = -F'(C_{op})e^{-\lambda \tau} \int_0^1 S'(s) \exp\left(-\int_x^1 \left(\lambda + \frac{PC^{e\prime}}{S'}\right) dy + \ln\left(\frac{S'(1)}{S'(x)}\right)\right) dx.\tag{5.30}$$

After minor rearrangements, we finally arrive at the characteristic equation

$$1 = -\gamma e^{-\lambda \tau} \int_0^1 e^{-\lambda(1-x)} \exp\left(-P \int_x^1 \frac{C^{e\prime}(y)}{S'(y)} dy\right) dx, \quad (5.31)$$

where $\gamma = F'(C_{op})S'(1)$ is the TGF gain.

5.6 Bifurcation Analysis

By relating λ to a number of parameters: γ, τ, P, S, C^e, $V_{\max}$ (implicitly through S'), the characteristic equation (5.31) can be used to make predictions about the stable solutions of the model equations, as a function of parameter values. This is done by computing λ, given all the other model parameters (γ, τ, P, etc.). Since $\lambda \in \mathbb{C}$, let $\lambda \equiv \rho + \iota\omega$. Because of the exponential term in Eq. (5.31), there is an infinite series of λ's (λ_1, λ_2, ...) that satisfy Eq. (5.31). If, for a particular set of parameters, $\rho_n < 0$ for all n, then the only stable solution is a time-independent steady state. If, on the other hand, $\rho_n > 0$ for one, and only one n, the only stable solution is a regular oscillation having frequency, for that n, of $\sim \omega_n/(2\pi)$. For cases where $\rho_n > 0$ for multiple values of n, there may be multiple stable oscillatory solutions. In such cases, the nature of the solutions must be investigated directly by solving the model equations to determine potential solution behaviors, behaviors which may depend on the initial conditions. The value of the gain γ that corresponds to the transition from a case where $\rho_n < 0$, for all n, to a case where, for at least one n, $\rho_n > 0$, is called a critical gain, denoted γ_c (thus, for that n, $\rho_n = 0$ at the point of transition). For the base-case parameters, $\gamma_c = 3.24$ where $\rho_1 = 0$.

We will consider two examples below.

5.6.1 A Model with Zero Chloride Permeability

We will first consider the simple case where the thick ascending limb actively pumps NaCl, but is impermeable to NaCl. That is, $P = 0$, which means that chloride does not leak back into the tubular lumen, however large the transmural electrochemical gradient. With $P = 0$, Eq. (5.31) simplifies (beautifully) to

$$1 = \gamma e^{-\lambda \tau} \left(\frac{e^{-\lambda} - 1}{\lambda}\right). \quad (5.32)$$

The question we ask is this: given $V_{\max}$, C^e (and thus S), what set of γ-τ values give rise to limit cycle oscillations when the system is given a transient perturbation? And what γ-τ values give rise to time-independent steady state solutions? Equivalently, we want to find boundaries in the γ-τ plane that separate

5.6 Bifurcation Analysis

regions which give rise to qualitatively different asymptotic behaviors. Now the asymptotic behavior of the solution is indicated by λ, or more specifically, by the sign of $\text{Re}(\lambda) = \rho$. Given this observation, we will compute curves in the γ-τ plan where $\rho = 0$.

Since τ is the TGF delay, we know that $\tau \geq 0$. Recall that $\gamma = F'(C_{op})S'(1)$. Since both $F'(C_{op})$ and $S'(1)$ are negative, we have $\gamma > 0$. Thus, we will focus on the first quadrant of the γ-τ plane. Setting $\rho = 0$ in Eq. (5.32), we obtain an equation that relates $\omega(= \text{Im}(\lambda))$, γ, and τ:

$$\frac{\omega}{2} = -\gamma \sin\left(\frac{\omega}{2}\right)\left(\cos\left(\omega\left(\tau + \frac{1}{2}\right)\right) - \iota \sin\left(\omega\left(\tau + \frac{1}{2}\right)\right)\right). \quad (5.33)$$

Consider the imaginary part of the above equation:

$$0 = \gamma \sin\left(\frac{\omega}{2}\right)\sin\left(\omega\left(\tau + \frac{1}{2}\right)\right). \quad (5.34)$$

This implies that

$$\frac{\omega}{2} = n\pi, \quad \text{or} \quad \omega\left(\tau + \frac{1}{2}\right) = n\tau, \quad (5.35)$$

where n is an integer. The first solution $\omega/2 = n\pi$ is rejected because upon substituting into Eq. (5.33) we realize that the equation isn't satisfied except for $n = 0$.

The real part of Eq. (5.33) is

$$\frac{\omega}{2} = -\gamma \sin\left(\frac{\omega}{2}\right)\cos\left(\omega\left(\tau + \frac{1}{2}\right)\right). \quad (5.36)$$

Substituting $\omega(\tau + \frac{1}{2}) = n\pi$ into the above equation, we get

$$\gamma = (-1)^{n+1}\frac{\frac{n\pi}{2}/(\tau + \frac{1}{2})}{\sin\left(\frac{n\pi}{2}/(\tau + \frac{1}{2})\right)}, \quad (5.37)$$

where $n = 1, 2, 3, \ldots$.

For a given n, Eq. (5.37) yields a γ–τ curve that corresponds to $\rho_n = 0$ and that separates the γ–τ plane into regions: γ and τ values that lie below the $\rho_n = 0$ curve correspond to solutions with $\rho_n < 0$ (i.e., damped solutions); conversely, γ and τ values that lie above the curve correspond to solutions with $\rho_n > 0$ (i.e., growing solutions). We have evaluated Eq. (5.37) for $n = 1, 2, 3$ and plotted those curves in Fig. 5.7. We show results only for gain and delay values that lie within the physiological ranges: $0 \leq \gamma \leq 10$ and $0 \leq \tau \leq 0.5$. For small values of γ and τ, the linear model predicts that all oscillatory modes are damped and the asymptotic solution is a time-independent steady-state solution. It is noteworthy that the curves

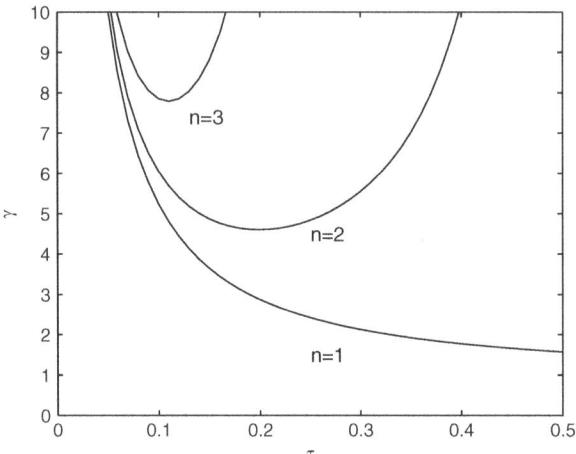

Fig. 5.7 Bifurcation diagram for TGF model with no backleak, i.e., $P = 0$. Each curve corresponds to $\rho_n = 0$

$\rho_2 = 0$, $\rho_3 = 0$, and $\rho_4 = 0$ (and in fact all $\rho_n = 0$ curves for $n \geq 2$) lie within the region where $\rho_1 > 0$. Thus, whenever $\rho_n > 0$, for any $n \geq 2$, we also have that $\rho_1 > 0$. In other words, whenever any of the higher frequency is growing, the fundamental mode is growing too.

5.6.2 A Model with Nonzero Chloride Permeability

The thick ascending limb has a small but nonzero permeability to chloride. This results in NaCl backleak and a steady-state chloride profile $S(x)$ that is different from the zero-permeability case. In fact, with nonzero backleak, static head now occurs at a nonzero luminal chloride concentration. Now with a different $S(x)$, we would expect the root curves to be different from the case with zero permeability. To compute a solution to Eq. (5.31) for $P \neq 0$, we substitute $\lambda = \iota \omega$ (ρ assumed to be 0), expand, and separate the real and imaginary parts of the equation:

$$1 = -\int_0^1 \gamma \cos(\omega(1 - x + \tau)) \exp\left(-P \int_x^1 \frac{C^{e\prime}(y)}{S'(y)} dy\right) dx, \quad (5.38)$$

$$0 = \int_0^1 \gamma \sin(\omega(1 - x + \tau)) \exp\left(-P \int_x^1 \frac{C^{e\prime}(y)}{S'(y)} dy\right) dx. \quad (5.39)$$

The unknowns for the above system of equations are γ, τ, and ω, and the solutions form curves in the γ–τ plane. Unlike the no-backleak case, however, there is no analytical expression like Eq. (5.37) that explicitly relates γ and τ. Instead, for a

5.6 Bifurcation Analysis

given value of τ, the coupled Eqs. (5.38) and (5.39) can be solved numerically to yield multiple pairs of γ_n–ω_n solutions, for $n = 1, 2, \ldots$, with each solution pair corresponding to difference oscillation frequencies. Different τ values yield different γ_n–ω_n solution pairs.

The procedure for approximating a γ_n–τ_n curve for some n deserves more discussion. Note that we have two Eqs. (5.38) and (5.39), and three unknowns (γ, τ, and ω). As a result, the solution is a curve in the γ–τ plane. Now how do we compute a γ–τ curve for some n? The way to do this is to sketch out the curve point by point. To approximate a segment of a γ_n–τ_n curve, say for $\tau \in [\tau_{\min}, \tau_{\max}]$, we discretize the τ interval. Then we loop over the τ values $\tau_{\min}, \tau_{\min} + \Delta\tau, \ldots \tau_{\min} + 2\Delta\tau, \ldots \tau_{\max}$. For each $\tau_j \equiv \tau_{\min} + j\Delta\tau$, we substitute $\tau = \tau_j$ into Eqs. (5.38) and (5.39). Now we have two equations and two unknowns: $\gamma(\tau_i)$ and $\omega(\tau_i)$; and we can numerically solve this 2-by-2 system. One popular method for solving a system of coupled nonlinear equations is the Newton's method. The solution of the system gives us one point on the γ–τ curve. After we've looped through $[\tau_{\min}, \tau_{\max}]$, we have points that can be connected to approximate that γ–τ segment.

Alternatively, the coupled equations can be solved for τ_n–ω_n with γ fixed. The same curve segment can be approximated by looping through $\gamma \in [\gamma_{\min}, \gamma_{\max}]$.

Here are a number of questions that you may (in fact, should) have:

1. *Question:* The system (5.38) and (5.39) has an infinite series of solutions $(\gamma_n, \tau_n, \omega_n)$, for $n = 1, 2, 3, \ldots$. Thus, for each τ_i (or γ_i), there may be multiple γ–ω (or τ–ω) solutions. So when we solve the system using Newton's method, which solution do we get? And how do we get the other solutions?
   Answer: Which solution Newton's method converges to depends on the initial guess that you supply. We will answer the second question of how to get the other solutions later.

2. *Question:* So how should we choose the initial guess?
   Answer: This is a good question, because not only does the initial guess determines which solution Newton's method converges to, frequently it also determines whether Newton's method converges at all!

   Suppose we are looping over $\tau \in [\tau_{\min}, \tau_{\max}]$ and we start at $\tau = \tau_{\min}$. We need to pick initial guesses for $\omega(\tau_{\min})$ and $\gamma(\tau_{\min})$. Recall that ω corresponds to the frequency of the solution, so a smaller ω (with the appropriate γ) will tend to yield a solution with a smaller n. Given a starting ω value, one can choose an initial guess for $\gamma_{\min}$ based on "experience" (e.g., knowledge of bifurcation curves of similar TGF systems).

   Now suppose we have already computed a portion of the γ–τ segment. We have just computed $(\tau_i, \gamma(\tau_i), \omega(\tau_i))$ and we are moving on to the solution corresponding to τ_{i+1}. Because the next solution triplet is likely close to the previous solution, $(\gamma(\tau_i), \omega(\tau_i))$ is generally a good initial guess when we wish to solve for $(\gamma(\tau_{i+1}), \omega(\tau_{i+1}))$. This approach is illustrated in Fig. 5.8.

3. *Question:* Back to the question of: how do we get the other solutions?
   Answer: By choosing different initial guesses. Note that ω corresponds to the frequency of the oscillations, so, when combined with appropriate γ or τ guesses, a larger ω may nudge Newton's method toward a higher-frequency mode.

Fig. 5.8 The γ and ω values of the computed solution pair (τ_i, γ_i) are used as an initial condition for the next point in the bifurcation curve, which corresponds to τ_{i+1}. If all goes well, the Newton iterations, denoted by the *open circle*, will converge to $(\tau_{i+1}, \gamma_{i+1})$

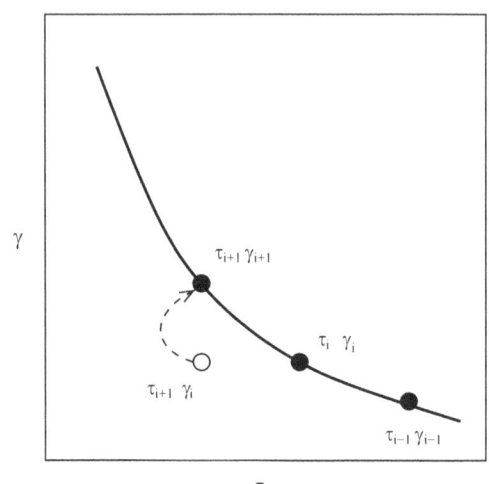

4. *Question:* To approximate a γ–τ curve segment, we could loop over τ, and solve for γ–ω; or we could loop over γ, and solve for τ–ω. Is one approach better than the other?
   Answer: Given an appropriate initial guess, the two approaches should yield the same curve segment. However, in practice, one approach sometimes works better than the other. In a portion of the γ–τ curve where $d\gamma/d\tau$ is large, then the difference between $\gamma(\tau)$ and $\gamma(\tau + \Delta\tau)$ may be huge. In that case, looping over τ is not advisable, because the previous solution $(\gamma(\tau_i), \omega(\tau_i))$ is no longer a good initial guess for computing $(\gamma(\tau_{i+1}), \omega(\tau_{i+1}))$ using Newton's method. However, this problem can be easily solved by switching to loops over γ, because $d\tau/d\gamma$ is small. Thus, the previous solution $(\tau(\gamma_i), \omega(\gamma_i))$ is a good initial guess for computing $(\tau(\gamma_{i+1}), \omega(\gamma_{i+1}))$.

Now that we have a better understanding of the computational procedures, we will compute bifurcation curves for the TGF model using the parameters in Table 5.1 and $P = 1.5 \times 10^{-5}$ cm/s. The results are shown in Fig. 5.9. A comparison between Fig. 5.7 ($P = 0$) and Fig. 5.9 indicates that the bifurcation behaviors of the TGF system may change dramatically when thick ascending limb permeability P is increased from $P = 0$ to $P = 1.5 \times 10^{-5}$ cm/s. It is particularly noteworthy that, in the zero permeability case (Fig. 5.7), the bifurcation curves for the conditions Re $\lambda_n = 0$, for $n > 1$, all lie above the Re $\lambda_1 = 0$ curve. In contrast, in the nonzero P case, the bifurcation curves for the conditions Re $\lambda_2 = 0$ and Re $\lambda_3 = 0$ cross the curve for Re $\lambda_1 = 0$. What does that mean in terms of the dynamic behaviors of the full model? Because the bifurcation diagrams are necessarily based on linearized forms of the model equations, actual model behavior must be investigated by means of simulations in which numerical solutions to the unaltered model equations are computed.

Numerous computations using the PDE model (Eqs. 5.15 and 5.16) with $P = 0$ reveal that, in the zero permeability model, only limit-cycle oscillations correspond-

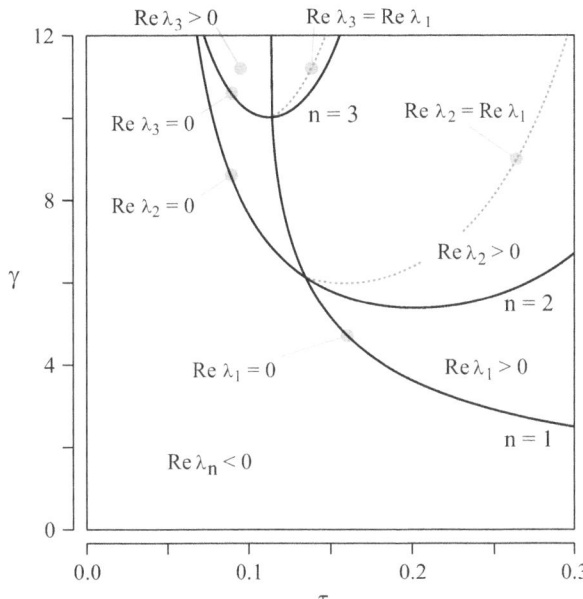

Fig. 5.9 Bifurcation diagram for TGF model with permeability $P = 1.5 \times 10^{-5}$ cm/s

ing to the fundamental frequency (i.e., $n = 1$) can be sustained. That is, given a transient flow perturbation, the TGF system either returns to steady state (for small τ and γ values), or develops sustained limit-cycle oscillations with frequency $\sim$30 mHz, which corresponds to the fundamental frequency. This full-model result is consistent with the bifurcation results, which indicate that when any of the $\rho_n > 0$, for $n > 1$, $\rho_1 > 0$ as well. The full model results suggest that the fundamental mode dominates all other modes.

As for the nonzero permeability case, extensive numerical simulations reveal that these crossings of the bifurcation curves have important consequences for the nature of the stable solutions. Because there are parameter regimes where $\rho_1 < 0$ but $\rho_n > 0$ for some $n > 1$, higher-frequency modes (i.e., limit-cycle oscillations with frequencies $\sim$60, $\sim$90 mHz, etc.) can now be sustained. For example, the point ($\tau = 0.11, \gamma = 9$) lies with the region where $\rho_2 > 0$ and $\rho_n < 0$ for all $n \neq 2$. Thus, we expect a limit-cycle oscillation with a frequency $\sim$60 mHz to be sustained with these parameter values.

5.7 Modeling Coupled TGF Systems

A rat kidney contains $\sim$35,000 nephrons; a human kidney contains 0.30–1.4 million nephrons. These nephrons do not act autonomously. Electrotonic conduction along the pre-glomerular vasculature gives rise to coupling between TGF systems in nearby nephrons. If two nephrons have afferent arterioles that are nearby on the cortical radial artery, the constrictions of one nephron's afferent arteriole tend to result in constrictions of the other afferent arteriole, thereby affecting that neighbor's TGF system. A system of coupled oscillators can yield many interesting dynamic behaviors, including a heightened tendency to oscillate, and synchronization. Synchronization of coupled oscillations has been observed in a number of biological systems, including networks of pacemaker cells in the heart, circadian pacemaker cells in the suprachiasmatic nucleus of the brain, metabolic synchrony in yeast cell suspensions, congregation of synchronously flashing fireflies, etc.

We will briefly describe how to expand the single-nephron TGF model to a set of N coupled TGF systems ($N > 1$). We assume that each TGF system is coupled, through the preglomerular vasculature, with the TGF systems of other model nephrons (each labeled by an index i). The N nephrons are allowed to have different parameters and thus their dynamic behaviors may differ.

In the ith model TGF system, thick ascending limb tubular fluid chloride concentration $C_i(x, t)$, thick ascending limb tubular fluid flow $\mathscr{F}_i(t)$, coupling with other nephrons, and a TGF signal delay are represented by the following equations:

$$A_i(x)\frac{\partial}{\partial t}C_i(x,t) = -\mathscr{F}_i(t)\frac{\partial}{\partial x}C_i(x,t) - 2\pi r_i(x) \times$$
$$\left(\frac{V_{\max}C_i(x,t)}{K_M + C_i(x,t)} + P\left(C_i(x,t) - C^e(x)\right)\right), \quad (5.40)$$

$$F_i(t) = F_0\left(1 + K_{1_i}\tanh\left(K_{2_i}\left(C_{\text{op}} - C_{\text{MD}_i}(t - \tau_i)\right)\right)\right), \quad (5.41)$$

$$\mathscr{F}_i(t) = F_i(t) + \sum_{j \neq i}\phi_{ij}(F_j(t) - F_0). \quad (5.42)$$

The solute conservation equation (5.40) is analogous to the single-nephron equation (5.15), except with $C(x, t)$ replaced by $C_i(x, t)$. For simplicity, we assume that all nephrons have the same transport properties. That assumption can certainly be relaxed, and in that case, the subscript i can be added to $V_{\max}$, K_M, and P.

Equation (5.42) gives $\mathscr{F}_i(t)$ as the sum of a nephron's own TGF-mediated thick ascending limb tubular flow response $F_i(t)$ and a term from the other model TGF systems; each summand in that term is a weighted difference between another system's TGF response $F_j(t)$ and the time-independent steady-state flow F_0. The weight, or coupling coefficient, ϕ_{ij} is a non-negative constant parameter that scales the influence of the j-th nephron on the i-th nephron. ϕ_{ij} takes on values between 0 and 1; if $\phi_{ij} = 0$, then the two nephrons are not coupled.

A bifurcation analysis can be done for the coupled nephron model; the procedure is analogous to that described in Sect. 5.6. For a two coupled-nephron model, where we allow the TGF delay and gain to be different for each nephron, and where we assume symmetrical coupling, i.e., $\phi_{12} = \phi_{21} \equiv \phi$, and zero permeability, the characteristic equation takes the form,

$$\left(\frac{\lambda}{\gamma_1 e^{\lambda \tau_1}(1-e^{-\lambda})}+1\right)\left(\frac{\lambda}{\gamma_2 e^{\lambda \tau_2}(1-e^{-\lambda})}+1\right)=\phi, \tag{5.43}$$

The derivation of the characteristic equation can be found in Layton et al. (2009).

5.8 Problems

Problem 5.1. Compute the solution to the delayed differential equation

$$\frac{dx}{dt}=-2x(t-1), \tag{5.44}$$

with initial history

$$x(t)=1, \quad t\leq 0, \tag{5.45}$$

for $t \in [0,3]$.

Problem 5.2. We will derive a reduced model that retains the time dependence, and its effects, of the PDE model, but eliminates the spatial dependence of the PDE model. The reduced model assumes zero permeability, i.e., $P=0$. We will assume that the spatial and time variables x and t are normalized by the thick ascending limb length and the transit time, respectively.

Consider the characteristic curves given by

$$\frac{d}{dt}x(t)=F(C(1,t-\tau)), \tag{5.46}$$

where $x(t)$ denotes the position of a fluid particle. We can write the solute conservation equation along the characteristic curves as

$$\frac{d}{dt}C(x(t),t)=-\frac{V_{\max}}{K_M+C(x(t),t)}. \tag{5.47}$$

Equations (5.46) and (5.47), which are in *characteristic form*, can be parameterized by t. To do this, define function $\mathscr{F}$ and $\mathscr{C}$ by

$$\mathscr{F}(t)=F(C(1,t-\tau)), \tag{5.48}$$

$$\mathscr{C}(t)=C(x(t),t). \tag{5.49}$$

(a) Let $T_x(t)$ be the thick ascending limb transit time from $x=0$ to position $x\in[0,1]$, i.e., the time required for a fluid particle to travel from the loop bend ($x=0$) to position x. Then $T_{\text{MD}}(t)$ denotes the transit time from loop bend to

the macula densa. Linearize $\mathscr{C}$ by means of a Taylor series expansion around $T_{MD} = 1$. Keep only the first-order terms.
(b) By using the linearization obtained in part (a), substitute into Eqs. (5.16) and (5.48) to obtain a linearization of $\mathscr{F}(t)$ around the steady-state value of 1 and in terms of K_1, K_2, and T_{MD}.
(c) Equation (5.46) can be rewritten as an implicit equation for T_x,

$$x(t) = \int_{t-T_x(t)}^{t} \mathscr{F}(s)\, ds, \tag{5.50}$$

where $t - T_x(t)$ is the time at which a fluid particle currently located at $x(t)$ enter the TAL. Linearize Eq. (5.50), again around $T_{MD} = 1$ and keep only the first-order terms. Then solve for T_{MD} to get

$$T_{MD}(t) = 1 + \frac{\int_{t-1}^{t}(1 - \mathscr{F}(s))\, ds}{\mathscr{F}(t-1)}. \tag{5.51}$$

(d) Substitute the above equation for T_{MD} into the equation you obtained in part (a) to derive the reduced model equation:

$$\mathscr{F}(t) = 1 + K_1 \tanh\left(\frac{\gamma \int_{t-\tau-1}^{t-\tau}(1 - \mathscr{F}(s))\, ds}{K_1 \mathscr{F}(t - \tau - 1)}\right). \tag{5.52}$$

Problem 5.3. Derive Eq. (5.23). Begin by expanding $F(S(L) + \epsilon c_\epsilon(L, t - \tau))$ and $K(S(x) + \epsilon c_\epsilon(x, t))$ (from Eq. 5.21) in terms of ϵ.

References

Layton, A.T., Moore, L.C., Layton, H.E.: Multistable dynamics mediated by tubuloglomerular feedback in a model of coupled nephrons. Bull. Math. Biol. **71**, 515–555 (2009)
Pitman, E.B., Zaritski, R.M., Kesseler, K.J., Moore, L.C., Layton, H.E.: Feedback-mediated dynamics in two coupled nephrons. Bull. Math. Biol. **66**(6), 1463–1492 (2004)

Chapter 6
Electrophysiology of Renal Vascular Smooth Muscle Cells

Abstract Vascular contraction in the kidney is an important mechanism for regulating renal blood flow. The contractility of vascular smooth muscle cells results from signaling cascades in which intracellular calcium plays a fundamental role. This chapter begins with an overview of cell electrophysiology, and the general properties of ion channels. We then focus on Ca^{2+} signaling in vascular smooth muscle cells, and formulate equations that represent Ca^{2+} transport via ion channels, Ca^{2+} buffering, and Ca^{2+} sequestration in intracellular stores. Finally, we describe models that link variations in intracellular Ca^{2+} to the contractile force.

6.1 Background

The delivery of blood flow to the kidney is regulated by several mechanisms, including tubuloglomerular feedback, the myogenic response, hormones and paracrine agents (such as the renin-angiotensin system), and renal sympathetic nerve activity. Most of these mechanisms act by modulating the contractility of renal blood vessels. This chapter focuses on the cellular-level signaling cascades by which vasoactive agents elicit the contraction or dilation of vascular smooth muscle cells (VSMC) in the kidney. Of particular relevance are the VSMCs of the afferent arteriole and the descending vasa recta (DVR) pericytes, which respectively control blood flow supply to the entire kidney and the medulla.

Smooth muscle cell contraction is usually triggered by a rise in the cytosolic concentration of calcium ions (Ca^{2+}). Increasing binding of Ca^{2+} to calmodulin (a calcium-binding messenger protein) activates myosin light chain kinase, an enzyme that stimulates the rate of actin-myosin cross-bridge formation, thereby generating the active contractile force. Spatial and temporal variations in cytosolic Ca^{2+} levels are tightly regulated, and result from enhanced Ca^{2+} influx from the extracellular space (via Ca^{2+} channels) and/or intracellular storage sites.

We begin this chapter with an overview of cell electrophysiology concepts. We then describe the general properties of ion channels, before focusing on Ca^{2+} signaling in VSMCs and the mechanisms underlying cellular contraction.

6.2 Overview of Cell Electrophysiology

What follows is with a very brief review of fundamental electrical concepts. Comprehensive descriptions can be found in two excellent books (Keener and Sneyd 1998; Hille 2001).

The charge of one proton (also known as the elementary charge) is $q_E = 1.6 \times 10^{-19}$ C (coulombs). Faraday's constant is the charge on one mole of protons, i.e., $F = N_A \; q_E = (6 \times 10^{+23}) \times (1.6 \times 10^{-19}) = 9.6 \times 10^4$ C/mol. The amount of charge carried by one mole of ions whose valence is z_S is $z_S F$. Thus, the charge on a mole of divalent anions such as dihydrogen phosphate (HPO_4^{2-}) is -2 F. The current is the flow of charge; it is measured in amperes (A), with $1 \text{ A} = 1$ C/s. The current density, or flux of charge, has units of A/m^2. The current density (I_S) is given by the product of the solute flux (J_S, in mol/m^2) and the amount of charge carried by the solute:

$$I_S = z_S F J_S. \tag{6.1}$$

The magnitude of the current between two points is a function of the path resistance to flow, and the potential difference. The electric potential difference between two points, or voltage, is the energy required to move a unit charge from one point to the other. It is measured in volts (V). Accordingly, 1 J of work is needed to move one coulomb across a 1V potential difference.

6.2.1 Electrical Circuit Model of the Cell Membrane

The cell membrane separates internal and external conducting solutions. The separation of charge gives rises to a potential difference across the membrane (denoted V_m). Thus, the membrane can be viewed as a capacitor, consisting of two conductors separated by an electrical insulator and characterized by a capacitance C_m (in units of farad, or F). The latter is defined as the ratio of the charge on each conductor to the potential difference between them:

$$C_m = \frac{Q}{V_m}. \tag{6.2}$$

6.2 Overview of Cell Electrophysiology

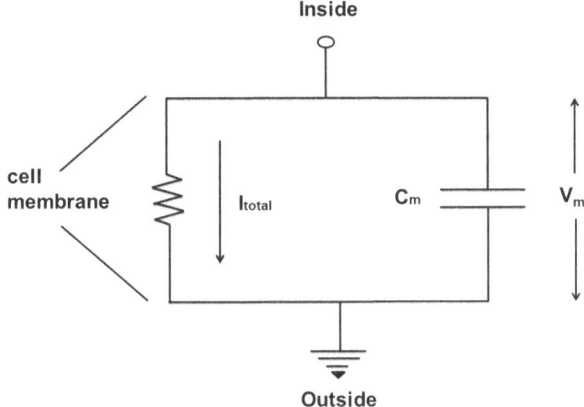

Fig. 6.1 Electrical circuit representation of the cell membrane

The rate of change of the transmembrane potential difference is therefore given by:

$$\frac{dV_m}{dt} = \frac{1}{C_m}\frac{dQ}{dt}. \qquad (6.3)$$

The specific (i.e., per unit area) capacitance of biological cell membranes is approximately 1 µF/cm². For example, the average cell capacitance of DVR pericytes has been measured as 12.1 ± 0.7 pF, so their capacitive membrane surface area is estimated as 1.21×10^{-5} cm².

In addition to acting as a capacitor, the cell membrane carries currents from one side of the membrane to the other, through a variety of ion channels and other transporters. The membrane can therefore be represented as an electrical circuit with a capacitor in parallel with a resistor, as shown in Fig. 6.1.

Note that V_m is defined as the potential within the cell minus that outside. I_{total} is the total current flowing across the cell membrane, from the inside to the outside. It must be equal and opposite to the rate of change of charge Q on the capacitor (i.e., dQ/dt). Hence the fundamental equation:

$$\frac{dV_m}{dt} = \frac{-I_{total}}{C_m}. \qquad (6.4)$$

As shown by Eq. 6.4, the larger the capacitance, the slower the response of the membrane potential to current.

6.2.2 Nernst Equilibrium Potential

Consider a semi-permeable membrane separating two compartments, as illustrated in Fig. 6.2. The membrane is impermeable to anion A but permeable to cation B.

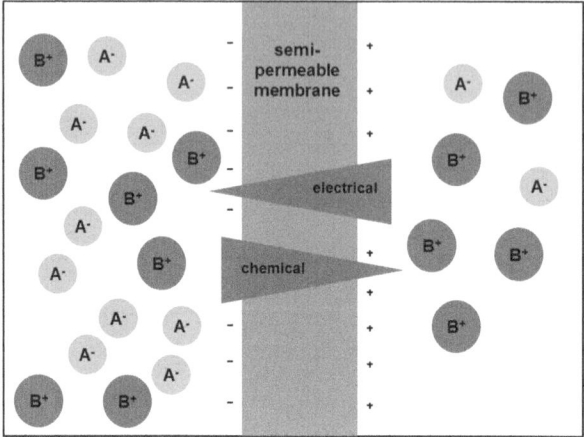

Fig. 6.2 Cations B, but not anions A, can cross the semi-permeable membrane that separates two compartments. As the cations diffuse from the left side (where they are more concentrated) to the right side, excess positive charge builds up on the dilute side. The resulting transmembrane potential difference acts to repel the cations from the right side. Equilibrium is reached when the electrical and diffusional fluxes of B balance each other

At time $t = 0$, a concentrated solution of salt AB is introduced on one side of the membrane, and a dilute solution of AB is introduced on the other side. Cations B then start to diffuse down their concentration gradient; since anions A cannot follow them, excess positive charge builds up on the dilute side, giving rise to an electric potential difference across the membrane. The electric field begins to exert an opposing force on the cations, which counters diffusion. Equilibrium is reached when the electric force that repels cations B is exactly counterbalanced by the diffusional force. The *Nernst (equilibrium) potential* of cations B (denoted E_B) is the value of the potential difference at equilibrium, when there is no more flow of B across the membrane. It can be determined by equating the electrochemical potential of B (μ_B) on both sides of the membrane.

The electrochemical potential of B (μ_B) on the internal (superscript "i") and external (superscript "e") sides is respectively given by:

$$\mu_B^i = RT \ln C_B^i + z_B F \psi^i, \tag{6.5}$$

$$\mu_B^e = RT \ln C_B^e + z_B F \psi^e, \tag{6.6}$$

where ψ denotes the electric potential, and z_B the valence of B. Equating μ_B^i and μ_B^e at equilibrium yields the Nernst potential of cations B:

$$E_B = \psi^i - \psi^e = \frac{1}{z_B F} \left(RT \ln C_B^e - RT \ln C_B^i \right), \tag{6.7}$$

6.2 Overview of Cell Electrophysiology

$$E_B = \frac{RT}{z_B F} \ln\left(\frac{C_B^e}{C_B^i}\right). \tag{6.8a}$$

Alternatively,

$$E_B = 2.303 \frac{RT}{z_B F} \log_{10}\left(\frac{C_B^e}{C_B^i}\right). \tag{6.8b}$$

It is useful to remember that 2.303 RT/F is approximately equal to 60 mV. Thus, if cation B has a valence of +1 and is 10 times more concentrated inside the cell than outside, its Nernst potential is roughly $60 \log_{10}(0.1) = -60$ mV.

To be more exact, RT/F equals 25.69 mV at 25 °C, and 26.73 at 37 °C. Typical intra- and extra-cellular concentrations of K^+ in smooth muscle are 150 and 5 mM, respectively, which yields $E_K = -90.9$ mV at 37 °C. Conversely, Na^+ and Cl^- are more concentrated in the extracellular medium (~140 mM) than intracellularly (~10 mM), and their Nernst potential is on the order of +70 and −70 mV, respectively. The extracellular concentration of Ca^{2+} is about 2 mM, versus 100 nM in the cytosol, and E_{Ca} is on the order of + 130 mV.

6.2.3 Ion Conservation Equations

Consider a smooth muscle cell surrounded by a homogeneous extracellular compartment (such as a large bath), the composition of which does not change with time. The intracellular amount of solute S will vary if there is a net flux of S between the cell and the surrounding medium, and/or if solute S is generated or consumed within the cell by chemical reaction. Let $V^i(t)$ and $C_S^i(t)$ respectively denote the volume and concentration of solute S in the intracellular compartment (superscript "i") at time t. The amount of solute S (in moles) that accumulates within V^i during the time interval $[t, t + dt]$ is given by:

$$\text{Accumulation} = V^i(t + dt)\, C_S^i(t + dt) - V^i(t)\, C_S^i(t).$$

By conservation of mass, this amount must equal the net amount of solute flowing into V^i, plus the net amount of solute formed by chemical reaction within V^i. The first term is expressed as:

$$\text{Net molar flow in} = -\int_t^{t+dt} A_m J_S^i(\tau)\, d\tau,$$

where J_S^i denotes the molar flux of S (per unit membrane area), which is taken to be positive if directed out of the cell (see below), and A_m is the surface area of the cell membrane. Solute formation is written in terms of the volumetric rate of net generation of solute S within the cell, denoted Φ^i_S:

$$\text{Net generation} = \int_t^{t+dt} V^i(\tau) \Phi^i_S(\tau) d\tau.$$

This source (or sink) term is zero for non-reacting ions such as Na^+, K^+, and Cl^-; for Ca^{2+}, it accounts for reactions with calcium buffers such as calmodulin. Combining the three previous terms, we have:

$$V^i(t+dt)\, C^i_S(t+dt) - V^i(t)\, C^i_S(t) = \\ -\int_t^{t+dt} A_m(\tau) J^i_S(\tau) d\tau + \int_t^{t+dt} V^i(\tau) \Phi^i_S(\tau) d\tau. \qquad (6.9)$$

The differential form of Eq. (6.9) is:

$$\frac{d\left(V^i C^i_S\right)}{dt} = -A_m J^i_S + V^i \Phi^i_S. \qquad (6.10)$$

This equation can be simplified if we assume that the cell volume remains constant, so that:

$$\frac{dC^i_S}{dt} = -\frac{A_m J^i_S}{V_i} + \Phi^i_S. \qquad (6.11)$$

Note that J^i_S represents the net efflux of S: in electrophysiological studies, the current is generally taken to be positive if it carries positive charge out of the cell. We may further rewrite Eq. (6.11) as:

$$\frac{dC^i_S}{dt} = \frac{-I^{net}_S}{z_S F V_i} + \Phi^i_S, \qquad (6.12)$$

where I^{net}_S denotes the net current of S across the cell membrane. Transmembrane currents are carried by a variety of ion channels, cotransporters or exchangers, and pumps. The next section focuses on currents through ion channels.

6.3 Ion Channels

Ion channels are macromolecular pores that passively carry specific ions across the membrane; the driving force for transport is the transmembrane potential difference and ionic concentration gradient. Ion channels are characterized by their current-voltage (I-V) relationship, the parameters of which depend on the biophysical

6.3 Ion Channels

properties of the channel. The current across a population of N channels can be written as:

$$I = NP_o(V_m, t) \, i \, (V_m, t), \tag{6.13}$$

where P_o is the fraction of open channels at time t ($0 \leq P_o \leq 1$), and i is the current across a single open channel. Note that both are a function of the transmembrane potential difference $V_m \equiv \psi^i - \psi^e$, hereafter referred to as the *membrane potential*. Below, we describe common models first for $i(V_m, t)$, and then for $P_o(V_m, t)$.

6.3.1 Current-Voltage Relationship of a Single Open Channel

The two most common models of I-V relationships are the modified form of Ohm's law, and the Goldman-Hodgkin-Katz (GHK) equation. Ohm's law, one of the fundamental relationships in electricity, was derived by the German physicist and mathematician Georg Simon Ohm (1789–1854) in the 1820s. The modified form of Ohm's law states that the flow of ions S across the channel is a linear function of the difference between the membrane potential and the equilibrium (Nernst) potential of S. It can be written as:

$$i_S = g_S (V_m - E_S), \tag{6.14}$$

where g_S is the channel conductance, in units of siemens (S). Note that the inverse of a conductance is a resistance, with units of ohms (Ω). As expected, Eq. (6.14) yields zero current when V_m equals the equilibrium potential of ions S. If V_m is higher than E_S, the current is positive, which means that S will be carried out of the cell if it is positively charged, and into the cell if it is negatively charged. Conversely, if V_m is lower than E_S, S will diffuse in if positively charged, and vice-versa. In VSMC, V_m is on the order of -60 mV, and K^+ channels carry potassium out ($E_K \sim -90$ mV) whereas Na^+ channels carry sodium in ($E_{Na} \sim +70$ mV).

The channel conductance is not necessarily constant; it can vary with concentration, voltage, or other factors. As an example, inward rectifying potassium channels (Kir) play an important role in maintaining the resting membrane potential. Inward-rectifying channels are so called because they carry current more easily inward (i.e., into the cell) than in the other direction; their conductance is a function of V_m. The activity of Kir channels is also modulated by the extracellular K^+ concentration (C_K^e). Experimentally, the Kir conductance is often found to increase with the square-root of C_K^e. Thus, the current across an inward rectifier K^+ channel, $i_{K,ir}$, can be expressed as:

$$i_{K,ir} = g_{Kir}(V_m - E_K), \tag{6.15}$$

$$g_{Kir} = \frac{g^o_{Kir}\sqrt{C^e_K}}{1 + \exp\left(\frac{V_m - V_{Kir}}{k_{Kir}}\right)}, \qquad (6.16)$$

where g^o_{Kir} is a constant, V_{Kir} is the half-activation potential, and k_{Kir} is a slope. The dependence of g_{Kir} on the membrane potential stems from the presence of gating charges, as described below.

Other channels are better represented by the *Goldman-Hodgkin-Katz (GHK) current equation*. Alan Lloyd Hodgkin was a British physiologist and biophysicist who, with Andrew Huxley, pioneered the use of the squid giant axon to measure ionic currents in the 1930s. Both were awarded the Nobel Prize in 1963. Bernard Katz was a German-born biophysicist who shared the Nobel Prize in 1970 for his work on synapses. The American David E. Goldman derived the GHK equation during his thesis work at Columbia University. He began by integrating the Nernst-Planck equation assuming a constant electric field across the membrane. The Nernst-Planck equation gives the flux of ions S when both concentration and electrical gradients are present:

$$J_S = -D_S\left(\nabla C_S + \frac{z_S F}{RT} C_S \nabla \psi\right). \qquad (6.17)$$

The first term corresponds to Fick's law, a constitutive equation that describes diffusion driven by a concentration gradient; D_S is the diffusivity of S. The second term corresponds to diffusion due to the electric field; the electric force exerted on a charged solute increases linearly with the electric field ($E = -\nabla \psi$).

At steady state, the flux of ions across a membrane is constant. Assuming that transport occurs in one direction only and that the electric field is constant across the membrane, it can be shown that (see Problem 6.1):

$$J_S = \frac{D_S}{L_m}\frac{z_S F V_m}{RT}\frac{C^i_S - C^e_S \exp(-z_S F V_m/RT)}{1 - \exp(-z_S F V_m/RT)}, \qquad (6.18)$$

where L_m is the membrane thickness; the ratio $P_S = D_S/L_m$ is the permeability of the membrane to S. To obtain the current density of ions S across the membrane, we multiply the flux by $z_s F$:

$$i_S = P_s \frac{z_S^2 F^2 V_m}{RT}\frac{C^i_S - C^e_S \exp(-z_S F V_m/RT)}{1 - \exp(-z_S F V_m/RT)}. \qquad (6.19)$$

Equation (6.19) is known as the GHK current equation. It is used for instance to determine the current across L-type Ca^{2+} channels and stretch-activated channels (see below). As expected, Eq. (6.19) also yields zero current when the membrane potential equals the Nernst potential of ions S:

$$i_S = 0 \Rightarrow C^i_S - C^e_S \exp(-z_S F V_m/RT) = 0 \Rightarrow V_m = \frac{RT}{z_S F}\ln\left(\frac{C^e_S}{C^i_S}\right) \equiv E_S.$$

6.3 Ion Channels

When the membrane is permeable to several types of ions, the potential at which the net current is zero, known as the reversal potential (V_{rev}), differs from the Nernst potential of individual ions. The reversal potential can easily be calculated analytically if we assume that all currents obey the GHK equation, and that the membrane is only permeable to ions of valence $z_s = +1$ or -1. In that case, the net current density is given by:

$$i_{net} = \sum_{z_j=+1} P_j \frac{F^2 V_m}{RT} \frac{C_j^i - C_j^e \exp(-FV_m/RT)}{1 - \exp(-FV_m/RT)}$$
$$+ \sum_{z_k=-1} P_k \frac{F^2 V_m}{RT} \frac{C_k^i - C_k^e \exp(+FV_m/RT)}{1 - \exp(+FV_m/RT)}. \quad (6.20)$$

And the reversal potential V_{rev} satisfies:

$$0 = \sum_{z_j=+1} P_j \frac{C_j^i - C_j^e \exp(-FV_{rev}/RT)}{1 - \exp(-FV_{rev}/RT)} + \sum_{z_k=-1} P_k \frac{C_k^i - C_k^e \exp(+FV_{rev}/RT)}{1 - \exp(+FV_{rev}/RT)}. \quad (6.21)$$

Equation (6.21) can be solved explicity for V_{rev}:

$$V_{rev} = -\frac{RT}{F} \ln \left(\frac{\sum_{z_j=+1} P_j C_j^i + \sum_{z_k=-1} P_k C_k^e}{\sum_{z_j=+1} P_j C_j^e + \sum_{z_k=-1} P_k C_k^i} \right). \quad (6.22)$$

Equation (6.22) is known as the *Goldman-Hodgkin-Katz voltage equation*. If the membrane is mainly permeable to Na$^+$, K$^+$, and Cl$^-$, the reversal potential is equal to:

$$V_{rev} = -\frac{RT}{F} \ln \left(\frac{P_{Na} C_{Na}^i + P_K C_K^i + P_{Cl} C_{Cl}^e}{P_{Na} C_{Na}^e + P_K C_K^e + P_{Cl} C_{Cl}^i} \right). \quad (6.23)$$

Excitable cells such as VSMCs are much more permeable to K$^+$ than to other ions; hence their resting potential is close to E_K.

6.3.2 Channel Gating

As stated above, the current flowing across a population of channels is equal to the number of open channels (NP_o) times the current across a given open channel. In excitable tissues such as smooth muscle, channels open in response to stimuli, such as ATP, Ca^{2+} concentration, or voltage. The simplest channel model assumes that the channel is either in the closed state C or in the open state O:

$$C \xleftrightarrow{\alpha/\beta} O$$

where α and β respectively denote the rates of conversion from C to O, and O to C. If n is the fraction of channels in the open state, $(1-n)$ is the fraction of channels in the closed stated, and we have:

$$\frac{dn}{dt} = \alpha(1-n) - \beta n = \alpha - (\alpha + \beta)n. \tag{6.24}$$

A quick analysis of Eq. (6.24) indicates that the characteristic time constant is $\tau = 1/(\alpha + \beta)$, and the steady-state value of n is $n_\infty = \alpha/(\alpha + \beta)$. The equation can be rewritten in terms of n_∞ and τ:

$$\frac{dn}{dt} = \frac{n_\infty - n}{\tau}. \tag{6.25}$$

In general, n_∞ and τ are voltage- or concentration-dependent, so that Eq. (6.25) cannot be solved analytically. Voltage-sensitive channels respond to electric potential variations; their voltage sensor consists of "gating" charges that move when V_m is altered, thereby resulting in a conformational change. For these channels, n_∞ obeys a Boltzmann distribution:

$$n_\infty = \frac{1}{1 + k_o \exp(-aFV_m/RT)}, \tag{6.26}$$

where a is a constant related to the number of gating charges on the channel and the distance over which they move during a change in conformation. The dependence of n_∞ on voltage is illustrated in Fig. 6.3. Note that most biological channels can exist in more than two states, and they display complex gating kinetics, characterized by delays, inactivation, or desensitization, as described in detail by Hille (2001).

6.3.3 *Current Across a Population of Channels*

Combining the expressions for $i(V_m, t)$ and $P_o(V_m, t)$ yields the overall current across a channel population. Some channels are permeable to several ions, so that the overall current includes the contribution of each type of permeating ions. For instance, some stretch-activated channels in vascular smooth muscle cells are permeable to K^+, Na^+ and Ca^{2+}. The overall current across these channels can be expressed as:

$$I_{M,total} = I_{M,K} + I_{M,Na} + I_{M,Ca}, \tag{6.27}$$

6.3 Ion Channels

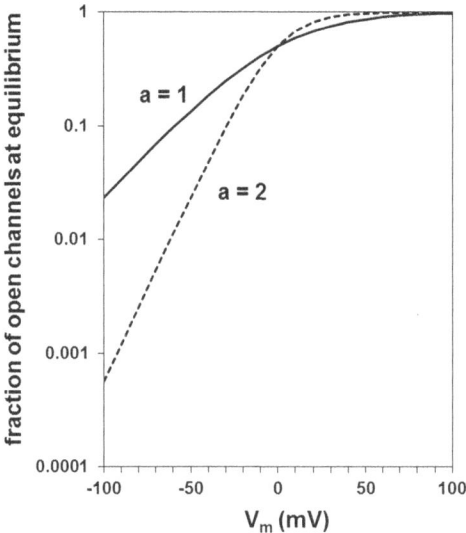

Fig. 6.3 Voltage dependence of the fraction of open channels at equilibrium (n_∞). As the gating charge on the channel becomes more negative, the voltage dependence is increasingly steep. Under resting conditions, V_m is on the order of -60 mV in VSMC, and n_∞ is approximately ten times lower in channels with $a = 2$ than with $a = 1$

where each current component is expressed using the GHK current equation:

$$I_{M,K} = A_m P_o \frac{F^2 V_m}{RT} P_K \frac{C_K^i - C_K^e \exp(-FV_m/RT)}{1 - \exp(-FV_m/RT)}, \quad (6.28a)$$

$$I_{M,Na} = A_m P_o \frac{F^2 V_m}{RT} P_{Na} \frac{C_{Na}^i - C_{Na}^e \exp(-FV_m/RT)}{1 - \exp(-FV_m/RT)}, \quad (6.28b)$$

$$I_{M,Ca} = A_m P_o \frac{4F^2 V_m}{RT} P_{Ca} \frac{C_{Ca}^i - C_{Ca}^e \exp(-2FV_m/RT)}{1 - \exp(-2FV_m/RT)}. \quad (6.28c)$$

A_m denotes the surface area of the membrane, and the open channel probability P_o varies with stretch. The physiological determinants of P_o have not been fully characterized. Some models assume that P_o is a Boltzmann function of the stress σ (i.e., the force per unit cross-sectional area) exerted on the membrane:

$$P_o = \frac{1}{1 + \exp\left[-(\sigma - \sigma_{1/2})/k_\sigma\right]}, \quad (6.29)$$

where $\sigma_{1/2}$ and k_σ are constants. The stress σ can be estimated using a cell mechanics model, as described in Sect. 6.5.

We now have the basic tools needed to determine currents, membrane potentials, and changes in intracellular concentrations. The remainder of this chapter centers on intracellular calcium, which plays an essential role in smooth muscle cell contraction.

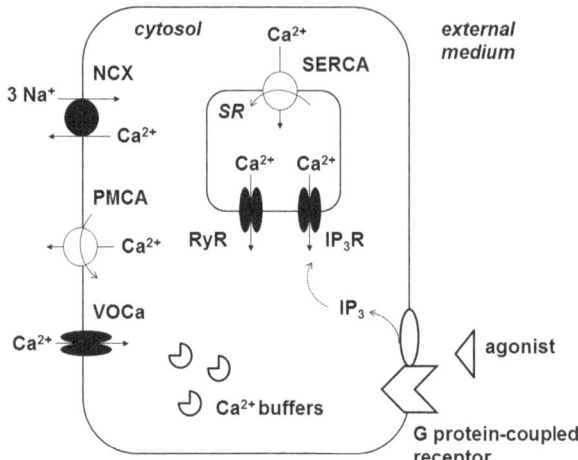

Fig. 6.4 Simplified representation of intracellular calcium signaling. Plasma membrane Ca^{2+} pumps (PMCA) and Na^+/Ca^{2+} exchangers (NCX) mediate Ca^{2+} efflux, whereas voltage-operated Ca^{2+} channels (VOCa) carry Ca^{2+} in when activated by membrane depolarization. Calcium stores in the sarcoplasmic reticulum (SR) are filled up by SR Ca^{2+} pumps (SERCA), and release Ca^{2+} into the cytosol via receptors that are sensitive to ryanodine (RyR) or inositol 1,4,5-trisphosphate (IP_3R). Agonist binding to G protein-coupled receptor leads to the formation of IP_3, thereby activating receptor-mediated Ca^{2+} release and triggering a signaling cascade

6.4 Calcium Signaling

Calcium is a key second messenger in many types of cells: stimuli such as hormones and neurotransmitters trigger signaling cascades in which temporal and spatial changes in the intracellular (cytosolic) concentration of calcium (C_{Ca}^{cyt}) ultimately generate a response such as cell contraction, differentiation, or growth. Herein we focus on the mechanisms by which increases in C_{Ca}^{cyt} result in vasoconstriction.

The resting concentration of Ca^{2+} in the cytosol is on the order of 100 nM, that is, several orders of magnitude lower than that in the systemic circulation (~2 mM). C_{Ca}^{cyt} is kept low due to the presence of (a) pumps that actively carry Ca^{2+} out of the cytosol, (b) high-affinity Ca^{2+} binding proteins (or buffers) in all intracellular compartments, and (c) Ca^{2+} stores in the sarcoplasmic reticulum (SR) that sequester most of the intracellular calcium. These processes are illustrated in Fig. 6.4.

Cell stimulation by a given agonist may lead to a steady increase in C_{Ca}^{cyt}, or to C_{Ca}^{cyt} oscillations characterized by their specific amplitude, frequency and spatial range (see below). The spatiotemporal complexity of calcium signaling, only briefly described herein, remains a very active area of study, both experimentally and theoretically.

6.4.1 Plasma Membrane Ca^{2+} Transporters

Two key transporters mediate Ca^{2+} efflux from the cell: the plasma membrane Ca^{2+} pump, and the sodium-calcium exchanger. Both are expressed in many different cell types. The Ca^{2+} current across plasma membrane Ca^{2+} pumps is generally determined using a Hill function:

$$I_{PMCA} = I_{PMCA}^{\max} \frac{C_{Ca}^{cyt}}{C_{Ca}^{cyt} + K_{m,PMCA}^{Ca}}. \tag{6.30}$$

In the equations below, "cyt" refers to the cytosol, and "e" to the external medium.

The Na^+/Ca^{2+} exchanger (NCX) exports 1 Ca^{2+} ion in exchange for 3 Na^+ ions. The entry of Na^+ into the cell is favored by its electrochemical potential gradient and thereby provides the energy needed to carry Ca^{2+} out, against its concentration gradient. The first kinetic model of NCX was developed by Mullins (1977). It assumes that the binding of Na^+ ions on one side of the carrier induces the formation of a Ca^{2+} binding site on the other side, and the subsequent translocation and dissociation of Ca^{2+}. The kinetic representation that we employ here, illustrated in Fig. 6.5, is identical to the original scheme but for one difference: whereas Mullins has posited a $1Ca^{2+}:4Na^+$ stoichiometry ratio based on studies on squid axons, we use the characteristic $1Ca^{2+}:3Na^+$ ratio found in mammalian cells. X and Y respectively denote the Na^+ and Ca^{2+} binding sites of the carrier.

Six of the reactions involve the association/dissociation of a sodium ion to/from the exchanger. Assuming that the binding of Na^+ to the external and cytosolic sides of the transmembrane carrier is much faster than translocation, these six reactions can be considered to be at equilibrium, and we have:

$$\begin{cases} k_3 C_{Na}^e C_X^e = k_{-3} C_{NaX}^e, \\ k_3 C_{Na}^e C_{NaX}^e = k_{-3} C_{Na2X}^e, \\ k_3 C_{Na}^e C_{Na2X}^e = k_{-3} C_{Na3X}^e, \end{cases} \tag{6.31}$$

$$\begin{cases} k_3 C_{Na}^{cyt} C_X^{cyt} = k_{-3} C_{NaX}^{cyt}, \\ k_3 C_{Na}^{cyt} C_{NaX}^{cyt} = k_{-3} C_{Na2X}^{cyt}, \\ k_3 C_{Na}^{cyt} C_{Na2X}^{cyt} = k_{-3} C_{Na3X}^{cyt}. \end{cases} \tag{6.32}$$

Similarly, assuming that the formation and subsequent occupancy of the Ca^{2+} binding site on both faces of the carrier are very fast, the four corresponding reactions are considered to be at equilibrium:

$$\begin{cases} k_4 C_{Na3X}^e = k_{-4} C_{Na3XY}^e, \\ k_5 C_{Na3XY}^e C_{Ca}^{cyt} = k_{-5} C_{Na3XYCa}^{e-cyt}. \end{cases} \tag{6.33}$$

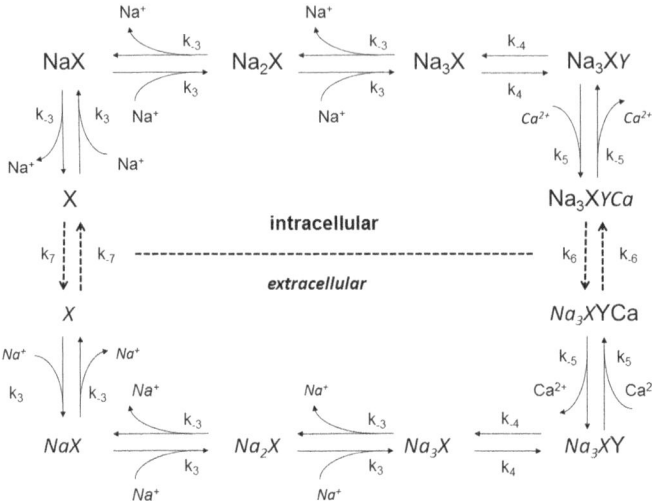

Fig. 6.5 Kinetic representation of the Na^+/Ca^{2+} exchanger, adapted from the model of Mullins (1977). X represents the Na^+ binding site of the transmembrane carrier, to which 3 Na^+ ions attach in succession during the first 3 steps. The Ca^{2+} binding site (denoted Y) is formed during step 4, and 1 Ca^{2+} ion attaches to the Na_3XY complex in step 5. The translocation of the fully loaded carrier (Na_3XYCa) from one side of the membrane to the other occurs in step 6. The model also considers the translocation of empty carrier (step 7). Extracellular species are denoted by italics

$$\begin{cases} k_4 C_{Na3X}^{cyt} = k_{-4} C_{Na3XY}^{cyt}, \\ k_5 C_{Na3XY}^{cyt} C_{Ca}^{e} = k_{-5} C_{Na3XYCa}^{cyt-e}, \end{cases} \quad (6.34)$$

where "cyt-e" and "e-cyt" apply to the fully loaded carrier with 3 Na^+ ions respectively on the intracellular and external sides. Combining Eqs. (6.31) and (6.33), and Eqs. (6.32) and (6.34), respectively, we obtain:

$$C_{Na3XYCa}^{e-cyt} = \frac{k_5}{k_{-5}} \frac{k_4}{k_{-4}} \left(\frac{k_3}{k_{-3}}\right)^3 C_X^e \left(C_{Na}^e\right)^3 C_{Ca}^{cyt}, \quad (6.35)$$

$$C_{Na3XYCa}^{cyt-e} = \frac{k_5}{k_{-5}} \frac{k_4}{k_{-4}} \left(\frac{k_3}{k_{-3}}\right)^3 C_X^{cyt} \left(C_{Na}^{cyt}\right)^3 C_{Ca}^e. \quad (6.36)$$

The translocation rates of the fully loaded carrier (namely, Na_3XYCa) are k_6 in the direction of Ca^{2+} influx, and k_{-6} in the opposite direction. Thus, the net flux of Ca^{2+} into the cytosol (J_{Ca}^{e-cyt}) is given by:

$$\begin{aligned} J_{Ca}^{e-cyt} &= k_6 C_{Na3XYCa}^{cyt-e} - k_{-6} C_{Na3XYCa}^{e-cyt} \\ &= \frac{k_5}{k_{-5}} \frac{k_4}{k_{-4}} \left(\frac{k_3}{k_{-3}}\right)^3 \left[k_6 C_X^{cyt} \left(C_{Na}^{cyt}\right)^3 C_{Ca}^e - k_{-6} C_X^e \left(C_{Na}^e\right)^3 C_{Ca}^{cyt}\right]. \end{aligned} \quad (6.37)$$

6.4 Calcium Signaling

The exchanger is electrogenic: each cycle is accompanied by the net movement of one positive charge into the cell. As described in more detail in Chap. 8, the exchanger reaches equilibrium when the Gibbs free energy of the system is zero, that is, when the transmembrane electrochemical potential gradient of 1 Ca^{2+} ion is exactly compensated by that of 3 Na^+ ions. Under these conditions, we have (see Problem 6.3):

$$\frac{C_{Ca}^{cyt}}{C_{Ca}^{e}} = \frac{\left(C_{Na}^{cyt}\right)^3}{\left(C_{Na}^{e}\right)^3} \exp\left(V_m F/RT\right). \tag{6.38}$$

By combining the two previous equations, we arrive at the general form of the Ca^{2+} flux across NCX (denoted J_{Ca}^{e-cyt} above):

$$J_{Ca}^{NCX} = k_{NCX} \left[\left(C_{Na}^{cyt}\right)^3 C_{Ca}^{e} \exp\left(V_m F/RT\right) - \left(C_{Na}^{e}\right)^3 C_{Ca}^{cyt} \right]. \tag{6.39}$$

As the complete equations of the Mullins model indicate, k_{NCX} is not a constant but a variable that depends on reaction rates as well as the external and internal concentrations of Na^+ and Ca^{2+}; it can be written as a polynomial of C_{Na}^{cyt}, C_{Na}^{e}, C_{Ca}^{e} and C_{Ca}^{cyt}. Subsequent models of NCX have taken into account the allosteric activation of the exchanger by cytosolic Ca^{2+} (Weber et al. 2001), as well as the shape of the energy barrier in the electric field (DiFrancesco and Noble 1985). In cardiac myocytes, the allosteric activation of NCX can be adequately represented by a Hill equation with a coefficient of 2:

$$allo = \frac{\left(C_{Ca}^{cyt}\right)^2}{\left(C_{Ca}^{cyt}\right)^2 + \left(K_{m,NCX}^{Ca}\right)^2}. \tag{6.40}$$

This allosteric effect is included as a multiplying factor in J_{Ca}^{NCX}. To date, there is no model of the specific renal isoform of NCX, and the current across the exchanger is usually determined using the prevalent cardiac model:

$$I_{NCX} = I_{NCX}^{max} \left(\frac{\left(C_{Ca}^{cyt}\right)^2}{\left(C_{Ca}^{cyt}\right)^2 + \left(K_{m,NCX}^{Ca}\right)^2} \right) \left(\frac{\Theta_F \left(C_{Na}^{cyt}\right)^3 C_{Ca}^{e} - \Theta_R \left(C_{Na}^{e}\right)^3 C_{Ca}^{cyt}}{\Gamma \left(1 + k_{sat} \Phi_R\right)} \right), \tag{6.41}$$

where I_{NCX}^{max} is the maximum current across NCX and:

$$\Theta_F = \exp\left[\gamma V_m F/RT\right], \tag{6.42}$$

$$\Theta_R = \exp\left[(\gamma - 1) V_m F/RT\right], \tag{6.43}$$

$$\Gamma = \left(C_{Na}^{e}\right)^{3} C_{Ca}^{cyt} + \left(C_{Na}^{cyt}\right)^{3} C_{Ca}^{e} + K_{mNae}{}^{3} C_{Ca}^{cyt} + K_{mCae} \left(C_{Na}^{cyt}\right)^{3}$$
$$+ K_{mNai}{}^{3} C_{Ca}^{e} \left(1 + C_{Ca}^{cyt}/K_{mCai}\right) + K_{mCai}\left(C_{Na}^{e}\right)^{3} \left(1 + \left(C_{Na}^{cyt}\right)^{3}/K_{mNai}{}^{3}\right). \qquad (6.44)$$

The parameter γ ($0 < \gamma < 1$) characterizes the energy barrier that controls the voltage dependence of the current, and k_{sat} accounts for exchanger saturation at very negative potentials. The constants K_{mNae}, K_{mNai}, K_{mCai}, and K_{mCae} represent binding affinities.

Voltage-Operated Calcium Channels

Another important class of Ca^{2+} channels in vascular smooth muscle consists of voltage-operated (or voltage-gated) Ca^{2+} channels. In contrast to plasma membrane Ca^{2+} pumps and NCX, these channels mediate Ca^{2+} influx into the cytosol, and they play an important role in cell contraction. They are normally closed at resting potential values, and are activated by membrane depolarization. There are several types of voltage-gated channels, which are distinguished by the toxins they respond to and the degree of voltage activation (high, intermediate, or low). High-voltage-activated L-type channels are predominantly expressed in skeletal, smooth, and cardiac muscle, and can be found in the afferent arteriole and DVR pericytes. They are inhibited by calcium channel blockers of the dihydropyridine class (such as nifedipine and nicardipine), which are used in the treatment of hypertension.

During sustained depolarization, L-type channels undergo a series of conformational changes: they first open and subsequently close. The process of channel closure during depolarization is known as inactivation. Once a channel is inactivated, it cannot be re-activated until the membrane has been repolarized. The fraction of open channels is therefore calculated as the product of two terms, one that corresponds to channel activation and the other to reversal of inactivation. Thus, L-type currents can be expressed as:

$$I_{Ca,L} = G_{Ca,L}^{max} d_L f_L (V_m - E_{Ca}), \qquad (6.45)$$

where $G_{Ca,L}^{max}$ is the maximum conductance (a constant), and d_L and f_L denote the voltage- and time-dependent activation and de-inactivation variables, respectively. As described above, the time variations of these variables are given by:

$$\frac{d(d_L)}{dt} = \frac{d_L^{\infty} - d_L}{\tau_d}, \qquad (6.46)$$

$$\frac{d(f_L)}{dt} = \frac{f_L^{\infty} - f_L}{\tau_f}, \qquad (6.47)$$

where the steady-state values (d_L^{∞}, f_L^{∞}) and time constants (τ_d, τ_f) depend on the membrane potential. Whereas d_L^{∞}, which represents the activation process, increases with depolarization, f_L^{∞}, which represents the de-inactivation process, decreases with increasing V_m, as illustrated in Fig. 6.6. The product $d_L^{\infty} \cdot f_L^{\infty}$, the fraction of open channels at equilibrium, is significantly above zero only in a narrow voltage window.

6.4 Calcium Signaling

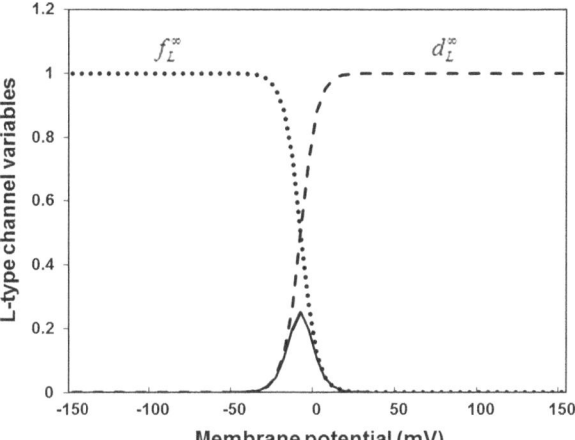

Fig. 6.6 Representative profiles of L-type channel activation (d_L^∞) and de-inactivation (f_L^∞) variables, as a function of the membrane potential (V_m). Also shown is the product of d_L^∞ and f_L^∞ (solid curve), which represents the open probability of the channel at steady state. In these simulations, $d_L^\infty = 1/(1 + \exp[-(V_m + 10)/5])$ and $f_L^\infty = 1/(1 + \exp[(V_m + 10)/5])$, where V_m is given in mV

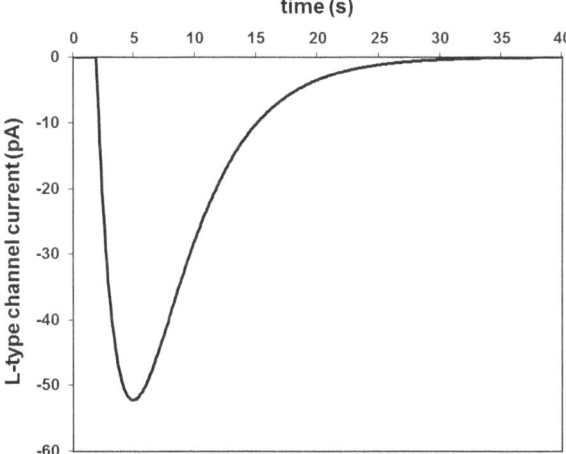

Fig. 6.7 Predicted effect of a step decrease in V_m from $+60$ to -60 mV at t = 2 s on the L-type channel current. The channel conductance is set to 1 nS, d_L^∞ and f_L^∞ are as given above (see Fig. 6.6), and the activation and inactivation time constants are taken as $\tau_d = 3 \exp[-((V_m - 5)/100)^2]$ and $\tau_f = 3 \exp[-((V_m + 5)/100)^2]$

To examine the behavior of L-type channels, consider a step change in the membrane potential, from $+60$ mV to -60 mV. As shown in Fig. 6.7, $I_{Ca,L}$ is initially zero at rest. Following a sudden decrease in V_m at t = 2 s, the channel opens rapidly, and then closes again, albeit more slowly, owing to inactivation. Note that $I_{Ca,L}$ is negative, as it mediates Ca^{2+} influx into the cell.

Passive Leak

The plasma membrane expresses other, unspecified channels that are permeable to Ca^{2+}. Models of calcium signaling thus incorporate a background current to account for the passive leak of Ca^{2+} across these channels, down its concentration gradient:

$$I_{Ca,leak} = G_{Ca,leak}(V_m - E_{Ca}). \qquad (6.48)$$

Similar background currents are generally included for the other ions considered in the model.

6.4.2 Calcium Buffers

As Ca^{2+} is exchanged between the cytosol and surrounding compartments, the extent to which it associates with intracellular buffers varies as well. The rates Φ_{Ca}^{cyt} and Φ_{Ca}^{SR} respectively characterize the Ca^{2+} binding reactions in the cytosol and SR. The nature of intracellular Ca^{2+} binding proteins depends on the cell type. In smooth muscle cells, the main Ca^{2+} buffers are calmodulin in the cytosol and calsequestrin in the SR. The chelation of Ca^{2+} by calsequestrin ("Seq") is described as a first-order dynamic process:

$$Ca^{2+} + Seq \underset{}{\overset{k_{Seq}^{on}/k_{Seq}^{off}}{\longleftrightarrow}} Seq \cdot Ca$$

If $C_{Seq.Ca}^{SR}$ denotes the concentration of the calcium-bound sites of calsequestrin, and $C_{Seq,tot}^{SR}$ the total concentration of calsequestrin in the SR, we have:

$$\frac{dC_{Seq.Ca}^{SR}}{dt} = -\Phi_{Ca}^{SR}, \qquad (6.49)$$

$$\Phi_{Ca}^{SR} = -k_{Seq}^{on} C_{Ca}^{SR} \left(C_{Seq,tot}^{SR} - C_{Seq.Ca}^{SR} \right) + k_{Seq}^{off} C_{Seq.Ca}^{SR}, \qquad (6.50)$$

where k_{Seq}^{on} and k_{Seq}^{off} are respectively the "on" and "off" calsequestrin rate constants.

Calmodulin (CaM) is a ubiquitous Ca^{2+} binding protein which plays a key role in VSMC contraction. The two terminal ends of CaM can each bind two Ca^{2+} ions. Activation of myosin light chain kinase (MLCK) by the CaM·Ca_4 complex increases the fraction of myosin light chains (MLC) that are phosphorylated and thereby stimulates cellular contraction, as described in more detail below. To predict vessel diameter changes, it is therefore necessary to determine the concentration of activated MLCK. Early models of MLCK activation assumed a simple 2-step process:

6.4 Calcium Signaling

$$CaM + 4\ Ca^{2+} \xrightleftharpoons{K_1} CaM \cdot Ca_4$$

$$MLCK + CaM \cdot Ca_4 \xrightleftharpoons{K_2} MLCK \cdot CaM \cdot Ca_4$$

If the first reaction is taken to be at equilibrium, then $\Phi_{Ca}^{cyt} = 0$ provided that CaM is the only cytosolic Ca^{2+} buffer that is being considered. Moreover, if both reactions are at equilibrium, the steady-state concentration of the MLCK·CaM·Ca$_4$ complex can easily be calculated as a function of C_{Ca}^{cyt}. Assuming that the 4 Ca^{2+} binding sites on CaM are independent and equivalent, the equilibrium concentrations of CaM·Ca$_4$ (denoted CaM*) and MLCK·CaM·Ca$_4$ (denoted MLCK*) are given by:

$$C_{CaM*}^{cyt} = \frac{C_{CaM,tot}^{cyt} - C_{MLCK*}^{cyt}}{\left(1 + \frac{K_1}{C_{Ca}^{cyt}}\right)^4}, \tag{6.51}$$

$$C_{MLCK*}^{cyt} = \frac{C_{MLCK,tot}^{cyt}}{1 + \frac{K_2}{C_{CaM*}^{cyt}}}, \tag{6.52}$$

where $C_{CaM,tot}^{cyt}$ and $C_{MLCK,tot}^{cyt}$ represent the total concentrations of CaM and MLCK, respectively, K_1 is the dissociation constant for the Ca^{2+} binding site on calmodulin, and K_2 is the dissociation constant for the MLCK·CaM·Ca$_4$ complex. To simplify the notation, we define the following non-dimensional variables and parameters $c = C_{Ca}^{cyt}/K_1$, $y = C_{CaM*}^{cyt}/C_{CaM,tot}^{cyt}$, $z = C_{MLCK*}^{cyt}/C_{MLCK,tot}^{cyt}$, $\gamma_1 = C_{CaM,tot}^{cyt}/K_2$, and $\gamma_2 = C_{MLCK,tot}^{cyt}/K_2$, and then rewrite Eqs. (6.51) and (6.52) as:

$$y = \frac{1 - C_{MLCK*}^{cyt}/C_{CaM,tot}^{cyt}}{(1 + 1/c)^4} = \frac{1 - (\gamma_2/\gamma_1)z}{(1 + 1/c)^4}, \tag{6.53}$$

$$z = \frac{1}{1 + \frac{K_2}{C_{CaM*}^{cyt}}} = \frac{1}{1 + \frac{1/\gamma_1}{y}}. \tag{6.54}$$

These two equations can be combined to eliminate y and solve for z. After rearrangement, we obtain the following dimensionless equation:

$$\gamma_2 z^2 - \left[\gamma_1 + \gamma_2 + (1 + 1/c)^4\right] z + \gamma_1 = 0. \tag{6.55}$$

Solving Eq. (6.55) yields the relative concentration of MLCK* as a function of C_{Ca}^{cyt}.

However, this simple approach does not consider the different binding rates of Ca^{2+} to the two terminal tails of CaM and neglects the possible binding of intermediate species (e.g., CaM, CaM.Ca, etc.) to MLCK. Complex kinetic schemes of the interactions between Ca^{2+}, CaM, and MLCK have since been developed, which can be used to more accurately determine both Φ_{Ca}^{cyt} and the concentration of activated MLCK (Fajmut et al. 2005).

6.4.3 Sarcoplamic Reticulum Calcium Stores

Elevations in C_{Ca}^{cyt} stem from increased Ca^{2+} influx across the plasma membrane, and/or from increased Ca^{2+} release from internal stores such as the SR. The amount of Ca^{2+} that is sequestered in the SR is tightly controlled by counteracting uptake and release mechanisms: SR Ca^{2+} pumps (known as SERCA) actively transport Ca^{2+} from the cytosol into the SR against its concentration gradient, whereas SR receptor-activated channels discharge Ca^{2+} into the cytosol in response to specific stimuli. There are two well-known families of SR Ca^{2+} channels: inositol 1,4,5-trisphosphate receptors (IP_3R) are ubiquitous, whereas ryanodine receptors (RyR) are expressed mostly in muscle fibers and cardiac myocytes. IP_3R are so called because they require the binding of IP_3, an intracellular second messenger, in order to open. IP_3 is generated following a signaling cascade triggered by the binding of agonists to plasma membrane G protein-coupled receptors (Fig. 6.4). RyR are so called because they are sensitive to ryanodine, a plant alkaloid that inhibits the channel. There is evidence that they are expressed in DVR pericytes.

SERCA Model

The sarco/endoplasmic reticulum calcium (SERCA) pumps allow for the accumulation of Ca^{2+} in the SR, against its electrochemical gradient. Calcium uptake by SERCA is usually described by a Hill equation:

$$I_{SERCA} = I_{SERCA}^{\max} \frac{(C_{Ca}^{cyt})^{n_{SERCA}}}{(C_{Ca}^{cyt})^{n_{SERCA}} + (K_{m,SERCA}^{Ca})^{n_{SERCA}}}, \quad (6.56)$$

where $I_{SERCA}^{\max}$ is the maximum current through the pump, and the Hill coefficient n_{SERCA} is generally taken as 1 or 2. More sophisticated models of SERCA kinetics, which account for possible bidirectional transport and the buffering effects of the pump, can be found elsewhere (Yano et al. 2004; Higgins et al. 2006).

The Goldbeter-Dupont-Berridge Model of SR Receptors

Some hormones and neurotransmitters generate repetitive spikes in C_{Ca}^{cyt}. These oscillations result from complex dynamic interactions, such as positive and negative feedback effects of calcium on SR receptors. Among these feedback loops is the phenomenon known as calcium-induced calcium release (CICR), whereby a small increase in C_{Ca}^{cyt} induces the release of a much larger amount of Ca^{2+} via SR receptors. The best known, early model of SR receptors that captured these features is that developed by Goldbeter, Dupont, and Berridge (1990). Their model assumes that IP_3 induces Ca^{2+} release from an IP_3-sensitive store into the cytosol (at a rate v_1), thereby activating Ca^{2+} pumping into an IP_3-insensitive pool (at a rate v_2); in

6.4 Calcium Signaling

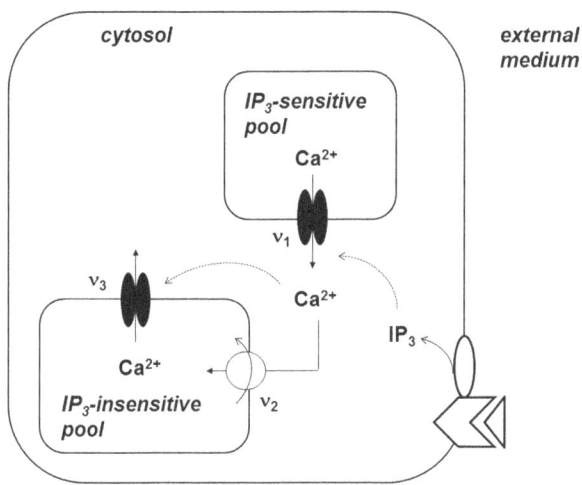

Fig. 6.8 Schematic representation of Ca^{2+} exchanges between intracellular compartments, according to the Goldbeter-Dupont-Berridge model. The generation of IP_3, which is triggered by agonist binding to G protein-coupled receptors, activates the release of Ca^{2+} from an IP_3-sensitive store. The resulting cytosolic Ca^{2+} increase enhances Ca^{2+} pumping into an IP_3-insensitive pool, while also stimulating Ca^{2+} release from that pool

turn, the latter releases Ca^{2+} into the cytosol (at a rate v_3) in a process activated by cytosolic Ca^{2+}. These processes are depicted in Fig. 6.8.

The rate of Ca^{2+} release from the IP_3-sensitive store is expressed as:

$$v_1 = v_{1M} \beta, \tag{6.57}$$

where v_{1M} is a constant, and β is a prescribed function of the cytosolic concentration of IP_3. The rate of Ca^{2+} pumping is a sigmoidal function of C_{Ca}^{cyt} with a Hill coefficient n_2 (as in Eq. 6.56):

$$v_2 = v_{2M} \frac{\left(C_{Ca}^{cyt}\right)^{n_2}}{K_2^{n_2} + \left(C_{Ca}^{cyt}\right)^{n_2}}. \tag{6.58}$$

Lastly, the rate of Ca^{2+} release from the IP_3-insensitive pool has two components: a release term which is a Michaelis-Menten function of the Ca^{2+} concentration in that pool (denoted C_{Ca}^{pool}), and an activation term which is a function of cytosolic Ca^{2+}. The model assumes that:

$$v_3 = v_{3M} \frac{\left(C_{Ca}^{pool}\right)^m}{K_R^m + \left(C_{Ca}^{pool}\right)^m} \frac{\left(C_{Ca}^{cyt}\right)^p}{K_A^p + \left(C_{Ca}^{cyt}\right)^p}, \tag{6.59}$$

where m and p are cooperativity coefficients, and K_R and K_A are threshold constants for release and activation. Importantly, this so-called minimal model demonstrates that periodic Ca^{2+} spikes can occur in the absence of IP_3 oscillations (Ca^{2+} oscillations are examined in more detail below). The Goldbeter-Dupont-Berridge model was widely used during the 1990s, but has since then been supplanted by binding models of IP_3R and RyR.

A Binding Model of IP$_3$R

Binding models of Ca^{2+} receptors are based upon kinetic diagrams, which serve to determine the open probability (P_o^R) of the receptor. The Ca^{2+} flux across the receptors is taken to be proportional to the open probability P_o^R, the receptor conductivity (ν_R), and the Ca^{2+} concentration difference between the SR and the cytosol (i.e., the driving force). A general expression for the Ca^{2+} current across SR receptors (I_R) is thus:

$$I_R = \nu_R P_o^R \left(C_{Ca}^{SR} - C_{Ca}^{cyt} \right) (2 F V_{SR}), \tag{6.60}$$

where V_{SR} is the SR volume, and the factor 2 accounts for the valence of the Ca^{2+} ion.

Binding models of IP$_3$R seek to account for the observation that the open probability of the IP$_3$ receptor is modulated by calcium in a biphasic manner: channel opening is stimulated by low C_{Ca}^{cyt} and inhibited by high C_{Ca}^{cyt}. The most influential IP$_3$R model to date remains that of De Young and Keizer (1992). This model assumes that the channel consists of 3 identical and independent subunits, and that each subunit has one IP$_3$ binding site (site # 1), one activating Ca^{2+} binding site (# 2), and one inhibiting Ca^{2+} binding site (# 3), as illustrated in Fig. 6.9. The fraction of subunits in state $S_{i_1 i_2 i_3}$ is denoted by $x_{i_1 i_2 i_3}$, where the jth binding site is occupied if $i_j = 1$ and free if $i_j = 0$. According to the model's hypothesis, the channel is open when all 3 subunits are in the state S_{110}, i.e., when each subunit is bound by one IP$_3$ ion ($i_1 = 1$), one activating Ca^{2+} ion ($i_2 = 1$), and no inhibiting Ca^{2+} ion ($i_3 = 0$). In other words, the open probability of the receptor is $P_o^R = (x_{110})^3$, and the IP$_3$R-mediated Ca^{2+} current is calculated as:

$$I_{IP3R} = \nu_{IP3R} (x_{110})^3 \left(C_{Ca}^{SR} - C_{Ca}^{cyt} \right) (2 F V_{SR}), \tag{6.61}$$

where ν_{IP3R} is the Ca^{2+} conductivity of IP$_3$R. The fractions $x_{i_1 i_2 i_3}$ are obtained by solving mass action kinetic equations. For example, as illustrated in Fig. 6.9, state S_{110} originates from the binding of one IP$_3$ ion to state S_{010}, or the dissociation of an inhibiting Ca^{2+} ion from state S_{111}, or the binding of an activating Ca^{2+} ion to state S_{100}. The kinetic equation for x_{110} is written accordingly:

$$\frac{dx_{110}}{dt} = \left(a_1 C_{IP3}^{cyt} x_{010} - b_1 x_{110} \right) - \left(a_2 C_{Ca}^{cyt} x_{110} - b_2 x_{111} \right) + \left(a_5 C_{Ca}^{cyt} x_{100} - b_5 x_{110} \right). \tag{6.62}$$

As these kinetic equations involve the cytosolic concentration of IP$_3$, the latter must be either specified or determined. If we assume simply that cytosolic IP$_3$ is generated at a constant rate ν_{IP3}, and consumed by a first-order reaction (with a rate constant I_r), we have:

$$\frac{dC_{IP3}^{cyt}}{dt} = \nu_{IP3} - I_r C_{IP3}^{cyt}. \tag{6.63}$$

6.4 Calcium Signaling

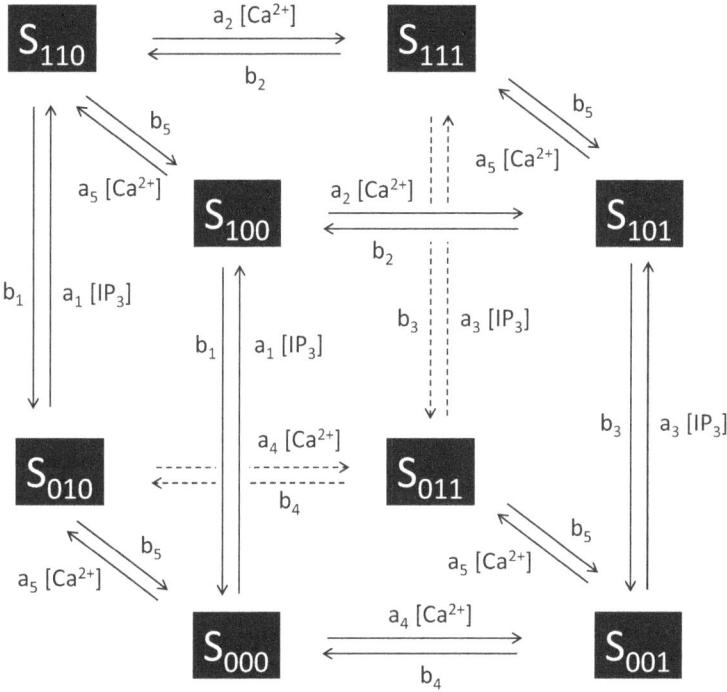

Fig. 6.9 Representation of one IP$_3$ receptor subunit in the De Young and Keizer model (1992). The receptor consists of 3 identical subunits

The model of DeYoung and Keiser includes an additional feedback mechanism, as it assumes that IP$_3$ generation is modulated by C_{Ca}^{cyt}, such that:

$$\frac{dC_{IP3}^{cyt}}{dt} = v_{IP3,\max} \left(\frac{C_{Ca}^{cyt} + (1 - \alpha_{IP3}) \, k_{IP3}}{C_{Ca}^{cyt} + k_{IP3}} \right) - I_r C_{IP3}^{cyt}, \quad (6.64)$$

where $v_{IP3,\max}$ is the maximum rate of IP$_3$ production, and α_{IP3} ($0 \leq \alpha_{IP3} \leq 1$) characterizes the extent to which Ca^{2+} affects IP$_3$ production. If α_{IP3} is zero, there is no feedback and Eq. (6.64) is equivalent to Eq. (6.63).

The system of differential equations for the eight unknown fractions ($x_{i_1 i_2 i_3}$) can be simplified by assuming that the binding of IP$_3$ is very rapid and that the corresponding reactions are at equilibrium. Under these conditions, we have (see Fig. 6.9):

$$a_1 C_{IP3}^{cyt} x_{0k0} = b_1 x_{1k0} \quad k = 0, 1, \quad (6.65a)$$

$$a_3 C_{IP3}^{cyt} x_{0k1} = b_3 x_{1k1} \quad k = 0, 1. \quad (6.65b)$$

With this hypothesis, the number of unknown fractions is reduced to 4, and the steady-state values of $x_{i_1 i_2 i_3}$ can be calculated analytically as a function of C_{Ca}^{cyt} and

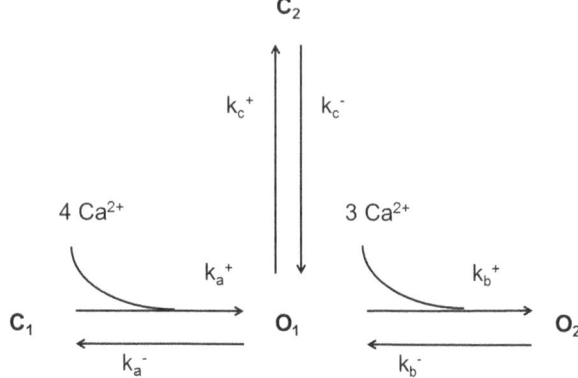

Fig. 6.10 Schematic representation of the four states of the ryanodine receptor, according to the Keizer-Levine model (1996). States O_1 and O_2 are open, whereas states C_1 and C_2 are closed

C_{IP3}^{cyt}. In particular, the steady-state value of x_{110} (which yields the open probability of the receptor at equilibrium) is given by:

$$x_{110} = \frac{d_2 C_{Ca}^{cyt} C_{IP3}^{cyt}}{\left(C_{Ca}^{cyt} C_{IP3}^{cyt} + d_2 C_{IP3}^{cyt} + d_1 d_2 + d_3 C_{Ca}^{cyt}\right)\left(d_5 + C_{Ca}^{cyt}\right)}, \quad (6.66)$$

where d_k is defined as b_k/a_k.

The model of De Young and Keizer adequately reproduces experimental data from the early 1990s, but not some of the more recent observations, such as the sequential binding of IP_3 and Ca^{2+}, and the tetrameric conformation of the receptor. These and other findings (e.g., the existence of different IP_3R subtypes) have since led to the development of second-generation models. A thorough review of early and recent models of IP_3R was published by Sneyd and Falcke (2005).

A Binding Model of RyR

Among the simpler and better-known models of RyR-mediated Ca^{2+} release is that built by Keizer and Levine (1996). As illustrated in Fig. 6.10, it assumes that the channel can exist in 2 open states (O_1 and O_2) and 2 closed states (C_1 and C_2), and that some transitions are Ca^{2+}-independent. The probability that the channel is in state J is denoted P_J.

As described above, the RyR-mediated Ca^{2+} current is given by:

$$I_{RyR} = \nu_{RyR} P_{RyR} \left(C_{Ca}^{SR} - C_{Ca}^{cyt}\right)(2FV_{SR}), \quad (6.67)$$

where ν_{RyR} is the Ca^{2+} conductivity of RyR, and P_{RyR}, the probability that the channel is in an open state, is equal to the sum of the probabilities P_{O1} and P_{O2} in this model. Based upon the kinetic scheme shown in Fig. 6.10, we have:

6.4 Calcium Signaling

$$\frac{dP_{O1}}{dt} = \left[k_a^+ \left(C_{Ca}^{cyt}\right)^4 P_{C1} - k_a^- P_{O1}\right] + \left[k_b^- P_{O2} - k_b^+ \left(C_{Ca}^{cyt}\right)^3 P_{O1}\right]$$
$$+ \left[k_c^- P_{C2} - k_c^+ P_{O1}\right], \tag{6.68}$$

$$\frac{dP_{O2}}{dt} = k_b^+ \left(C_{Ca}^{cyt}\right)^3 P_{O1} - k_b^- P_{O2}. \tag{6.69}$$

Similar equations can be written for P_{C1} and P_{C2}. The four differential equations are solved simultaneously to determine P_{RyR} and then I_{RyR}. To simplify the calculations, it is sometimes assumed that the transitions between states O_1, O_2, and C_1 are much faster than that between state O_1 and C_2. With this hypothesis, P_{RyR} can be approximated as (see Problem 6.4):

$$P_{RyR} = \frac{\omega \left[1 + \left(C_{Ca}^{cyt}/K_b\right)^3\right]}{1 + \left(K_a/C_{Ca}^{cyt}\right)^4 + \left(C_{Ca}^{cyt}/K_b\right)^3}, \tag{6.70}$$

where $K_a^4 \equiv k_a^-/k_a^+$, $K_b^3 \equiv k_b^-/k_b^+$, $K_c \equiv k_c^-/k_c^+$, and ω, the fraction of channels not in state C_2, is given by:

$$\frac{d\omega}{dt} = \frac{k_c^- (\omega^\infty - \omega)}{\omega^\infty}, \tag{6.71}$$

$$\omega^\infty = \frac{1 + \left(K_a/C_{Ca}^{cyt}\right)^4 + \left(C_{Ca}^{cyt}/K_b\right)^3}{1 + 1/K_c + \left(K_a/C_{Ca}^{cyt}\right)^4 + \left(C_{Ca}^{cyt}/K_b\right)^3}. \tag{6.72}$$

Note that there are many other models of RyR-mediated Ca^{2+} release, as briefly reviewed elsewhere (Sneyd and Falcke 2005).

Figure 6.11 illustrates the dependence of the open probability at equilibrium of IP_3R (P_{IP3R}) and RyR (P_{RyR}) on C_{Ca}^{cyt}. P_{IP3R} and P_{RyR} are calculated using the De Young-Keizer and Keizer-Levine models, respectively. Under resting conditions, when $C_{Ca}^{cyt} \sim 100$ nM $= 10^{-7}$ M, P_{RyR} is significantly lower than P_{IP3R}. As C_{Ca}^{cyt} rises above 100 nM, P_{RyR} and P_{IP3R} both increase at first. However, when C_{Ca}^{cyt} exceeds 200 nM, P_{IP3R} starts to fall, because IP_3R is inhibited by high Ca^{2+} concentrations. In contrast, P_{RyR} continues to increase and approaches 1 when $C_{Ca}^{cyt} \sim 10$ μM $= 10^{-5}$ M. Thus, the P_{RyR} curve illustrates in a simple manner the phenomenon of calcium-induced calcium release, whereby an increase in C_{Ca}^{cyt} induces RyR to release more calcium from the SR.

6.4.4 Temporal Variations in Calcium Concentration

Having explicitly described the major Ca^{2+} currents and buffering reactions, we can now express the conservation of Ca^{2+} in the cytosol as:

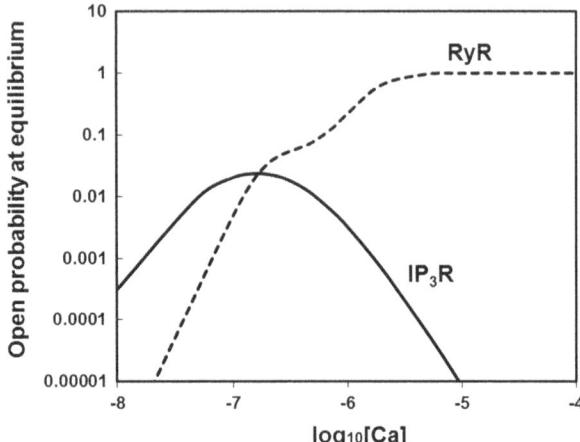

Fig. 6.11 Fraction of open ryanodine and IP$_3$ receptors at equilibrium, as a function of C_{Ca}^{cyt}. P_{IP3R} (i.e., x_{110}^3) is calculated assuming that C_{IP3}^{cyt} = 240 nM. Other parameters can be found in De Young and Keizer (1992) and Keizer and Levine (1996)

$$\frac{dC_{Ca}^{cyt}}{dt} = \frac{-I_{Ca}^{net}}{2FV^{cyt}} + \Phi_{Ca}^{cyt}$$

$$= \frac{-\left(I_{PMCA} - I_{NCX} + I_{Ca.L} + I_{Ca.leak} - I_{IP3R} - I_{RyR} + I_{SERCA}\right)}{2FV^{cyt}} + \Phi_{Ca}^{cyt}. \quad (6.73)$$

Similarly, conservation of Ca^{2+} in the SR is expressed as:

$$\frac{dC_{Ca}^{SR}}{dt} = \frac{-\left(I_{IP3R} + I_{RyR} - I_{SERCA}\right)}{2FV^{SR}} + \Phi_{Ca}^{SR}. \quad (6.74)$$

If the plasma membrane expresses other Ca^{2+} channels, such as store-operated channels (which are activated by SR Ca^{2+} store depletion) or stretch-sensitive channels, the corresponding currents need to be included in Eq. (6.73).

Spatial Variations

We need to acknowledge at this point that representing the cytosol as a homogeneous compartment is an oversimplification. In reality, Ca^{2+} is unevenly distributed throughout the cell, and highly localized elevations of Ca^{2+} concentration can occur. For instance, it is thought that Ca^{2+} levels are significantly higher in subplasmalemmal microdomains than in the cytosol. These microdomains, formed through close association of the SR with the overlying plasma membrane, express specific transporters that are not present in the membrane that lies directly above the bulk cytosol (Moore et al. 1993). Blaustein and colleagues (2006) postulated that modulation of microdomain Na^+ concentration by ouabain (an endogenous hormone) regulates Ca^{2+} loading into SR stores as well as C_{Ca}^{cyt} variations, and that this

6.4 Calcium Signaling

mechanism plays a key role in regulating vascular contraction and blood pressure. A VSMC model that accounts for the presence of subplasmalemmal microdomains suggests that modulation of Ca^{2+} signaling by transport events in microdomains is indeed feasible, provided that there is a high degree of isolation from the cytosol (Edwards and Pallone 2007). In addition, spontaneous, RyR-mediated localized C_{Ca}^{cyt} transients, known as Ca^{2+} sparks, may sometime fuse and trigger Ca^{2+} waves that propagate throughout the cell; such transients allow for both local and global regulation of cell function. A few mathematical models of Ca^{2+} dynamics incorporate this spatial heterogeneity (Spiro and Othmer 1999; Sneyd et al. 2003).

Calcium Oscillations

Some stimuli raise C_{Ca}^{cyt} in a peak and plateau manner, whereas others evoke repetitive C_{Ca}^{cyt} spikes. In fact, angiotensin II (Ang II) induces C_{Ca}^{cyt} elevations in some DVR pericytes, and C_{Ca}^{cyt} oscillations in others. Why does C_{Ca}^{cyt} oscillate? To answer this question, we can use a simplified model of Ca^{2+} dynamics, following the approach of Somogyi and Stucki (1991). Let x be the concentration of Ca^{2+} in the cytosol, and y that in the SR. We assume that PMCA and SERCA pump Ca^{2+} at linear rates (β and γ, respectively), and we consider two passive (leak) Ca^{2+} fluxes into the cell, one from the extracellular compartment (rate k_o) and one from the SR (rate k_s). Finally, we assume that receptor-mediated Ca^{2+} release into the cytosol is represented by a function $f(x)$. With these hypotheses, the temporal Ca^{2+} concentration variations are written as:

$$\begin{cases} \frac{dx}{dt} = -\beta x - \gamma x + k_o + k_s y + f(x)y, \\ \frac{dy}{dt} = +\gamma x - k_s y - f(x)y. \end{cases} \quad (6.75)$$

The analysis of this system is the object of Problem 6.5. Here we further simplify the problem by assuming that $f(x) = x^2$. Moreover, since the passive leak of Ca^{2+} from the SR is generally negligible relative to the receptor-mediated release of Ca^{2+}, k_s is taken as zero. The resulting system of equations is known as the *Brusselator*, a theoretical model for certain types of autocatalytic reactions developed by Prirogine and colleagues. In our case, it is written as:

$$\begin{cases} \frac{dx}{dt} \equiv \dot{x} = -\beta x - \gamma x + k_o + x^2 y, \\ \frac{dy}{dt} \equiv \dot{y} = +\gamma x - x^2 y. \end{cases} \quad (6.76)$$

The key concepts of oscillation theory were introduced in Chap. 5. Whether this system exhibits oscillations depends on the stability of the steady-state values of x and y (denoted x_{ss} and y_{ss}, respectively). The latter are easily obtained by setting the time derivatives to zero in Eqs. (6.76):

$$x_{ss} = k_o/\beta, \quad y_{ss} = \beta\gamma/k_o. \quad (6.77)$$

Oscillatory behavior depends on the eigenvalues λ of the characteristic equation, $\det(J - \lambda I) = 0$, where J is the Jacobian matrix of the system at (x_{ss}, y_{ss}). More specifically, the system will be unstable if the real part of λ, $\text{Re}(\lambda)$, is positive. The Jacobian matrix is given by:

$$J = \begin{bmatrix} \frac{\partial \dot{x}}{\partial x} & \frac{\partial \dot{x}}{\partial y} \\ \frac{\partial \dot{y}}{\partial x} & \frac{\partial \dot{y}}{\partial y} \end{bmatrix}_{x_{ss}, y_{ss}} = \begin{bmatrix} -\beta - \gamma + 2xy & x^2 \\ \gamma - 2xy & -x^2 \end{bmatrix}_{x_{ss}, y_{ss}}, \quad (6.78)$$

$$J = \begin{bmatrix} -\beta + \gamma & (k_0/\beta)^2 \\ -\gamma & -(k_0/\beta)^2 \end{bmatrix}. \quad (6.79)$$

The matrix $(J - \lambda I)$ is then given by:

$$J - \lambda I = \begin{bmatrix} -\beta + \gamma - \lambda & (k_0/\beta)^2 \\ -\gamma & -(k_0/\beta)^2 - \lambda \end{bmatrix}. \quad (6.80)$$

We can now compute the characteristic equation:

$$\begin{aligned} \det(J - \lambda I) &= (-\beta + \gamma - \lambda)(-(k_0/\beta)^2 - \lambda) - \left(k_0/\beta\right)^2(-\gamma) \\ &= \lambda^2 - \left(\gamma - \beta - (k_0/\beta)^2\right)\lambda + \gamma\left(k_0/\beta\right)^2. \end{aligned} \quad (6.81)$$

Let $b \equiv \gamma - \beta - (k_0/\beta)^2$, $c \equiv \gamma(k_0/\beta)^2$. Equation (6.81) is rewritten as:

$$\det(J - \lambda I) = \lambda^2 - b\lambda + c. \quad (6.82)$$

The solutions for λ are:

$$\lambda = \frac{b \pm \sqrt{b^2 - 4c}}{2}. \quad (6.83)$$

Since $c > 0$, we must consider the sign of the discriminant $(b^2 - 4c)$ to determine $\text{Re}(\lambda)$.

- If $b^2 > 4c$, then λ is real and both solutions have the same sign as b. Hence, the system is stable if $b < 0$, and unstable if $b > 0$.
- If $b^2 < 4c$, the solutions of the characteristic equations are a pair of complex conjugates, whose real part equals b. Here again, the system is stable if $b < 0$, and unstable if $b > 0$.

The boundary of stability in the three-dimensional parameter space can thus be calculated by setting $b = 0$. To illustrate the behavior of this system, we examine two specific cases: we set $\beta = k_o = 1$ in both cases, and $\gamma = 1$ in case A, $\gamma = 3$ in case B. Thus, $b = -1 < 0$ in case A, and $b = +1 > 0$ in case B. The temporal variations of x and y for both scenarios are shown in Fig. 6.12. As expected, Ca^{2+}

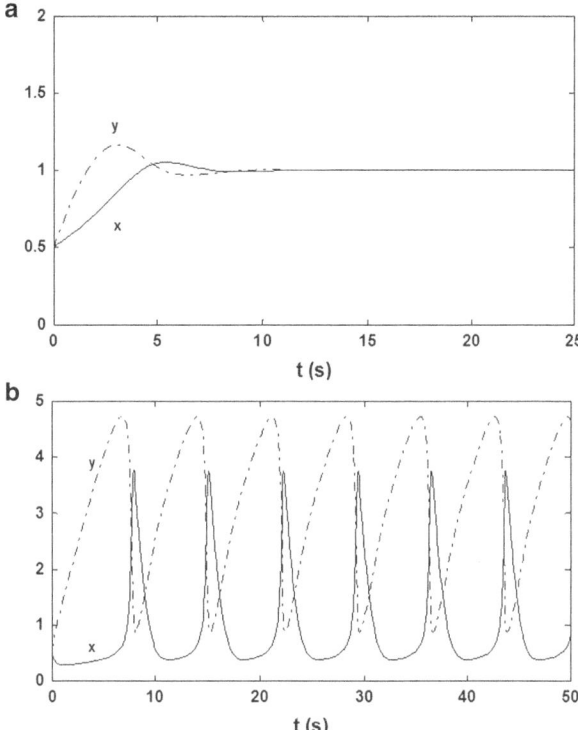

Fig. 6.12 Ca^{2+} concentrations in the cytosol (x) and the SR (y), with $x(t=0) = y(t=0) = 0.5$. (Panel **a**, case A), $\beta = k_o = \gamma = 1$. (Panel **b**, case B), $\beta = k_o = 1$ and $\gamma = 3$

concentrations in the cytosol and the SR oscillate in case B, but not in case A. Remember that γ characterizes the SERCA pump rate. These results thus indicate that the rate at which Ca^{2+} is pumped into the SR must be sufficiently high to raise the SR concentration of Ca^{2+} (i.e., the variable y) above the threshold beyond which it induces the rapid release of Ca^{2+} into the cytosol. As shown in Fig. 6.12, this rapid release is accompanied by a partial emptying of SR Ca^{2+} stores, and these are subsequently refilled via SERCA pumps. As a result, repetitive Ca^{2+} spikes occur in the cytosol and SR.

6.5 Kinetic Model for Cellular Contraction

Once the intracellular concentrations of Ca^{2+} and related species are known, the effects of calcium (more specifically, the MLCK·CaM·Ca_4 complex) on cellular machinery can be determined.

The elastic and contractile properties of muscle are imparted by myosin light chains (MLC). Myosins are ATP-dependent motor proteins that attach to actin filaments to form cross-bridges. The contraction process involves several steps,

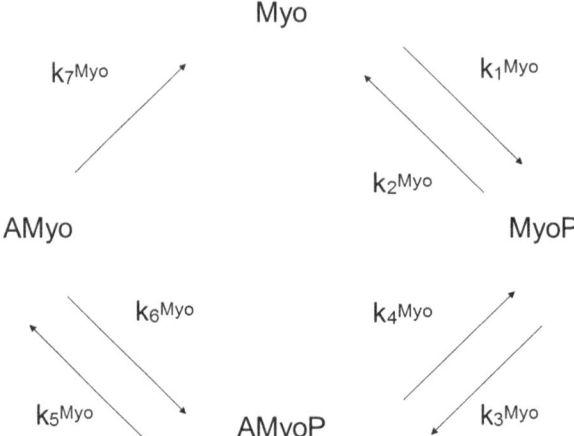

Fig. 6.13 Kinetic model of myosin light chain phosphorylation and cross-bridge formation, adopted from the model of Hai and Murphy (1988). Four species are considered: free cross-bridges (Myo), phosphorylated cross-bridges (MyoP), attached phosphorylated, cycling cross-bridges (AMyoP), and attached dephosphorylated, non-cycling cross-bridges (AMyo). The rate constants k_1^{Myo} and k_6^{Myo} depend on the fraction of fully activated MLCK. Note that the $AMyo \rightarrow Myo + A$ reaction is assumed to be irreversible, that is, cross-bridges cannot attach to actin filaments unless they are first phosphorylated

known as myosin-actin cycling: myosin moves forward, attaches to the binding sites on actin, contracts, detaches from actin, and moves forward anew to initiate a new cycle. Note that only phosphorylated cross-bridges can bind to actin, and that ATP hydrolysis is required to dissociate the myosin-actin complex.

During sustained contractions, calcium levels begin to drop, leading to inactivation of MLCK and reducing the number of phosphorylated cross-bridges. Yet, in smooth muscle, some dephosphorylated cross-bridges remain latched together, and continue to sustain contraction without consuming ATP. This so-called latch mechanism allows the smooth muscle cell to expand less energy.

Hai and Murphy (1988) proposed a simple kinetic model for cross-bridge interactions in smooth muscle that accounts for the latch mechanism. Their model considers four myosin light chain species: free cross-bridges (Myo), phosphorylated cross-bridges (MyoP), attached phosphorylated, cycling cross-bridges (AMyoP), and attached dephosphorylated, non-cycling cross-bridges (AMyo). The corresponding 4-state kinetic model is illustrated in Fig. 6.13.

The concentration of the 4 MLC species is determined by solving the following set of equations:

$$\frac{dC_{Myo}^{cyt}}{dt} = -k_1^{Myo} C_{Myo}^{cyt} + k_2^{Myo} C_{MyoP}^{cyt} + k_7^{Myo} C_{AMyo}^{cyt}, \qquad (6.84)$$

6.5 Kinetic Model for Cellular Contraction

$$\frac{dC_{MyoP}^{cyt}}{dt} = +k_1^{Myo} C_{Myo}^{cyt} - k_2^{Myo} C_{MyoP}^{cyt} - k_3^{Myo} C_{MyoP}^{cyt} + k_4^{Myo} C_{AMyoP}^{cyt}, \quad (6.85)$$

$$\frac{dC_{AMyoP}^{cyt}}{dt} = +k_3^{Myo} C_{MyoP}^{cyt} - k_4^{Myo} C_{AMyoP}^{cyt} - k_5^{Myo} C_{AMyoP}^{cyt} + k_6^{Myo} C_{AMyo}^{cyt}, \quad (6.86)$$

$$C_{Myo}^{cyt} + C_{MyoP}^{cyt} + C_{AMyoP}^{cyt} + C_{AMyo}^{cyt} = C_{Myo,tot}^{cyt}. \quad (6.87)$$

where $C_{Myo,tot}^{cyt}$ is the total cytosolic concentration of MLC. The rate constants k_1^{Myo} and k_6^{Myo} represent the activity of MLCK, and are taken to be proportional to the concentration of the fully activated form of the enzyme, namely the MLCK·CaM·Ca$_4$ complex. The rate constants k_2^{Myo} and k_5^{Myo} represent the activity of MLCP and are taken to be constant; k_3^{Myo}, k_4^{Myo}, and k_7^{Myo} are also fixed.

Once the proportion of attached cross-bridges is determined, several approaches can be used to estimate the strength of the contractile force. The simplest way is to employ an empirical relationship. Lee et al. (1997) correlated the percentage of phosphorylated myosin (i.e., $P_{Myo} = (C_{MyoP}^{cyt} + C_{AMyoP}^{cyt})/C_{Myo,tot}^{cyt} \times 100\%$) with the contractile force (F_{cont}) in arterial smooth muscle, using a third-degree polynomial:

$$F_{cont} = 0.56 - 0.69 P_{Myo} + 0.046 \left(P_{Myo}\right)^2 - 0.00029 \left(P_{Myo}\right)^3, \quad (6.88)$$

where F_{cont} is expressed relative to the maximum force, as measured by a force transducer. Equation (6.88) can serve to assess the extent to which the contractile force varies following changes in cytosolic myosin light chain levels.

To illustrate these concepts, let us examine the effects of a step increase in C_{Ca}^{cyt} on the relative contractile force: C_{Ca}^{cyt} is set to 120 nM at rest, and is increased to 300 nM at t = 100 s. To determine F_{cont}, we first calculate the concentration of the MLCK·CaM·Ca$_4$ complex (i.e., MLCK*) using Eq. (6.55). The kinetic rates k_1^{Myo} and k_6^{Myo} are then calculated assuming that:

$$k_1^{Myo} = k_6^{Myo} = \kappa\, C_{MLCK*}^{cyt}, \quad (6.89)$$

where κ is a constant (set to 4×10^{-6} M$^{-1} \cdot$s^{-1}). The concentrations of the 4 MLC species are subsequently obtained by integrating the set of differential-algebraic Eqs. (6.84), (6.85), (6.86) and (6.87), and the force F_{cont} is computed using Eq. (6.88). Results are displayed in Fig. 6.14. Following the step increase in C_{Ca}^{cyt}, the concentration of MLCK* increases by a factor of 35, and so do k_1^{Myo} and k_6^{Myo}. The fraction of phosphorylated myosin thus rises from 2 to 42 %, and the relative force reaches 31 %.

Implicit in this approach for calculating F_{cont} is the assumption that C_{Ca}^{cyt}-dependent cross-bridge phosphorylation by MLCK is the main determinant of the contractile force. We should nevertheless acknowledge that VSMC contraction is also regulated by other mechanisms, such as PKC-dependent signaling pathways (Christova et al. 1997).

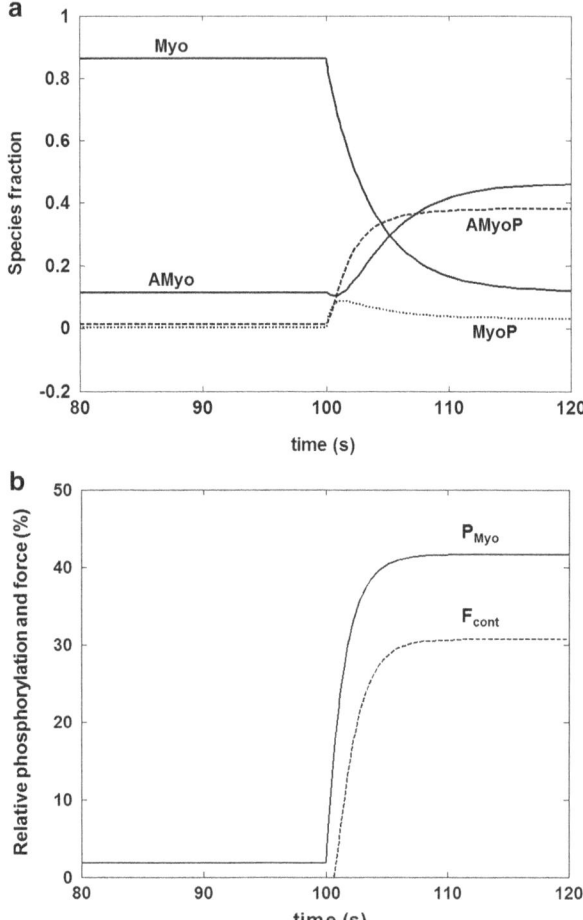

Fig. 6.14 Changes in the relative abundance of myosin species (panel **a**), the fraction of phosphorylated myosin, and the relative contractile force (panel **b**), following a step increase in C_{Ca}^{cyt} from 120 to 300 nM at t = 100 s. Parameter values:
$K_1 = 10^{-5}$ M,
$K_2 = 10^{-9}$ M,
$C_{CaM,tot}^{cyt} = 10^{-5}$ M,
$C_{MLCK,tot}^{cyt} = 10^{-6}$ M,
$k_2^{Myo} = k_5^{Myo} = 0.4$ s^{-1},
$k_3^{Myo} = 1.8$ s^{-1},
$k_4^{Myo} = 0.1$ s^{-1}, and
$k_7^{Myo} = 0.045$ s^{-1}

6.6 Problems

Problem 6.1. Derive Equation (6.18) for the flux of ions S when both concentration and electrical gradients are present.

Problem 6.2. Consider an ion channel, the open fraction of which obeys Eqs. (6.25) and (6.26), with $k_o = a = 1$. The transmembrane potential is initially maintained at -60 mV. At time t = 0, V_m is suddenly increased to $+60$ mV for a duration of 5 τ, after which it returns to its initial value.

(a) Plot the time course of the fraction of open channels n from 0 to 10 τ.
(b) Assume now that the channel consists of four identical subunits, each of which has a probability n of being in the open configuration. The probability that the full channel is open is n^4. Compare the time courses of n and n^4, and comment.

Problem 6.3. Derive Equation (6.38). NCX is at equilibrium when the Gibbs free energy of the transport process is zero, i.e., when the internal-to-external electrochemical potential difference of 1 Ca^{2+} ion equals that of 3 Na^{2+} ions.

Problem 6.4. Derive Equations (6.70), (6.71) and (6.72) from the RyR model developed by Keizer and Levine (1996). The schematic representation of the 4 RyR states is shown in Fig. 6.10. Assume that steps a and b are much faster than step c. Note that $K_a^4 \equiv k_a^-/k_a^+$, $K_b^3 \equiv k_b^-/k_b^+$, $K_c \equiv k_c^-/k_c^+$.

Problem 6.5. Conduct a stability analysis of a simplified model of Ca^{2+} dynamics. Assume that the cytosolic and SR concentration of Ca^{2+} obey Eq. (6.75), with $f(x) = \frac{x^n}{x^n + a^n}$.

(a) Derive the corresponding characteristic equation.
(b) Let $n = 4$, $\beta = 1$, $\gamma = 1$, $k_s = 0.05$, and $k_o = 1$. Determine the values of the parameter a ($0 \le a \le 10$) for which the steady state is unstable.

References

Blaustein, M.P., Zhang, J., et al.: How does salt retention raise blood pressure? Am. J. Physiol. Regul. Integr. Comp. Physiol. **290**(3), R514–R523 (2006)
Christova, T., Duridanova, D., et al.: Protein kinase C and smooth muscle contraction. Biomed. Rev. **8**, 87–100 (1997)
De Young, G., Keizer, J.: A single-pool inositol 1,4,5-trisphosphate-receptor-based model for agonist-stimulated oscillations in Ca2+ concentrations. Proc. Natl. Acad. Sci. U. S. A. **89**, 9895–9899 (1992)
DiFrancesco, D., Noble, D.: A model of cardiac electrical activity incorporating ionic pumps and concentration changes. Philos. Trans. R. Soc. Lond. B. Biol. Sci. **307**, 353–398 (1985)
Edwards, A., Pallone, T.L.: Modification of cytosolic calcium signaling by subplasmalemmal microdomains. Am. J. Physiol. Renal Physiol. **292**(6), F1827–F1845 (2007)
Fajmut, A., Brumen, M., et al.: Theoretical model of the interactions between Ca2+, calmodulin and myosin light chain kinase. FEBS Lett. **579**(20), 4361–4366 (2005)
Goldbeter, A., Dupont, G., Berridge M.J.: Minimal model for signal-induced Ca^{2+} oscillations and for their frequency encoding through protein phosphorylation. Proc. Natl. Acad. Sci. U.S.A. **87**, 1461–1465 (1990)
Hai, C.-M., Murphy, R.A.: Regulation of shortening velocity by cross-bridge phosphorylation in smooth muscle. Am. J. Physiol. Cell Physiol. **255**, C86–C94 (1988)
Higgins, E.R., Cannell, M.B., et al.: A buffering SERCA pump in models of calcium dynamics. Biophys. J. **91**(1), 151–163 (2006)
Hille, B.: Ion channels of excitable membranes. Sinauer Associates, Sunderland (2001)
Keener, J., Sneyd, J.: Mathematical physiology. Springer, New York (1998)
Keizer, J., Levine, L.: Ryanodine receptor adaptation and Ca2+(−)induced Ca2+ release-dependent Ca2+ oscillations. Biophys. J. **71**(6), 3477–3487 (1996)

Lee, M.R., Li, L., et al.: Cyclic GMP Causes Ca2+ Desensitization in Vascular Smooth Muscle by Activating the Myosin Light Chain Phosphatase. J. Biol. Chem. **272**(8), 5063–5068 (1997)

Moore, E.D.W., Etter, E.F., et al.: Coupling of the Na+/Ca2+ exchanger, Na+/K+ pump and sarcoplasmic reticulum in smooth muscle. Nature **365**, 657–660 (1993)

Mullins, L.J.: A mechanism for Na/Ca transport. J. Gen. Physiol. **70**(6), 681–695 (1977)

Sneyd, J., Falcke, M.: Models of the inositol trisphosphate receptor. Prog. Biophys. Mol. Biol. **89**, 207–245 (2005)

Sneyd, J., Tsaneva-Atanasova, K., et al.: A model of calcium waves in pancreatic and parotid acinar cells. Biophys. J. **85**, 1392–1405 (2003)

Somogyi, R., Stucki, J.W.: Hormone-induced calcium oscillations in liver cells can be explained by a simple one pool model. J. Biol. Chem. **266**, 11068–11077 (1991)

Spiro, P.A., Othmer, H.G.: The effect of heterogeneously-distributed RyR channels on calcium dynamics in cardiac myocytes. Bull. Math. Biol. **61**, 651–681 (1999)

Weber, C.R., Ginsburg, K.S., et al.: Allosteric regulation of Na/Ca exchange current by cytosolic Ca in intact cardiac myocytes. J. Gen. Physiol. **117**(2), 119–132 (2001)

Yano, K., Petersen, O.H., et al.: Dual sensitivity of sarcoplasmic/endoplasmic Ca2+−ATPase to cytosolic and endoplasmic reticulum Ca2+ as a mechanism of modulating cytosolic Ca2+ oscillations. Biochem. J. **383**, 353–360 (2004)

Chapter 7
Vasomotion and Myogenic Response of the Afferent Arteriole

Abstract In this chapter we introduce techniques for modeling the vasomotion and myogenic response of the afferent arteriole, which supplies blood to the nephron. We develop a mathematical model that simulates the spontaneous rhythmic activities exhibited by the renal afferent arteriole. That model consists of a system of coupled nonlinear ODEs, and is based on the well-known Morris-Lecar model. The afferent arteriole responds to luminal pressure elevation with constriction, and to pressure reduction with dilation. That response, which is called the myogenic response, can be modeled by incorporating into the above model a hypothesis that allows changes in hydrostatic pressure to cause appropriate changes in intracellular calcium concentration, thereby inducing vasoconstriction or vasodilation.

7.1 The Afferent Arteriole

Using the tools that we have learned in the preceding chapter, we will study the electrophysiology of a specific type of vascular smooth muscle cells in the kidney: the afferent arteriole. The afferent arterioles are a group of blood vessels that supply blood to the nephrons. The afferent arterioles arise from the renal artery, and later branch into glomerular capillaries. A portion of the blood delivered by the afferent arteriole is filtered through the glomerulus into the nephron. The amount of blood that enters the nephron as filtrate depends, in part, on the afferent arteriolar pressure, and glomerular filtration rate (GFR) impacts tubular reabsorption and other renal functions. Indeed, normal renal functions require GFR to stay within a narrow window despite changes in arterial pressure. That goal is accomplished by autoregulatory mechanisms, in which the afferent arteriole participates via vasodilation or vasoconstriction in response to several signals, including blood flow pressure and tubuloglomerular signal from the macula densa.

The renal afferent arteriole, like most other small arteries and arterioles, exhibits spontaneous rhythmic activity, a.k.a. vasomotion. Vasomotion is *spontaneous* in the sense that vascular tone oscillates independently of heart beat, innervation, or respiration. The driving stimulus of vasomotion is believed to be the oscillations of the same frequency intrinsically appearing on the electrical activity of the smooth muscle cells that form part of the arteriolar walls.

Vascular smooth muscle responds to increased stretch with active force development, a phenomenon termed the *myogenic response*. This response enables arterial blood vessels to constrict as intraluminal pressure increases under physiological conditions. In the arteriolar system, myogenic responses are thought to be important for local autoregulation of blood flow and regulation of capillary pressure. Note that another type of renal vascular smooth muscle cells, the pericytes, do not exhibit the myogenic response. The myogenic response is blocked by the same blockers (such as Ca^{2+} and K^+ membrane channels blockers) that eliminate the spontaneous vasomotion, which is believed to be functionally related.

An afferent arteriole is composed of an interior layer of endothelial cells that come in direct contact with the blood stream. The endothelium is wrapped around by a layer of smooth muscle cells. Vascular smooth muscle cells are responsible for vasomotion and for myogenic tone in vascular beds. In this chapter, we present a mathematical model that describes the ionic transport and membrane potential of an afferent arteriole smooth muscle cell, and we introduce the mathematical tools that assist in the analysis of that model.

7.2 Nonlinear ODEs

Let's first study a simple model that describes the changes in membrane potential as a function of a voltage-gated calcium channel. Despite its relative simplicity, the analysis of this model is not trivial, in large part owing to its nonlinearity. If all differential equations were linear, the mathematician's life would be much easier but also less interesting. Indeed, it is the nonlinearities inherent in many model equations that describe physical and biological systems that give rise to a broad range of interesting behaviors including oscillations and chaos.

We will learn how to compute the solution of a nonlinear ODE and analyze its behaviors by studying an equation that describes the electric potential difference (v) across a membrane:

$$C\frac{dv}{dt} = -g_L(v - v_L) - g_{Ca}m_\infty(v)(v - v_{Ca}) + I. \qquad (7.1)$$

The first term on the right-hand side is the leak current, where v_L denotes the associated reversal potential. The leak current was discussed in Eq. (6.48). The second term is the calcium current, where g_{Ca} is the maximum whole-cell membrane conductance for the calcium current. This calcium current arises from the voltage-operated calcium channels discussed in Chap. 6. In that chapter, the L-type currents are given by a system of ODEs (6.45)–(6.47). Here we assume that the calcium channels operate at a much faster time-scale than the membrane voltage, and that

7.2 Nonlinear ODEs

Table 7.1 Model parameters used in the bifurcation study. Units are included but are omitted elsewhere in the chapter

v_L	-60 mV
v_{Ca}	120 mV
g_L	2 nS
g_{Ca}	4 nS
C	20 pF
v_1	-1.2 mV
v_2	18 mV

the ODEs (6.46) and (6.47) are at steady state, so that we only need to deal with one ODE. With this assumption, one can see that m_∞, which represents the fraction of open calcium channels at steady state, corresponds to the product $d_L^\infty f_L^\infty$, by comparing the term $g_{Ca} m_\infty(v)(v_\infty - v_{Ca})$ with Eq. (6.45). For simplicity we ignore inactivation here, so that in fact m_∞ corresponds to d_L^∞ only. Based on experimental data, m_∞ is described as a function of membrane potential v

$$m_\infty(v) = 0.5\left(1 + \tanh\left(\frac{v - v_1}{v_2}\right)\right), \tag{7.2}$$

where v_1 is the voltage at which half of the channels are open, and v_2 determines the spread of the distribution. For very negative v, $\tanh((v - v_1)/v_2) \to -1$ and $m_\infty \to 0$, which implies that almost all calcium channels are closed. For large (more positive) v, $\tanh((v - v_1)/v_2) \to 1$ and $m_\infty \to 1$, which implies that most calcium channels are now open.

When we say we study the nonlinear dynamics of a system, we usually mean that we want to understand how that system's behaviors depend on parameters. For now we will fix all but one of the parameters in the system (7.1). The fixed parameter values are shown in Table 7.1. In a biological membrane, the current I represents all other currents, i.e., besides leak currents and the calcium current through voltage-activated channels. Thus, I includes potassium currents (which are among the largest currents in vascular smooth muscle cells) but also other ionic (e.g., sodium and chloride) currents, and potentially an input current (as in the Morris-Lecar model below, as in patch-clamp studies). We will let the current I vary and study how the system's steady-state solution v changes.

Suppose we start with a polarizing current of $I = -90$, and then slowly increase I. We will investigate how the steady-state membrane potential v changes. By solving Eq. (7.1) with the left-hand-side set to 0, we find that the steady-state v increases, along the dashed curve segment in Fig. 7.1. All goes smoothly, until we hit $I = 36.8$ (marked by the asterisk in Fig. 7.1). Suddenly, the potential v jumps from -32 to $+64$ mV, and then increases along the dashed-dotted curve segment, as I further increases.

Alternatively, if we start with a polarizing current of $I = 80$, and slowly decrease I, then v decreases along the dashed-dotted curve segment, until we cross $I = -201.5$ (marked by the square), at which point the potential drops precipitously.

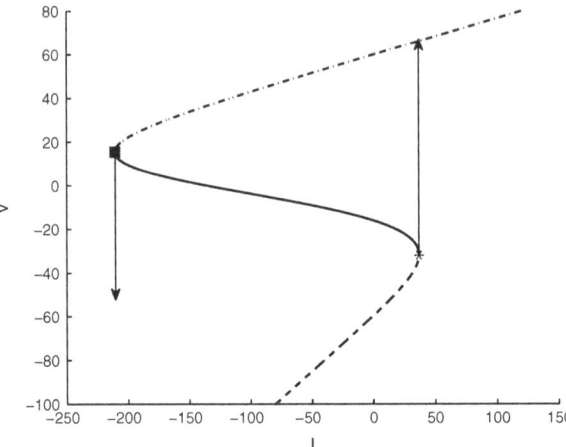

Fig. 7.1 Steady-state solution curve of Eq. (7.1)

To understand why the solution jumps abruptly when we cross $I = 36.8$ and $I = -201.5$, we show all the steady-state solutions in Fig. 7.1. For $-201.5 < I < 36.8$, there are three steady states. Two of these are stable solutions (the dashed-dotted and dashed curves); the one in-between (the solid curve) is an unstable steady state. (You might wonder how we computed the unstable steady-state solution. Instead of specifying a value for I and solving for the steady-state potential v, we set a value for v and then solved for I.)

The two points, marked by an asterisk and a square, across which the potential jumps, are called saddle-nodes bifurcations. They represent a point in parameter space where a pair of solutions come together to form one solution. It is noteworthy that the steady-state potential corresponding to some current $-201.5 < I < 36.8$ depends on its past environment. This phenomenon, which is known as hysteresis, arises from the appearance of two stable steady states. This hysteresis in the I–V curve can give rise to oscillatory behavior.

7.3 The Morris-Lecar Model

The preceding model explicitly tracks only the calcium channel. Since potassium currents are known to play a role in the spontaneous vasomotion of the afferent arteriole, we will explicitly add a voltage-gated potassium channel. That results in a system that is represented by the Morris-Lecar model.

The Morris-Lecar model grew out of an experimental study of the excitability of the giant muscle fiber of the huge Pacific barnacle, *balanus nubilis* (named by Charles Darwin, who probably meant to call it *balanus nobilis*). Synaptic depolarizations of these muscle cells lead to the opening of Ca^{2+} channels, allowing

7.3 The Morris-Lecar Model

external Ca^{2+} ions to enter deep into the cell interior to activate muscle contraction. The Morris-Lecar model describes this membrane with two conductances, Ca^{2+} and K^+, the interplay of which yields qualitative phase portrait changes with small changes in experimental parameters, such as the relative densities of Ca^{2+} and K^+ channels or the relative relaxation times of the conducting systems. This simple model was capable of simulating the entire panoply of (two-dimensional) oscillation phenomena that had been observed experimentally. Parameter maps in phase-space can be drawn to identify and classify the parametric regions having different types of stability.

7.3.1 Model Equations

Morris and Lecar's eponymous two-dimensional equations appeared in the middle of a longish paper. The real barnacle fiber exhibited many phenomena that required a third dimension, such as bursting oscillations and variable-duration plateaus, which terminated abruptly. Nonetheless, owing to the simplicity of the 2-D model, and the joys of studying the phase plane, the Morris-Lecar equations seemed to have taken on a life of their own as a prototypical model for excitability in a wide variety of systems.

The model equations are

$$C\frac{dv}{dt} = -g_L(v - v_L) - g_{Ca}m_\infty(v)(v - v_{Ca}) - g_K n(v - v_K) + I, \qquad (7.3)$$

$$\frac{dn}{dt} = \phi_n \cosh\left(\frac{v - v_3}{2v_4}\right)(n_\infty(v) - n). \qquad (7.4)$$

The new term $-g_K n(v - v_K)$ in Eq. (7.3) represents the transmembrane potassium current induced by the opening of potassium channels; n denotes the fraction of open K^+ channels. In Eq. (7.4), n_∞ denotes the fraction of open K^+ channels at steady state; this fraction depends on the membrane potential v:

$$n_\infty(v) = 0.5\left(1 + \tanh\left(\frac{v - v_3}{v_4}\right)\right), \qquad (7.5)$$

which has a form similar to the equilibrium distribution of open Ca^{2+} channel states in Eq. (7.2). The potential v_3 determines the voltage at which half of the potassium channels are open, and v_4 characterizes the spread of the distribution of n_∞.

Note also that both the potassium current (which we denote $I_K = -g_K n(v - v_K)$) and the calcium current (denoted $I_{Ca} = -g_{Ca}m_\infty(v)(v - v_{Ca})$) depend on the membrane potential v, and both currents in turn change the membrane potential. Parameters for this model are given in Tables 7.1 and 7.2. Note that we assume that the Nernst potentials (v_{Ca} and v_K) are constant, whereas in fact they vary with concentrations, which themselves vary with membrane potential.

Table 7.2 Additional parameters needed for the Morris-Lecar model

v_K	−85
g_K	8
v_3	12
v_4	17
ϕ	0.0667

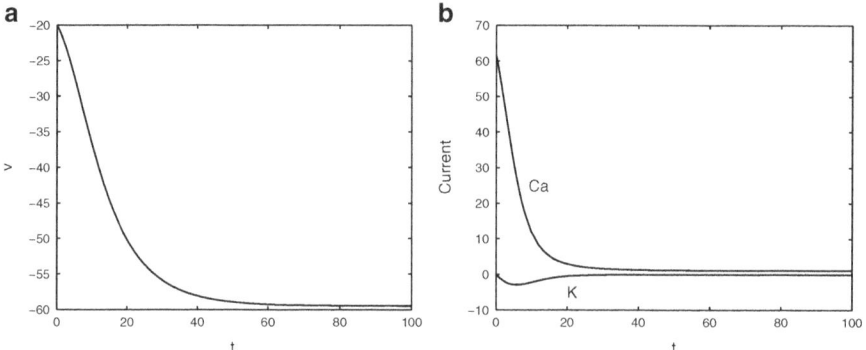

Fig. 7.2 Solution to the Morris Lecar model, with v initialized to -20 mV. (**a**) Voltage; (**b**) K^+ and Ca^{2+} currents, The voltage and current both decay to zero

7.3.2 Simulations, Nullclines

To understand the interactions between I_K, I_{Ca}, and v, we numerically integrated the ODEs Eqs. (7.3) and (7.4). The input current I was set to 0, membrane potential v was initialized to -20 mM, and n was initialized to 0. We plot v, and the currents I_K and I_{Ca} as functions of time in Fig. 7.2. With these parameters and these initial conditions, the voltage and currents decay to rest.

Let's try a different initial condition, with $v(0) = -10$ mV. Now the system behaves very differently: the voltage rises substantially before decaying to rest (see Fig. 7.3a). This behavior is qualitatively different from what we previously got using $v(0) = -20$ mV, so what is going on? To gain insight, we consider the currents, which are shown in Fig. 7.3b. The magnitude of both currents increases before decaying to rest. As you can see, an interesting feature of this system is that the two currents go in opposite directions: I_K is outward-directed thus hyperpolarizes the cell, whereas I_{Ca} is inward-directed and depolarizes the cell. Because the calcium channels are voltage-gated, once the voltage crosses a threshold there is a large inward-directed calcium current. (Thus this is an example of an excitable cell.) The current causes the voltage to increase and eventually the current slows down and reaches its peak. Then the large outward-directed potassium current comes into play and repolarizes the cell.

7.3 The Morris-Lecar Model

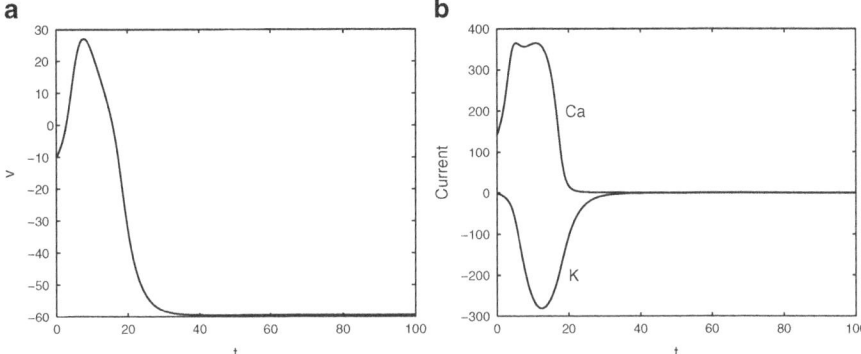

Fig. 7.3 Solution to the Morris Lecar model, with v initialized to -10 mV. (**a**) voltage; (**b**) K$^+$ and Ca^{2+} currents. The solution exhibits an initial bump (or crest) before decaying to rest

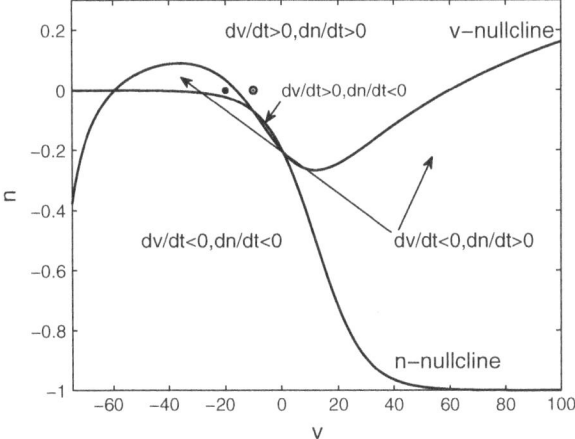

Fig. 7.4 The v- and n-nullclines divide the v-n space into regions where v and n are increasing or decreasing

So what causes this threshold behavior for excitable cells? Let's study the nullclines of the system, which are curves where $dv/dt = 0$ and $dn/dt = 0$. The nullclines are graphed in Fig. 7.4. The first thing to note is that the two nullclines intercept at three equilibrium points. If the system is initialized at those v and n values, then the system will remain at equilibrium.

The two nullclines divide the v–n space into several regions, in which v and n are increasing or decreasing. These regions are labeled in Fig. 7.4. The two previous simulations that produce qualitatively different behaviors correspond to initial v and n values that lie in different regions. With $v(0) = -20$ mV and $n(0) = 0$ (indicated by the closed circle in Fig. 7.4), the system lies in the region where $dv/dt < 0$ and $dn/dt > 0$, so the voltage decays to rest (see Fig. 7.2a), whereas the gating variable

n, after an initial increase, also decays to 0. With $v(0) = -10$ mV (indicated by the open circle in Fig. 7.4), however, the system lies in the region where $dv/dt > 0$ and $dn/dt > 0$, so the voltage rises to a peak before decaying to rest (see Fig. 7.3a).

It is noteworthy that since neither of these nullclines is linear, the two curves can intersect in a variety of ways as the conductance parameters are varied. The intersections of the v- and n-nullclines, of course, give the singular points for each different parameter set. As an example, the v-nullcline can be altered systematically by taking a progression of values for g_{Ca}. For the high and low values of g_{Ca}, the nullclines intersect once. For a narrow intermediate range of g_{Ca}, the nullclines can intertwine and intersect at three points. Our choice of g_{Ca} falls into this range, just barely (note the small region where $d/dt > 0$ and $dn/dt < 0$ in Fig. 7.4). We will study the nullclines arising from different values of g_{Ca}, and also g_K, in Problem 7.2(c).

7.4 Spontaneous Vasomotion

So far we have studied the dynamic behaviors of generic ODE models. The rest of this chapter will focus on the afferent arteriole. Like a number of other blood vessels, the afferent arteriole engages in spontaneous vasomotion, where the vascular smooth muscles exhibit periodic and spontaneous constriction and dilation. The phenomenon of vasomotion was first reported more than 150 years ago, when T. Wharton Jones described rhythmic contractility in the veins of bat wing. Since then, vasomotion has been reported in many different vascular beds, from many different species, both in vivo and in vitro. The observation of vasomotion in vitro suggests that the initiating mechanism is inherent to the vascular wall (although it by no means precludes its modulation through extravascular mechanisms including neural influences).

The physiological role of vasomotion is still controversial. Several hypotheses have been advanced. Increased flow is one possibility: a vessel with an oscillating diameter may conduct more flow than a vessel with a static diameter. Vasomotion could also be a mechanism to increase the reactivity of a blood vessel by avoiding the "latch state," which is a low ATP cycling state of prolonged force generation common in vascular smooth muscle.

We will use the Morris-Lecar model to illustrate how the interaction of Ca^{2+} fluxes, which are mediated by voltage-gated channels, and K^+ fluxes, mediated by voltage- and calcium-gated channels, gives rise to periodicity in the transport of the two ions. This results in a time-periodic cytosolic calcium concentration, myosin light chain phosphorylation, and crossbridges formation with the attending muscle stress. And spontaneous vasomotion results. We will take the Morris-Lecar equations (7.3) and (7.4) and set the external current I to 0. But now we assume that the potassium channel opening probability depends both on membrane voltage and free cytosolic calcium concentration $[Ca^{2+}]$. Specifically, we modify the distribution of open potassium channels (Eq. 7.5) so that v_3, the voltage at which

7.4 Spontaneous Vasomotion

Table 7.3 Arteriolar membrane parameters for vasomotion model in Sect. 7.4

Parameter	Value	Unit
v_1	−22.5	mV
v_2	25.0	mV
v_4	14.5	mV
v_5	8.00	mV
v_6	−15.0	mV
v_L	−70.0	mV
v_K	−95.0	mV
v_{Ca}	80.0	mV
Ca_3	400	nM
Ca_4	150	nM
ϕ_n	0.925	s^{-1}

half of the channels are open, is not fixed but instead depends on $[Ca^{2+}]$

$$v_3 = -\frac{v_5}{2}\tanh\left(\frac{[Ca^{2+}] - Ca_3}{Ca_4}\right) + v_6, \tag{7.6}$$

where v_5, v_6, Ca_3, and Ca_4 are constants.

The rate of change of $[Ca^{2+}]$ is given by

$$\frac{d[Ca^{2+}]}{dt} = \left(-\alpha g_{Ca} m_\infty (v - v_{Ca}) - k_{Ca}[Ca^{2+}]\right)\left(\frac{(K_d + [Ca^{2+}])^2}{(K_d + [Ca^{2+}])^2 + K_d B_T}\right). \tag{7.7}$$

The first term in the first pair of parentheses accounts for calcium flux through the open channels; the second term represents cytosolic calcium extrusion. The term in the second pair of parentheses arises from the distribution of cytosolic calcium between free and buffer-bound states. More specifically, $\alpha = 1/(z_{Ca}\beta V_{cell}F)$, $z_{Ca} = 2$ is the valence of the calcium ion, β is the fraction of cell volume occupied by the cytosol, V_{cell} is the cell volume, F is the Faraday constant, g_{Ca} is the maximum whole-cell membrane conductance for the calcium current, k_{Ca} is the first-order rate constant for cytosolic calcium extrusion, K_d is the ratio of the forward and backward reaction rates of the calcium-buffer system, and B_T is the total buffer concentration.

Model parameters, which are based on the afferent arteriole in the rat kidney, are given in Tables 7.3 and 7.4. With these parameters, the model predicts limit-cycle oscillations. Figure 7.5a depicts the oscillations of electrical current across the membrane carried by Ca^{2+} and by K^+ (i.e., $I_K = -g_K n(v - v_K)$ and $I_{Ca} = -g_{Ca} m_\infty(v)(v - v_{Ca})$) and the corresponding transmembrane potential v. The frequency of those oscillations is approximately 175 mHz, consistent with experimental measurements. The asynchrony between the ionic currents I_{Ca} and I_K gives rise to the oscillations of the membrane potential. The inward-directed

Table 7.4 Arteriolar cell parameters for vasomotion model in Sect. 7.4

Parameter	Value	Unit
g_L	7.85×10^{-14}	$C \cdot s^{-1} \cdot mV^{-1}$
g_K	3.14×10^{-13}	$C \cdot s^{-1} \cdot mV^{-1}$
g_{Ca}	1.57×10^{-13}	$C \cdot s^{-1} \cdot mV^{-1}$
C	7.85×10^{-14}	$C \cdot mV^{-1}$
K_d	10^3	nM
B_T	10^5	nM
α	8.00×10^{15}	$nM \cdot C^{-1}$
β	0.550	Dimensionless
k_{Ca}	190	s^{-1}

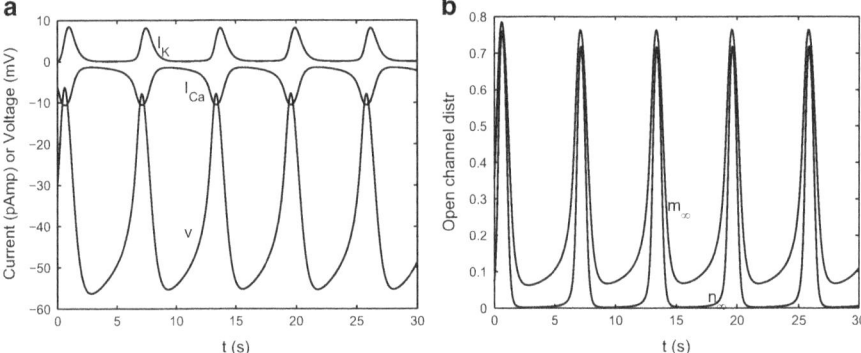

Fig. 7.5 Vasomotion model predicts oscillations in membrane potential v, potassium and calcium currents I_K and I_{Ca} (**a**) and in opening of potassium and calcium channels (**b**)

Ca^{2+} current depolarizes the cell, which results in an increase in the membrane potential. The outward-directed K^+ current then follows and repolarizes the cell, resulting in a decrease in the membrane potential. Because both the Ca^{2+}- and K^+-channels are voltage dependent, variations in membrane electric potential v affect those currents. As v decreases, the equilibrium distributions of open Ca^{2+} and K^+ channel states (denoted m_∞ and n_∞; see Eqs. 7.2 and 7.5) both decrease. Consequently, the magnitudes of currents I_{Ca} and I_K decrease, which results in periodic oscillations in the transmembrane potential and the ionic currents.

Oscillations in I_{Ca} result in oscillations in the intracellular free calcium concentration, $[Ca^{2+}]$; see Fig. 7.6. To relate oscillations in $[Ca^{2+}]$ to variations in vascular diameter, we adopt a simple model. Changes in $[Ca^{2+}]$ vary the phosphorylation rate of the 20 k-Da myosin light chains (MLC), which are involved in the formation of crossbridges between overlapping myosin and actin filaments. The formation of crossbridges develops stress. The deviation of vascular diameter from its equilibrium value also gives rise to an restoring force. We model the changes in vascular diameter as:

$$\frac{d^2 D}{dt^2} = -K([Ca^{2+}] - [\bar{Ca}^{2+}]) - T_0 * (D - \bar{D}). \tag{7.8}$$

7.5 Myogenic Response

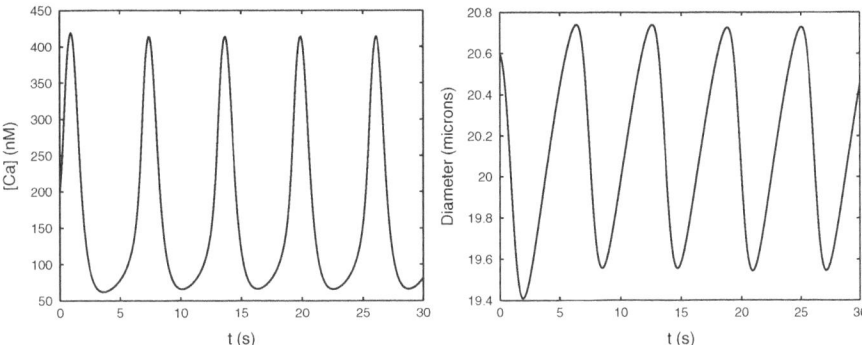

Fig. 7.6 Vasomotion model predicts oscillations in intracellular calcium concentration (*left*) and in vascular diameter (*right*)

The first term on the right hand side represents the contractile force arising from changes in $[Ca^{2+}]$; the second term represents the elastic force. We set both K and T_0 to 0.01, $[\bar{Ca}^{2+}]$ to 211 nM, and $\bar{D}$ to 20.6 μm. With these parameters, the model predicts an average diameter of $\sim$20 μm and an oscillation amplitude of $\sim$1 μm.

Equation (7.8) is a simplistic, empirical representation of the relation between vascular diameter and intracellular $[Ca^{2+}]$. In fact variations in $[Ca^{2+}]$ induce changes in vascular diameter through a number of steps, as discussed in Chap. 6: phosphorylation of myosin, formation of crossbridges, development of hoop stresses, etc. More complex models that represent these details can be found in Chen et al. (2011) and Gonzalez-Fernandez and Ermentrout (1994).

7.5 Myogenic Response

Unlike a passive tube, the afferent arterioles respond to transmural pressure elevations with constriction and to pressure reductions with dilation. This behavior, termed the myogenic response, is inherent to most smooth muscles and is independent of neural, metabolic, and hormonal influences. A typical example of myogenic behavior, in response to step changes in pressure, is illustrated in Fig. 7.7. After the pressure step-increase, the vessel exhibits an initial, passive distension, followed by vascular constriction. Upon release of the pressure step, the arteriole first transiently collapses, then dilates. The myogenic response is sometimes referred to as the *Bayliss effect*, since its discovery was credited to physiologist Sir William Bayliss in 1902.

The transduction mechanisms, by which an increase in pressure leads to vascular constriction, are not fully understood. Nonetheless, the current prevailing thought is that a myogenic constriction is initiated by the depolarization of the vascular smooth muscle cell (via mechanisms that remain controversial), which then activates Ca^{2+}

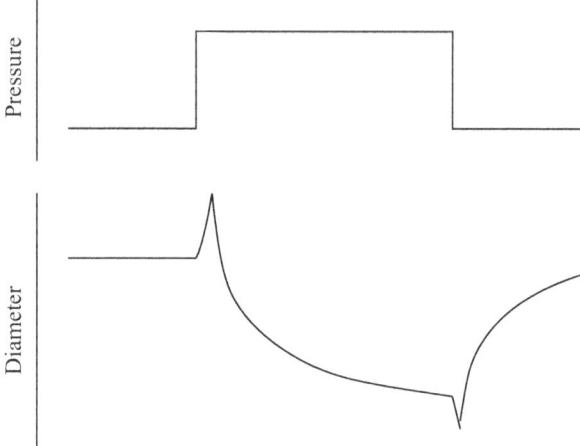

Fig. 7.7 Example of myogenic response in arterioles

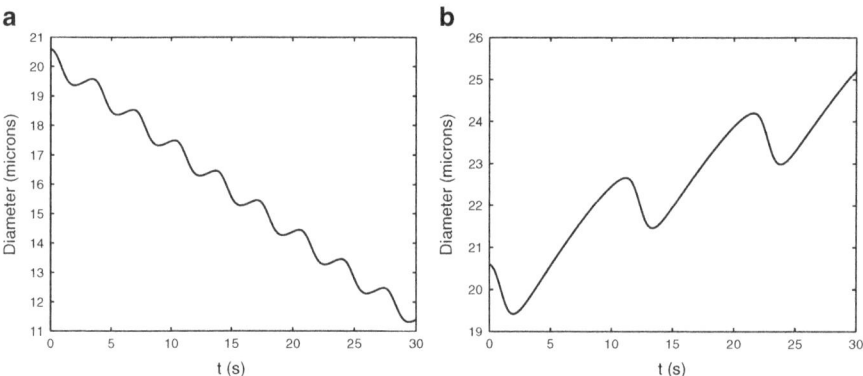

Fig. 7.8 (a) Vasoconstriction induced by $I = 10$. (b) Vasodilation induced by $I = -2$

entry through voltage-gated Ca^{2+} channels. A high cytosolic Ca^{2+} concentration facilitates the formation of crossbridges which causes smooth muscle constriction.

One hypothesis for the myogenic response mechanism is that changes in hydrostatic pressure induce changes in the activity of non-selective cation channels. The resulting changes in membrane potential then affect calcium influx through changes in the activity of the voltage-gated calcium channels. In this model, this hypothesis can be represented by treating I in Eq. (7.3) as a pressure-dependent current $I(p)$. When hydrostatic pressure exceeds its equilibrium value, then the opening of cation channels and the resulting cation influx can be represented by a positive current $I(p) > 0$, which gives rise to membrane depolarization. That results in the entry of Ca^{2+} via the voltage-gated Ca^{2+} channels and causes muscle constriction. Figure 7.8a shows vasoconstriction induced by setting $I = 10$.

Vascular diameter decreases from ~20 to ~11 μm over 30 s. Conversely, when pressure dips below its equilibrium value, we set $I(p) < 0$ which repolarizes the membrane and yields muscle dilation. Vasodilation induced by setting $I = -2$ is shown in Fig. 7.8b. Note that I also has an effect on the frequency of the oscillations.

7.6 Problems

Problem 7.1. Consider the Morris-Lecar model. Write a code to numerically integrate Eqs. (7.3) and (7.4). Make sure you can reproduce the results in Figs. 7.2 and 7.3. Then,

(a) Construct the phase-plane plot of the currents $I_{Ca} = -g_{Ca}m_\infty(v)(v - v_{Ca})$ and $I_K = -g_K n(v - v_K)$. Do this first with v initialized to -20 mV. Can you relate your phase-plane curve to the current curves in Fig. 7.2?
(b) Repeat (a) but with v initialized to -10 mV. Relate your result to Fig. 7.3.
(c) One can obtain oscillatory solution by applying a current. Set $I = 120$ and initialize v to -10 mV. Integrate Eqs. (7.3) and (7.4) again. You should see that the solution exhibits damped oscillations.

Problem 7.2. Let's continue studying the Morris-Lecar model.

(a) Set $I = 120$. Construct the nullclines in the v–n plane. How many times do the nullclines intercept? Locate the point $(v, n) = (-10, 0)$. Which region is it in? By considering the signs of dv/dt and dn/dt in that region, would you predict v to simply decay or exhibit an initial rise? Does you answer agree with your results in Problem 7.1(c)?
(b) What if v is initialized to -20 mV, with $I = 120$? Do you expect the system to decay as it does with $I = 0$?
(c) Besides varying I, we can change the number of times the v- and n-nullclines intercept by changing other parameters such as g_{Ca} or g_K, which affect the relative strength of the Ca^{2+} and K^+ currents. Try decreasing and increasing each of these parameters, and compute the resulting nullclines. Can you find values of g_{Ca} and g_K that yield only one intercept?

Problem 7.3. Extend your Morris-Lecar model to a model of the afferent arteriole smooth muscle cell by incorporating the dependence of the open K-channels distribution on free cytoplasmic $[Ca^{2+}]$ (i.e., Eq. 7.6), and adding the $[Ca^{2+}]$ and vascular diameter evolution equations (i.e., Eqs. 7.7 and 7.8). Verify that you can reproduce the limit-cycle oscillations shown in Figs. 7.5 and 7.6.

Another hypothesis for the myogenic mechanism is that the dependence of calcium-channel openings on voltage (i.e., Eq. 7.2) is shifted by the changes in transmural pressure, such that vessel diameter decreases with increasing pressure and vice versa. In other words, v_1, which is the voltage at which half of the channels are open, may vary as a function of pressure. Vary v_1 (say by ± 2 mV) and observe the effect on vascular diameter.

References

Chen, J., Sgouralis, I., Moore, L.C., Layton, H.E., Layton, A.T.: A mathematical model of the myogenic response to systolic pressure in the afferent arteriole. Am. J. Physiol. Ren. Physiol. **300**, F669–F681 (2011)

Gonzalez-Fernandez, J.M., Ermentrout, B.: On the origin and dynamics of the vasomotion of small arteries. Math. Biosci. **119**, 127–167 (1994)

Chapter 8
Transport Across Tubular Epithelia

Abstract The kidney regulates the composition of the final urine by modulating the reabsorption and secretion of water and solutes across the specialized epithelium of each nephron segment. This chapter begins with an overview of epithelial barriers, including their permeability properties and main classes of transporters. We then derive the conservation and flux equations that are needed to represent the dynamic exchange of water and solutes across tubular epithelia. Lastly, we describe how to formulate a complete, cell-based model of transport across renal tubules.

8.1 Fundamental Aspects of Transepithelial Transport

Renal tubular transport plays an essential role in maintaining homeostasis. As the filtrate flows along the nephron, the tubular epithelium secretes or reabsorbs water and solutes so that ultimately, urinary excretion matches daily intake. The kidney adapts to variations in blood volume and composition by modulating the expression and/or activity of its epithelial transporters. These changes are mediated by a variety of hormonal and neural signals and involve complex signaling cascades. The heterogeneity of the different nephron segments is crucial for this adaptive capacity. Whereas the proximal tubules reabsorb large amounts of water and solutes iso-osmotically, other tubular epithelia have more specialized functions. In the distal nephron for example, principal cells regulate the reabsorption of sodium and potassium, whereas intercalated cells act mostly to maintain the acid-base balance. A detailed description of the specificities of each segment is beyond the scope of this chapter. We provide here a general framework to represent transepithelial transport at the cellular level.

The main objectives of mathematical models of renal tubular function are to elucidate the mechanisms of water and solute reabsorption (or secretion) along a given nephron segment, to predict transepithelial fluxes and tubular fluid composition,

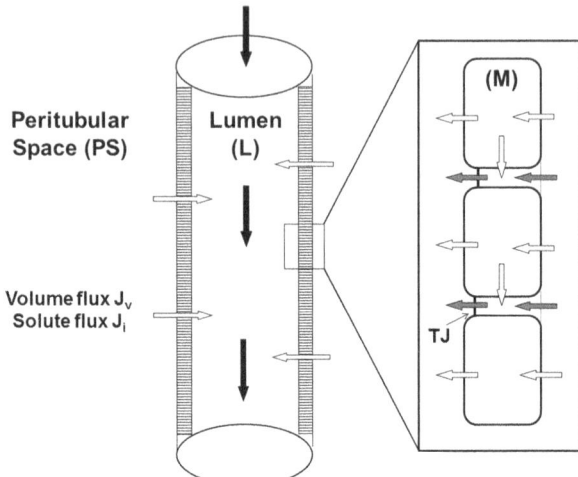

Fig. 8.1 Schematic representation of transport along a renal tubule. The tubule is idealized as a straight cylinder. As fluid flows along the tubular lumen (*L*), water and solutes are either secreted from or reabsorbed into the peritubular space (*PS*). The epithelial barrier consists of two pathways in parallel: the transcellular route, across the cell cytosol (*M*), and the paracellular route, via tight junctions (*TJ*)

and to investigate the effects of variations in transporter expression or activity on tubular transport. The models can be used to simulate specific diseases, targeted gene deletion, hormonal or drug delivery, etc. We begin this chapter with a characterization of epithelial barriers and their properties. The main classes of epithelial transporters are described in the following section. The last parts of this chapter are devoted to model formulation.

8.1.1 Paracellular and Transcellular Pathways

Transepithelial transport can proceed via transcellular and/or paracellular pathways, as depicted in Fig. 8.1. Solutes moving across the paracellular route must traverse tight junctions (also known as zonula occludens), junctional structures that mediate adhesion between cells. The main components of tight junctions are claudins and occludins, which together determine the permeability of the paracellular barrier.

Epithelia are characterized as tight or leaky depending on their transmembrane resistance. In an epithelial monolayer, the paracellular and transcellular routes form resistances in parallel. The transcellular pathway itself consists of two resistances in series (viz., the apical and the basolateral membranes), and it is typically much less conductive (i.e., more resistant) than the paracellular pathway, even in the presence of specialized transcellular transporters. Hence, the transepithelial resistance predominantly reflects the resistance of the tight junction. In leaky epithelia such as the proximal tubule, the tight junctional resistance is low, on the order of 10 $\Omega \cdot cm^2$. The resistance of tight epithelia, such as that of the collecting tubule, is about 100 times higher, that is, on the order of 1,000 $\Omega \cdot cm^2$.

8.1 Fundamental Aspects of Transepithelial Transport

The resistance of the tight junction is related to its permeability as follows. The conductance (i.e., the inverse of the resistance) of a barrier to a charged solute S is equal to:

$$G_S = \frac{P_S z_S^2 F^2 \overline{C}_S}{RT}, \tag{8.1}$$

where P_S is the membrane permeability to S, and $\overline{C}_S$ is a mean transmembrane concentration, generally calculated as:

$$\overline{C}_S = \frac{\Delta C_S}{\Delta \ln C_S} = \frac{C_S^e - C_S^i}{\ln C_S^e - \ln C_S^i}, \tag{8.2}$$

where the superscripts "e" and "i" respectively refer to the extra- and intracellular compartments. Equation (8.1) can be derived from the Goldman-Hodgkin-Katz (GHK) current equation (Eq. 6.19 in Chap. 6):

$$i_S = P_S \frac{z_S^2 F^2 V_m}{RT} \frac{C_S^i - C_S^e \exp(-z_S F V_m/RT)}{1 - \exp(-z_S F V_m/RT)}.$$

Taking the limit $\Delta C_S \to 0$, $i_S \approx P_S z_S^2 F^2 \overline{C}_S V_m/RT$, which subsequently leads to Eq. (8.1). The overall transepithelial conductance is thus calculated as:

$$G_{TJ} = \sum_S G_S = \frac{F^2}{RT} \sum_S z_S^2 P_S \overline{C}_S. \tag{8.3}$$

The transepithelial resistance is then given by $R_{TJ} = 1/G_{TJ}$. Since conductance is proportional to concentration, we may consider only the dominant ions (i.e., Na$^+$, K$^+$, and Cl$^-$) in determining G_{TJ}. As an illustration, consider the outer medullary collecting duct epithelium. Reported estimates of the rabbit tight junctional permeability to Na$^+$, K$^+$ and Cl$^-$ in that segment are 3.9, 5.9 and 4.8×10^{-6} cm/s (Weinstein 2000). To calculate G_{TJ}, we first compute mean transmembrane concentrations based on typical levels in blood and tubular fluid (the latter at the outer medullary collecting duct inlet):

$$\overline{C}_{Na} \sim \frac{140 - 70}{\ln(140/70)} \sim 100 \ mM,$$

$$\overline{C}_K \sim \frac{5 - 45}{\ln(5/45)} \sim 18 \ mM,$$

$$\overline{C}_{Cl} \sim \frac{115 - 95}{\ln(115/95)} \sim 105 \ mM.$$

The overall transepithelial conductance is then estimated as:

$$G_{TJ} = \frac{(96.5 \ C/mEq)^2}{(2.57 \ J/mmol)} [100(3.9) + 18(5.9) + 105(4.8)]$$

$$\times \left[10^{-3} mmol/cm^3\right] \left[10^{-6} cm/s\right],$$

$$G_{TJ} = 3.6 \ mS/cm^2, \quad \text{or} \quad R_{TJ} = 275 \ \Omega \cdot cm^2.$$

This estimate closely matches the experimental measurements of Koeppen (1986), who reported an average R_{TJ} of 28.5 kΩ·cm, that is, 272 Ω·cm^2 assuming a tubule diameter of 30.4 μm.

8.1.2 Passive and Active Transport

Passive transport by definition does not require energy, as opposed to *active transport*. You may recall that energetically favorable processes are those that decrease the Gibbs free energy (G) of the system. Thus, the spontaneous (or passive) direction of a transport process is that which reduces G. In open systems at constant temperature and pressure, ΔG is proportional to the change in the electrochemical potentials of the system components. By definition, the electrochemical potential of solute S in compartment j (μ_S^j) is:

$$\mu_S^j \equiv \left[\frac{\partial(n_{tot}G)}{\partial n_S}\right]_{P,T,n_k}, \tag{8.4}$$

where n_S is the number of moles of S and n_{tot} is the total number of moles. Multiple phases (or compartments) at the same temperature and pressure are in equilibrium when the chemical potential of each species is the same in all phases, that is, when ΔG is zero. As derived from thermodynamics, in dilute solutions in which solute-solute interactions are negligible, μ_S^j is given by (Job and Herrmann 2006):

$$\mu_S^j = \mu_S^o + RT \ln C_S^j + z_S F \psi^j. \tag{8.5}$$

In this equation, μ_S^o denotes the chemical potential of the pure solute in a reference state, z_S is the solute valence, and ψ^j is the electric potential in compartment j. Solute is transported spontaneously from compartment j to compartment k if this process lowers the Gibbs free energy of the system, that is, if:

$$\Delta \mu_S = \mu_S^k - \mu_S^j < 0, \quad \text{i.e.,} \quad \mu_S^j > \mu_S^k. \tag{8.6}$$

8.1 Fundamental Aspects of Transepithelial Transport

In other words, passive transport is the movement of solute down its electrochemical potential gradient. In contrast, active transport involves the movement of solute against an electrochemical gradient and necessitates energy. Three forms of passive transport can be distinguished:

- Simple diffusion is the diffusion of solute across the membrane without the aid of an integral membrane protein. To cross the hydrophobic core of the lipid bilayer "unassisted", the solute must be substantially hydrophobic. Examples include small gas molecules such as oxygen and carbon dioxide.
- Channel diffusion: ion channels are transmembrane proteins with a hydrophilic pore. They are selectively permeable to certain solutes, and their opening is regulated (or gated) by different factors, such as the transmembrane voltage or specific ligands (see Chap. 6).
- Facilitated diffusion occurs through passive carriers, transmembrane proteins that lack a hydrophobic pore and that are solute-specific. Facilitated diffusion proceeds in three steps: the solute binds to the carrier, the carrier then undergoes a conformational change that moves the solute across the membrane, finally the solute dissociates from the carrier. Note that carrier-mediated transport is several orders of magnitude slower than channel-mediated transport, and it is also more rapidly saturated.

We must also distinguish between *primary* and *secondary active transport*. Primary, or direct, active transport uses the energy stored in chemical bonds to move solutes across membranes. Most of the enzymes that mediate primary active transport are transmembrane ATPases, enzymes that catalyze the hydrolysis of adenosine triphosphate (ATP) into adenosine diphosphate (ADP) and phosphate. The energy that is released by this reaction allows solute transport to proceed in an energetically unfavorable direction.

Secondary transport also uses energy to move solutes across membranes, but the source of energy is not ATP but the electrochemical potential gradient generated by primary transport. Specifically, secondary transporters couple the energy of the transmembrane potential difference of one solute to that of another and thereby move the latter uphill. Secondary active transporters are either cotransporters (i.e., symporters) or exchangers (i.e., antiporters): in symport, the two species of solutes are carried in the same direction, whereas in antiport the two species move in opposite directions. A well-known example of antiporter is the sodium-calcium exchanger, which couples the (energetically unfavorable) efflux of one Ca^{2+} ion to the (energetically favorable) entry of 3 Na^+ ions into the cell. By similarly harnessing the Na^+ electrochemical potential gradient (or simply the Na^+ gradient), the glucose symporter SGLT1 co-transports glucose and sodium into the cell.

8.1.3 Acid-Base Balance

Cells need to maintain their intracellular pH within very tight bounds (around 7.2), since intracellular pH affects the ionization of a very large number of intracellular components, including all peptides and proteins. Thus, preserving a stable pH is fundamental for a number of intracellular processes such as gene and protein synthesis, muscle contractility, and cell division. Metabolic acidosis, an acid-base imbalance characterized by too much acid in body fluids, is often accompanied by rapid breathing, confusion or lethargy; severe cases may lead to coma and death.

Cells control their pH with the help of intracellular buffers, each of which consists of a weak acid and its conjugate weak pair. The most common intracellular buffers are the ammonium/ammonia pair (NH_4^+/NH_3), the dihydrogen/hydrogen phosphate pair ($H_2PO_4^-/HPO_4^{2-}$), and the carbonic acid/bicarbonate pair (H_2CO_3/HCO_3^-). Boron (2004) wrote a thorough review on the mechanisms of intracellular pH regulation, which we succinctly summarize below.

As can be shown (Problem 8.2), protons and NH_4^+ passively penetrate into cells, whereas OH^- and HCO_3^- passively diffuse out. To counteract this chronic acid load, the cell is equipped with so called "acid extruders", which require energy to extrude H^+ or to accumulate weak bases such as bicarbonate. The main acid extruders found in the kidney are vacuolar-type H^+-ATPase (or v-ATPase) pumps, Na^+/H^+ exchangers, and Na^+-HCO_3^- cotransporters (with a 1:2 stoichiometry). The v-ATPase pumps hydrolyze ATP to generate the energy needed to carry protons against their electrochemical potential gradient (an example of primary active transport). The other two types of acid extruders use the energy of the sodium gradient to export H^+ or import HCO_3^-, and thus constitute secondary active transporters.

Cells are sometimes confronted with an alkali load (e.g., after administration of bicarbonates or a diet rich in fruits and vegetables), to which they respond by enhancing the passive exit of OH^- and HCO_3^-, as well as the passive entry of H^+. Some cells also express additional "acid-loaders" such as Cl^-/HCO_3^- exchangers. Interestingly, in the proximal tubule, the Na^+-HCO_3^- cotransporter, which is expressed basolaterally, functions as an acid-loader: it operates with a 1:3 stoichiometry that thermodynamically favors the export of Na^+ and HCO_3^- (Problem 8.3). This exchanger is the main basolateral pathway for HCO_3^- reabsorption in the proximal tubule.

8.2 Principal Classes of Transepithelial Transporters

In this section, we briefly describe the major categories of transepithelial transporters, with a focus on flux calculations.

8.2.1 Aquaporins

Aquaporins (AQP) are a family of small water-permeable channels that are essential in the maintenance of body fluid homeostasis. These transmembrane proteins were discovered by Peter C. Agre, who received the 2003 Nobel Prize in Chemistry for his work. According to him, aquaporins can be viewed as blueprints for cellular plumbing systems. In the kidney, aquaporins play a major role in the formation of concentrated urine; deletion of AQP in transgenic mice markedly reduces their urinary concentrating capacity.

Whereas AQP1, AQP3 and AQP4 are constitutively expressed, AQP2 is inducible, which means that its trafficking between intracellular vesicles and the cell membrane is dynamically and tightly controlled. It is no coincidence that AQP2 is found in cortical and medullary collecting ducts, that is, in those segments where urinary water excretion is finely regulated. The principal cells of the collecting duct express AQP2 in the apical membrane, which is the rate-limiting barrier for water reabsorption, and AQP3 and AQP4 on the basolateral side. When the body detects a decrease in blood volume or an increase in blood osmolality, it releases the hormone vasopressin (also known as the anti-diuretic hormone, ADH) from the posterior pituitary gland. Vasopressin then binds to its basolateral (V2R) receptors in principal cells, thereby triggering a signaling cascade that leads to the increased exocytosis (i.e., insertion into the plasma membrane) and the decreased endocytosis (i.e., retrieval from the membrane) of AQP2. As a result, the water permeability of the collecting duct is significantly enhanced and the body is able to retain more water.

Water transport across aquaporins is predominantly osmotically driven, since these channels are essentially permeable to water only. Hydraulic (ΔP) and oncotic ($\Delta \Pi$) pressure differences may both be significant across epithelial membranes. Thus, the water flux across AQP is determined as (see Eq. 4.29):

$$J_V^{AQP} = L_p^{AQP} \left(\Delta P - \Delta \Pi - RT \sum_{ss} \gamma_{ss} \Delta C_{ss} \right), \qquad (8.7)$$

where L_p^{AQP} is the permeability of AQP to water, the superscript "ss" denotes small solutes, and γ is a solute activity coefficient.

8.2.2 Na,K-ATPase Pumps

The Na,K-ATPase, also known as the sodium pump, is a ubiquitous transmembrane enzyme. It was discovered by the Danish scientist Jens Christian Skou, a recipient of the Nobel Prize in Chemistry in 1997. The Na,K-ATPase actively moves 3 Na$^+$ ions out of the cell for every 2 K$^+$ ions pumped into the cell. Without it, the cell wouldn't be able to maintain high intracellular levels of K$^+$ and low levels of Na$^+$. The pump is therefore essential for maintaining the resting potential and regulating cellular volume. It also provides most of the energy needed for secondary active transport.

We can compute ionic fluxes across the Na,K-ATPase by viewing the binding of each ion to the enzyme as an independent process. Assume that the binding of one intracellular Na⁺ ion to the free enzyme (denoted E) to form the complex NaE is a first-order, reversible reaction:

$$Na^+ + E \underset{k_{NaE}^{off}}{\overset{k_{NaE}^{on}}{\longleftrightarrow}} NaE$$

The rate of NaE formation is given by:

$$\frac{dC_{NaE}}{dt} = k_{NaE}^{on} C_{Na}^i C_E - k_{NaE}^{off} C_{NaE}, \qquad (8.8)$$

where k_{NaE}^{on} and k_{NaE}^{off} are respectively the association and dissociation kinetic constants for this reaction. As the total concentration of enzyme ($C_E^{tot} = C_E + C_{NaE}$) remains constant, Eq. (8.8) can be rewritten as:

$$\begin{aligned}\frac{dC_{NaE}}{dt} &= k_{NaE}^{on} C_{Na}^i \left(C_E^{tot} - C_{NaE}\right) - k_{NaE}^{off} C_{NaE}, \\ &= k_{NaE}^{on} C_{Na}^i C_E^{tot} - \left(k_{NaE}^{on} C_{Na}^i + k_{NaE}^{off}\right) C_{NaE}.\end{aligned} \qquad (8.9)$$

At steady state, we thus have:

$$C_{NaE} = \frac{C_E^{tot} C_{Na}^i}{C_{Na}^i + K_{Na}^i}, \qquad (8.10)$$

where $K_{Na}^i = k_{NaE}^{off}/k_{NaE}^{on}$ is the apparent dissociation constant of the NaE complex. Eq. (8.10) means that the probability (p_{Na}) of having one Na⁺ ion bound to one pump unit is proportional to $C_{Na}^i/(C_{Na}^i + K_{Na}^i)$. If all the Na⁺ binding sites have the same affinity and there is no cooperativity between them, the probability of having 3 intracellular Na⁺ ions bound to the pump is simply p_{Na}^3. Similarly, the probability of having 2 extracellular K⁺ ions bound to the pump is p_K^2, where p_K is proportional to $C_K^e/(C_K^e + K_K^e)$, C_K^e is the external K⁺ concentration, and K_K^e denotes the apparent dissociation of the KE complex. Thus, the flux of Na⁺ ions across the pump can be expressed as:

$$J_{Na}^{NaK} = J_{Na}^{NaK,\max} \left[\frac{C_{Na}^i}{C_{Na}^i + K_{Na}^i}\right]^3 \left[\frac{C_K^e}{C_K^e + K_K^e}\right]^2, \qquad (8.11)$$

and that of K⁺ ions as:

$$J_K^{NaK} = -(2/3) J_{Na}^{NaK}. \qquad (8.12)$$

$J_{Na}^{NaK,\max}$ is the maximum efflux of Na⁺ ions at steady state. Garay and Garrahan (1973) found that the apparent Na⁺ affinity of the pump increases linearly with intracellular K⁺ levels:

$$K_{Na}^i = K_{Na}^{NaK}\left(1 + C_K^i/a_{NaK}\right), \tag{8.13}$$

where K_{Na}^{NaK} and a_{NaK} are both constants. Similarly, the apparent K^+ affinity is altered by extracellular Na^+ (Strieter et al. 1992), such that:

$$K_K^e = K_K^{NaK}\left(1 + C_{Na}^e/b_{NaK}\right). \tag{8.14}$$

In the kidney, K_{Na}^{NaK} and K_K^{NaK} are taken as 0.2 and 0.1 mM, respectively, and a_{NaK} as b_{NaK} as 8.33 and 18.5 mM, respectively. Thus, under typical conditions ($C_K^i \sim C_{Na}^e \sim 150$ mM), the apparent affinity of the pump for Na^+ and K^+ is on the order of 4 and 1 mM, respectively.

8.2.3 An Antiport System: The Na^+/H^+ Exchanger

Many types of antiporters are expressed in the kidney. We use as an example the luminal Na^+/H^+ exchanger of the proximal tubule (an acid-extruder), for which Alan Weinstein, a professor of physiology and biophysics at Cornell University, developed a model that served as a basis for representing similar transporters later on. The kinetic diagram of Na^+/H^+ exchanger, shown in Fig. 8.2, accounts for the competitive binding of NH_4^+ and H^+. Following the original notation (Weinstein 1995), the solutes A, B, and C respectively represent Na^+, H^+ and NH_4^+, and X is the empty transporter. The superscript "i" denotes the internal face of the membrane, and "e" the external face. The key assumption of the model is that ion binding is very rapid relative to membrane translocation. It is also assumed that the internal and external binding affinities are identical, but the equations can be easily modified to account for non-symmetric binding (see Problem 8.6). To simplify the notation below, concentrations are denoted by lower case letters; for example, a represents the concentration of A, and ax that of the complex AX.

Assuming that the binding reactions are instantaneous, we have:

$$K_a = \frac{a^i x^i}{(ax)^i} = \frac{a^e x^e}{(ax)^e}, \quad K_b = \frac{b^i x^i}{(bx)^i} = \frac{b^e x^e}{(bx)^e}, \quad K_c = \frac{c^i x^i}{(cx)^i} = \frac{c^e x^e}{(cx)^e}, \tag{8.15}$$

where K_a, K_b, and K_c represent equilibrium constants. The total amount of carrier (x_T) is conserved, so that:

$$x^i + (ax)^i + (bx)^i + (cx)^i + x^e + (ax)^e + (bx)^e + (cx)^e = x_T. \tag{8.16}$$

In addition the flux of carrier in one direction must be counterbalanced by that in the other direction, so that there is zero net flux:

$$T_a(ax)^i + T_b(bx)^i + T_c(cx)^i = T_a(ax)^e + T_b(bx)^e + T_c(cx)^e, \tag{8.17}$$

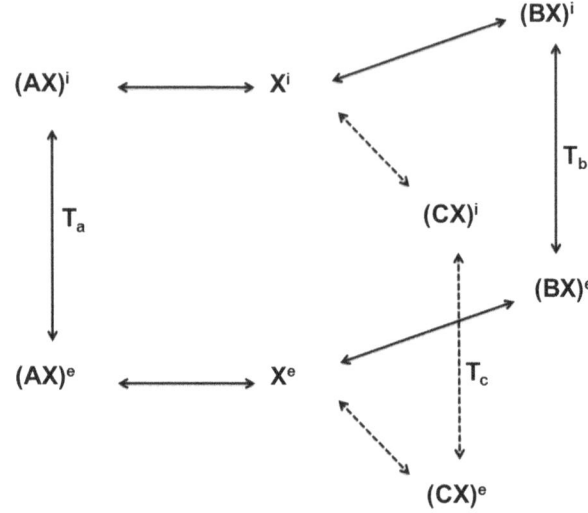

Fig. 8.2 Model representation of the Na$^+$/H$^+$ exchanger. Na$^+$ (A), H$^+$ (B) and NH$_4^+$ (C) bind to the empty carrier (X), and the resulting complexes are translocated across the membrane. The model assumes sequential translocation (also known as the ping-pong mechanism)

where T_k represents the translocation rate of solute k. Here, the forward and backward rates for a given solute are taken to be equal, and there is no translocation of empty carrier. Henceforth, it is helpful to use the following non-dimensional concentrations:

$$\alpha \equiv \frac{a}{K_a}, \quad \beta \equiv \frac{b}{K_b}, \quad \gamma \equiv \frac{c}{K_c}.$$

Note that $(ax)^i = a^i x^i / K_a = \alpha^i x^i$, $(bx)^i = \beta^i x^i$, and so on. Equations (8.16) and (8.17) are then rewritten as:

$$x^i \left[1 + \alpha^i + \beta^i + \gamma^i\right] + x^e \left[1 + \alpha^e + \beta^e + \gamma^e\right] = x_T, \quad (8.18)$$

$$-x^i \left[T_a \alpha^i + T_b \beta^i + T_c \gamma^i\right] + x^e \left[T_a \alpha^e + T_b \beta^e + T_c \gamma^e\right] = 0. \quad (8.19)$$

This 2×2 system can easily be solved for x^i and x^e. The determinant equals:

$$\Sigma = \left(1 + \alpha^i + \beta^i + \gamma^i\right)\left(T_a \alpha^e + T_b \beta^e + T_c \gamma^e\right) + \left(1 + \alpha^e + \beta^e + \gamma^e\right)\left(T_a \alpha^i + T_b \beta^i + T_c \gamma^i\right). \quad (8.20)$$

And we have:

$$x^i = x_T \left(T_a \alpha^e + T_b \beta^e + T_c \gamma^e\right) / \Sigma, \quad (8.21)$$

$$x^e = x_T \left(T_a \alpha^i + T_b \beta^i + T_c \gamma^i\right) / \Sigma. \quad (8.22)$$

We can now calculate the flux of each ion across the carrier. The net outward flux of solute A is given by:

$$J_a = T_a(ax)^i - T_a(ax)^e = T_a\left(\alpha^i x^i - \alpha^e x^e\right). \tag{8.23}$$

Substituting Eqs. (8.21) and (8.22) into Eq. (8.23) and rearranging, we obtain:

$$J_a = \frac{x_T T_a}{\Sigma}\left[T_b\left(\alpha^i \beta^e - \alpha^e \beta^i\right) + T_c\left(\alpha^i \gamma^e - \alpha^e \gamma^i\right)\right]. \tag{8.24}$$

Similarly, the net outward fluxes of B and C are equal to:

$$J_b = \frac{x_T T_b}{\Sigma}\left[T_a\left(\beta^i \alpha^e - \beta^e \alpha^i\right) + T_c\left(\beta^i \gamma^e - \beta^e \gamma^i\right)\right], \tag{8.25}$$

$$J_c = \frac{x_T T_c}{\Sigma}\left[T_a\left(\gamma^i \alpha^e - \gamma^e \alpha^i\right) + T_b\left(\gamma^i \beta^e - \gamma^e \beta^i\right)\right]. \tag{8.26}$$

Thus, knowing the binding equilibrium constants, the translocation rates, and the total amount of carrier, the fluxes are calculated as a function of internal and external concentrations. In practice, the model parameters (particularly translocation rates) are seldom directly measured. Instead, they are obtained by fitting the model equations to experimental kinetics data. Since the number of parameters frequently exceeds the number of independent measurements, additional assumptions must be made. For instance, one of the translocation rates may be fixed. Alternatively, internal and external binding affinities may be taken to be equal (as in the model described above), if experimental observations support the latter hypothesis.

This type of kinetic characterization can be easily expanded not only to other exchangers, but also to cotransporters. Examples include the Na^+-K^+-$2Cl^-$ (NKCC2) cotransporter and the K^+-Cl^- (KCC) cotransporter of the thick ascending limb.

8.2.4 A Symport System: The Na^+-Cl^- Cotransporter

Without the assumption of rapid binding on both sides of the membrane, model equations cannot be solved as easily. Consider the model of Chang and Fujita (1999) for the thiazide-sensitive NaCl cotransporter depicted on Fig. 8.3. Thiazides (denoted by D on the figure) are widely prescribed diuretics that inhibit NaCl reabsorption in the distal convoluted tubule, where the NaCl cotransporter is expressed apically. The model assumes that they compete with chloride ions for the same binding sites. The rates of formation of the ENa and ENaCl complexes are expressed as:

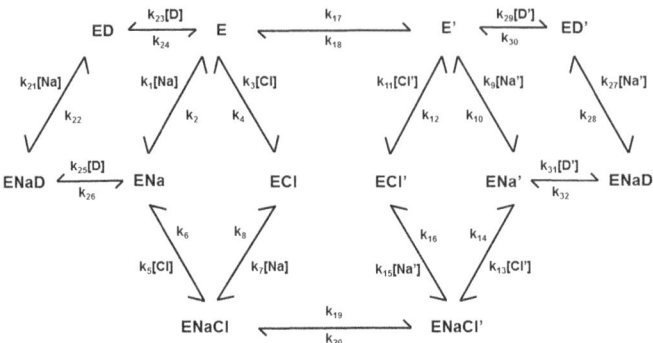

Fig. 8.3 Representation of the thiazide-sensitive NaCl cotransporter found in the distal tubule. Thiazide (D) competes with Cl⁻ for the same binding sites on the empty carrier (E), whereas Na⁺ binds to different sites (Reproduced from Chang and Fujita (1999))

$$\frac{dC_{ENa}}{dt} = (k_1 C_E C_{Na} - k_2 C_{ENa}) + (k_6 C_{ENaCl} - k_5 C_{ENa} C_{Cl})$$
$$+ (k_{26} C_{ENaD} - k_{25} C_D C_{ENa}), \qquad (8.27)$$

$$\frac{dC_{ENaCl}}{dt} = (k_5 C_{ENa} C_{Cl} - k_6 C_{ENaCl}) + (k_7 C_{ECl} C_{Na} - k_8 C_{ENaCl})$$
$$+ (k_{20} C_{ENaCl'} - k_{19} C_{ENaCl}). \qquad (8.28)$$

Similar equations can be written for the ten other species shown in Fig. 8.3: E, ECl, ED, ENaD on the intracellular side, and E′, ECl′, ENa′, ED′, ENaCl′ and ENaD′ on the extracellular side. In total, there are 12 independent equations with 32 rate constants. Chang and Fujita (1999) assumed that all the substrate and inhibitor binding rates (i.e., k_{2n+1}, $n = 0-10$) are diffusion-limited (that is, the reaction occurs so quickly that the reaction rate is almost equal to the rate of diffusion in the medium) and equal to 10^5 mM^{-1}·s^{-1}. Five other rate constants were determined using the principle of detailed balance (see Problem 8.4), which is described immediately below. The remaining rates were obtained by fitting the steady-state model equations to experimental data.

The principle of detailed balance is a thermodynamic requirement that applies to any set of reactions that form a loop. As an illustration, consider the subset of NaCl cotransporter reactions shown in Fig. 8.4; this loop corresponds to the state diagram of the cotransporter in the absence of thiazide and translocation across the membrane. If the system is in thermodynamic equilibrium, each elementary reaction is equilibrated by its reverse reaction. Proceeding counter clock-wise, this means that:

$$k_1 C_E C_{Na} = k_2 C_{ENa}, \qquad (8.29a)$$

8.2 Principal Classes of Transepithelial Transporters

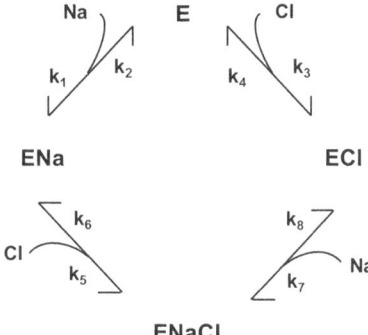

Fig. 8.4 Subset of reactions from the state diagram for the thiazide-sensitive NaCl cotransporter. These four reactions form a loop that must satisfy the principle of detailed balance

$$k_5 C_{ENa} C_{Cl} = k_6 C_{ENaCl}, \tag{8.29b}$$

$$k_8 C_{ENaCl} = k_7 C_{ECl} C_{Na}, \tag{8.29c}$$

$$k_4 C_{ECl} = k_3 C_E C_{Cl}. \tag{8.29d}$$

If we multiply all these equations, we obtain:

$$k_1 k_4 k_5 k_8 C_E C_{Na} C_{Cl} C_{ECl} C_{ECl} C_{ENaCl} = k_2 k_3 k_6 k_7 C_E C_{Na} C_{Cl} C_{ENa} C_{ECl} C_{ENaCl}. \tag{8.30}$$

That is:

$$k_1 k_4 k_5 k_8 = k_2 k_3 k_6 k_7. \tag{8.31}$$

This relationship is independent of concentrations, and thus applies not only under thermodynamic equilibrium but at all times. More generally, the principle of detailed balance states that the product of the rate constants in one direction around the loop must equal the product of the rate constants in the other direction.

8.2.5 Non-equilibrium Thermodynamic Formalism

When there is no available kinetic model for the transporter being considered because it hasn't been characterized experimentally, the non-equilibrium thermodynamic formalism can be used to determine fluxes. This approach was first adapted to renal tubular transport models by Alan Weinstein (1983). Briefly, the diffusive component of the flux of solute S is written as:

$$J_S^{diff} = \sum_{k=1,n} L_{Sk} \Delta\mu_k, \qquad (8.32)$$

where n is the number of solutes, and $\Delta\mu_k$ is the electrochemical potential difference of solute k across the membrane (see Eq. 8.5):

$$\Delta\mu_k = RT\Delta \ln C_k + z_k F\Delta\psi. \qquad (8.33)$$

The coefficient L_{Sk} couples the flux of solute S to the driving force exerted on species k. It is zero when there are no interactions between S and k. It can be shown that L_{SS} is related to the membrane permeability to solute S (P_S) as:

$$L_{SS} = \frac{RTP_S}{\overline{C}_S}, \qquad (8.34)$$

where $\overline{C}_S$ is the mean transmembrane concentration defined above (Eq. 8.2). Consider for example an electroneutral Cl^-/HCO_3^- exchanger, with a 1:1 stoichiometry. Using the non-equilibrium thermodynamic formalism, the Cl^- and HCO_3^- fluxes across the exchanger are given by:

$$\begin{bmatrix} J_{Cl}^{ex} \\ J_{HCO3}^{ex} \end{bmatrix} = L_{Cl/HCO3} \begin{bmatrix} +1 & -1 \\ -1 & +1 \end{bmatrix} \begin{bmatrix} \Delta\mu_{Cl} \\ \Delta\mu_{HCO3} \end{bmatrix}. \qquad (8.35)$$

The fluxes are therefore calculated as:

$$\begin{aligned} J_{Cl}^{ex} &= L_{Cl/HCO3} \left(\Delta\mu_{Cl} - \Delta\mu_{HCO3} \right), \\ J_{HCO3}^{ex} &= L_{Cl/HCO3} \left(\Delta\mu_{HCO3} - \Delta\mu_{Cl} \right). \end{aligned} \qquad (8.36)$$

Those equations illustrate a concept that we discussed above, namely that the energy provided by the electrochemical potential gradient of one of the ions serves to drive the transport of the other ion. For the Na_2-HPO_4 (NaP) cotransporter which has a 2:1 stoichiometry, the non-equilibrium thermodynamic formalism yields:

$$\begin{bmatrix} J_{Na}^{NaP} \\ J_{HPO4}^{NaP} \end{bmatrix} = L_{Na-HPO4} \begin{bmatrix} +4 & +2 \\ +2 & +1 \end{bmatrix} \begin{bmatrix} \Delta\mu_{Na} \\ \Delta\mu_{HPO4} \end{bmatrix}. \qquad (8.37)$$

The non-equilibrium thermodynamic formalism is very helpful in the absence of kinetic measurements. The resulting equations satisfy thermodynamic requirements while requiring specification of only one parameter, namely the coupling coefficient L_{Sk}. But some important limitations of this approach should be kept in mind: it does not distinguish between transporter expression and activity, it cannot account for ion-specific binding affinities and translocation rates, and it does not consider internal and external asymmetries.

8.3 Fundamental Equations of Epithelial Models

To construct a complete epithelial transport model, we must first specify the structural details of the tubule being considered. We then derive the fundamental conservation equations for luminal and epithelial compartments.

8.3.1 Morphological Properties

The tubule lumen is modeled as a cylinder of inner radius r. Some tubules express one cell type, other express several cell types, such as the principal and intercalated cells of the connecting tubule. For each cell type, baseline morphological properties need to be quantified, including the cytosolic volume and the surface areas of the apical, basal, and lateral membranes. The latter are usually expressed in units of cm^2 epithelium, since many experimental measurements are reported as such. The baseline dimensions of the lateral space between cells are also needed: its volume, and the surface areas of the tight junction on the luminal side and the basement membrane on the opposite side.

8.3.2 Time-Dependent Conservation Equations for Water and Solute

In order to predict transport rates across the tubular epithelium, we must determine solute concentrations, volume, and electric potential along tubules, both in the tubular lumen and in the adjacent epithelial cells. These variables are obtained by solving conservation equations for mass, volume, and charge, respectively. In this section, we derive a more general form of the conservation equations for water (i.e., volume) and solutes in different types of renal compartments, without assuming that the system is at equilibrium. The fluid in the tubular lumen is usually taken to be incompressible, with a constant density. Let $F_v(x, t)$ and $C_S^L(x, t)$ respectively denote the fluid flow and the concentration of solute S in the tubular lumen at position x and time t.

Volume. We begin by writing mass balances for the volume of fluid comprised between x and $x + dx$, i.e.,

$$dV = \int_x^{x+dx} \pi \, r^2 ds.$$

If the cylinder is not rigid, that is, if its radius may vary, the amount of fluid volume accumulated in dV during the time interval $[t, t + dt]$ is given by:

$$\text{Accumulation} = dV(t+dt) - dV(t) = \int_{x}^{x+dx} \pi\, r^2(s, t+dt)\, ds - \int_{x}^{x+dx} \pi\, r^2(s, t)\, ds.$$

By the law of conservation of mass, the amount of fluid that accumulates within dV must equal the net amount of fluid flowing into dV during dt. Fluid can enter dV both axially (by bulk motion) and radially (via transmembrane transport), and the net amount of fluid entering dV is the sum of two contributions:

$$\text{Net axial flow in} = \int_{t}^{t+dt} [F_V(x,\tau) - F_V(x+dx,\tau)]\, d\tau,$$

$$\text{Net radial flow in} = \int_{t}^{t+dt} \int_{x}^{x+dx} 2\pi\, r(s,\tau)\, J_V(s,\tau)\, ds\, d\tau,$$

where J_V denotes the volume flux (per unit membrane area), taken positive into the tubule. Note that the flux accounts for both transcellular and paracellular transport. Combining the last three equations, we have:

$$\int_{x}^{x+dx} \pi\, r^2(s, t+dt)\, ds - \int_{x}^{x+dx} \pi\, r^2(s,t)\, ds =$$
$$\int_{t}^{t+dt} [F_V(x,\tau) - F_V(x+dx,\tau)]\, d\tau + \int_{t}^{t+dt} \int_{x}^{x+dx} 2\pi\, r(s,\tau)\, J_V(s,\tau)\, ds\, d\tau.$$
(8.38)

Equation (8.38) may be rewritten as:

$$\int_{t}^{t+dt} \int_{x}^{x+dx} \pi\, \frac{\partial r^2(s,\tau)}{\partial \tau}\, ds\, d\tau =$$
$$-\int_{t}^{t+dt} \int_{x}^{x+dx} \frac{\partial F_V(s,\tau)}{\partial s}\, ds\, d\tau + \int_{t}^{t+dt} \int_{x}^{x+dx} 2\pi\, r(s,\tau)\, J_V(s,\tau)\, ds\, d\tau.$$
(8.39)

The differential form of Eq. (8.39) is the equation for the conservation of volume:

$$\pi\, \frac{\partial r^2}{\partial t} = -\frac{\partial F_V}{\partial x} + 2\pi\, r\, J_V.$$
(8.40)

If the tubule is rigid, Eq. (8.40) takes the usual form (see Eq. 2.5):

$$\frac{\partial F_V}{\partial x} = 2\pi\, r\, J_V.$$
(8.41)

8.3 Fundamental Equations of Epithelial Models

Solute. Similarly, the amount of a given solute S that accumulates in dV during the time interval $[t, t + dt]$ is given by:

$$\text{Accumulation} = \int_x^{x+dx} \pi\, r^2(s, t+dt)\, C_S^L(s, t+dt)\, ds - \int_x^{x+dx} \pi\, r^2(s,t)\, C_S^L(s,t)\, ds.$$

The amount of accumulated solute (in moles) must equal the net amount of solute flowing into dV, plus the net amount of solute formed by chemical reaction within dV. The first term, which includes both axial and radial solute flows, is expressed as:

$$\text{Net axial flow in} = \int_t^{t+dt} \left[F_V(x, \tau)\, C_S^L(x, \tau) - F_V(x+dx, \tau)\, C_S^L(x+dx, \tau) \right] d\tau,$$

$$\text{Net radial flow in} = \int_t^{t+dt} \int_x^{x+dx} 2\pi\, r(s, \tau)\, J_S(s, \tau)\, ds\, d\tau,$$

where J_S denotes the molar flux of solute S (per unit membrane area) into the tubule. The reaction term is written in terms of the volumetric rate of net generation of solute S in the tubular lumen, denoted Φ_S^L:

$$\text{Net generation} = \int_t^{t+dt} \int_x^{x+dx} \pi\, r^2(s, \tau)\, \Phi_S^L(s, \tau)\, ds\, d\tau.$$

Combining all terms, we obtain:

$$\int_x^{x+dx} \pi\, r^2(s, t+dt)\, C_S^L(s, t+dt)\, ds - \int_x^{x+dx} \pi\, r^2(s,t)\, C_S^L(s,t)\, ds =$$
$$\int_t^{t+dt} \left[F_V(x, \tau)\, C_S^L(x, \tau) - F_V(x+dx, \tau)\, C_S^L(x+dx, \tau) \right] d\tau +$$
$$\int_t^{t+dt} \int_x^{x+dx} 2\pi\, r(s, \tau)\, J_S(s, \tau)\, ds\, d\tau + \int_t^{t+dt} \int_x^{x+dx} \pi\, r^2(s, \tau)\, \Phi_S^L(s, \tau)\, ds\, d\tau.$$
(8.42)

Following the same approach as above, we obtain the equation for the conservation of solute:

$$\pi \frac{\partial \left(r^2 C_S^L \right)}{\partial t} = -\frac{\partial \left(F_V C_S^L \right)}{\partial x} + 2\pi\, r\, J_S + \pi\, r^2\, \Phi_S^L. \tag{8.43}$$

At steady state, and for a non-reacting solute (i.e., $\Phi_S^L = 0$), Eq. (8.43) takes the usual form (Eq. 2.13):

$$\frac{\partial \left(F_V C_S^L\right)}{\partial x} = 2\pi\, r\, J_S. \qquad (8.44)$$

These conservation equations were written for the tubule lumen. We now derive corresponding equations for epithelial cells. Epithelial cells exchange with the tubular lumen on the apical side, and with the peritubular fluid (or interstitium) and the lateral space between cells on the basolateral side. We denote by M the epithelial cell cytosolic compartment, and by N its surrounding compartments (e.g., the lumen and peritubular space for the tubule represented in Fig. 8.1). The volume of the cell cytosol (V^M) can expand and contract, and the amount of fluid accumulated during the time interval $[t, t+dt]$ is equal to the net amount of volume flowing into the cytosol from all adjacent compartments during dt:

$$V^M(t+dt) - V^M(t) = \int_t^{t+dt} \sum_N A^{NM}(\tau) J_V^{NM}(\tau)\, d\tau, \qquad (8.45)$$

where A^{NM} is the surface area at the interface between compartments N and M, and J_V^{NM} is the flux of volume from N to M. The differential form of Eq. (8.45) yields the intracellular volume conservation equation:

$$\frac{\partial V^M}{\partial t} = \sum_N A^{NM} J_V^{NM}. \qquad (8.46)$$

Similarly, the amount of a given solute S that accumulates within the cell cytosol during the time interval $[t, t+dt]$ equals the net flow of S into the cell, plus the net amount of S formed by chemical reaction within the cell during dt:

$$V^M(t+dt)\, C_S^M(t+dt) - V^M(t) C_S^M(t) =$$
$$\int_t^{t+dt} \sum_N A^{NM}(\tau) J_S^{NM}(\tau)\, d\tau + \int_t^{t+dt} V^M(\tau) \Phi_S^M(\tau)\, d\tau, \qquad (8.47)$$

where J_S^{NM} is the molar flux of solute S from N to M, and Φ_S^M is the volumetric rate of net generation of S within the cytosol. The differential form of Eq. (8.47) yields the intracellular solute conservation equation:

$$\frac{\partial \left(V^M C_S^M\right)}{\partial t} = \sum_N A^{NM} J_S^{NM} + V^M \Phi_S^M. \qquad (8.48)$$

The conservation equations for the lateral space between cells (i.e., the paracellular pathway) are similar to those for the cell cytosol.

8.3 Fundamental Equations of Epithelial Models

8.3.3 Rate of Solute Generation and Proton Conservation

For non-reacting solutes such as Na^+, K^+, Cl^-, and urea, the generation rate is zero. For an acid-base pair denoted HA/A^- (such as NH_4^+/NH_3 and $H_2PO_4^-/HPO_4^{2-}$), the reaction can be represented as:

$$HA \underset{k_a}{\overset{k_d}{\longleftrightarrow}} A^- + H^+$$

The net generation rate of HA (per unit volume) is written as:

$$\Phi_{HA} = -\Phi_A = -k_d C_{HA} + k_a C_A C_H, \qquad (8.49)$$

where superscripts have been dropped for simplicity, and k_d and k_a are the rates of dissociation and association, respectively. Buffer protonation reactions are generally very rapid and considered to be at equilibrium; setting the net generation rate to zero, we obtain:

$$\frac{C_A C_H}{C_{HA}} = k_d/k_a \equiv K_a. \qquad (8.50)$$

You may recognize the more familiar logarithmic form of this equation:

$$pH = pK_a + \log_{10}\left[\frac{C_A}{C_{HA}}\right], \qquad (8.51)$$

where $pK_a = -\log_{10}(K_a)$.

The CO_2/HCO_3^- buffer needs to be considered separately. The dissociation of CO_2 into bicarbonate is a two-step process that begins with the conversion of CO_2 and water into carbonic acid (H_2CO_3):

$$CO_2 + H_2O \underset{k_{dh}}{\overset{k_h}{\longleftrightarrow}} H_2CO_3 \underset{k_s}{\overset{k_{ds}}{\longleftrightarrow}} HCO_3^- + H^+$$

Most textbooks assume that both reactions are instantaneous, and use the Henderson-Hasselbalch equation to relate the concentrations of CO_2 and HCO_3^-:

$$pH = pK_a + \log_{10}\left[\frac{C_{HCO3}}{s_{CO2} P_{CO2}}\right], \qquad (8.52)$$

where P_{CO2} is the partial pressure of CO_2 in the gas phase with which the fluid is in equilibrium (40 mmHg in the atmosphere), and s_{CO2} is the C_{O2} solubility coefficient ($\sim$0.03 mM/mmHg in plasma). However, the inter-conversion of CO_2 and H_2O into H_2CO_3 is catalyzed by a family of enzymes known as carbonic anhydrases, the expression of which varies significantly between the tubular fluid and the cytosol (and from one cell type to another). Consequently, it is more accurate to determine the net generation rates as:

$$\Phi_{CO2} = -k_h C_{CO2} + k_{dh} C_{H2CO3}, \tag{8.53}$$

$$\Phi_{HCO3} = -k_s C_{HCO3} C_H + k_{ds} C_{H2CO3}, \tag{8.54}$$

$$\Phi_{H2CO3} = -\Phi_{CO2} - \Phi_{HCO3}, \tag{8.55}$$

where the rate constants for CO_2 hydration (k_h) and dehydration (k_{dh}) depend on the amount of carbonic anhydrase in the compartment being considered. Since the protonation of HCO_3^- is extremely rapid, the reaction rate Φ_{HCO3} is usually taken to be zero. The concentrations of HCO_3^- and H_2CO_3 are then related using a relationship such as Eq. (8.51).

Once all the acid-base reaction rates have been specified, conservation equations can be written for protons (H^+) in the tubular lumen and cytosol:

$$\frac{\partial \left(\pi r^2 C_H^L\right)}{\partial t} = -\frac{\partial F_v C_H^L}{\partial x} + 2\pi r J_H + \pi r^2 \sum_{base\ A} \Phi_A^L, \tag{8.56}$$

$$\frac{\partial \left(V^M C_H^M\right)}{\partial t} = \sum_N A^{NM} J_H^{NM} + V^M \sum_{base\ A} \Phi_A^M. \tag{8.57}$$

The last summation term on the right-hand side corresponds to the net production of protons from acid-base reactions. These equations serve to determine the pH in the tubular lumen fluid and in the cytosol of epithelial compartment M.

8.3.4 Conservation of Electric Charge

As described in Chap. 6, the cell membrane can be represented as an electrical circuit with a capacitor in parallel with a resistor, and variations in the membrane potential are inversely proportional to the membrane capacitance (C_m). The electric potential of the peritubular space (superscript "P") is always taken to be the ground potential (i.e., $\psi^P = 0$). Assuming that the capacitance of the tight junction is zero, the apical (ψ^{ML}) and basolateral (ψ^{MP}) transmembrane electric potentials obey:

$$C_m^{ML} \frac{\partial \psi^{ML}}{\partial t} = -\sum_{solute\ S} z_S F \left(A^{ML} J_S^{ML} + A^{PL} J_S^{PL}\right), \tag{8.58}$$

$$C_m^{MP} \frac{\partial \psi^{MP}}{\partial t} = -\sum_{solute\ S} z_S F \left(A^{MP} J_S^{MP} - A^{PL} J_S^{PL}\right), \quad (8.59)$$

where the capacitance C_m is assumed to be proportional to the surface area, with a proportionality constant of 1 µF/cm². Because capacitance values are very small, these electrical potential equations give rise to a stiff system. To circumvent this issue, most epithelial transport models use approximations instead, and determine membrane potentials based upon (a) electroneutrality within each epithelial compartment M, and (b) open-circuit conditions (i.e., no net current into the lumen). In other words:

$$\sum_{solute\ S} z_S C_S^M = 0, \quad (8.60)$$

$$\sum_{solute\ S} z_S F \left(A^{ML} J_S^{ML} + A^{PL} J_S^{PL}\right) = 0. \quad (8.61)$$

8.4 Full Model Specification

We are now ready to construct a complete tubular transport model. In the previous section, we derived the conservation equations that yield concentrations, volumes, and electrical potential, as a function of time and position, in the tubular lumen and epithelial cells. We must now provide a full description of water and solute fluxes, one that builds upon the concepts and equations given in Sect. 8.2. Next, we touch upon solution methods. Finally, we note some important limitations of current modeling approaches.

8.4.1 Determinants of Volume Flux

In its most general form, the volume flux from compartment M to compartment N is written as:

$$J_V^{MN} = L_p^{MN} \left(\Delta P^{MN} - \Delta \Pi^{MN} - RT \sum_{ss} \gamma_{ss} \sigma_{ss}^{MN} \left(C_{ss}^M - C_{ss}^N\right)\right), \quad (8.62)$$

where L_p^{MN} is the water permeability of the membrane between M and N, and ΔP^{MN} and $\Delta \Pi^{MN}$ are respectively the transmembrane hydraulic and oncotic pressure differences. The third term on the right hand side represents the osmotic pressure exerted by small solutes. As described above, transcellular water transport is usually mediated by aquaporins, which are impermeable to most solutes. Thus, reflection coefficients (σ^{MN}) are equal to 1 for apical and basolateral membranes. They are usually taken to be zero for the non-selective interspace basement membrane, and between 0 and 1 for tight junctions.

Oncotic pressures are exerted by large proteins that do not cross epithelial barriers. In the tubular lumen and peritubular space, they depend on the composition of the fluid and are generally specified at the outset. In a given cell M, Π^M is calculated based on the concentration of impermeants ("imp"), the number of moles of which remains constant:

$$\Pi^M = RTC_{imp}^M = RTC_{imp,o}^M \left(V_o^M / V^M \right), \tag{8.63}$$

where the subscript "o" denotes reference (baseline) conditions. The variations in hydraulic pressure in the lumen (P^L) are generally determined assuming Poiseuille flow in the tubule:

$$\frac{\partial P^L}{\partial x} = -\frac{8\eta F_V}{\pi r^4}, \tag{8.64}$$

where η is the luminal fluid viscosity (6.4×10^{-6} mmHg/s). The intracellular hydraulic pressure (P^M) is assumed equal to the luminal pressure, and the peritubular hydraulic pressure (P^S) is fixed. Based on observations in the gallbladder, the hydraulic pressure in the lateral space (P^E) is related to the area of the basement membrane (S^{bm}) by a compliance relation:

$$P^E = P^S + \frac{1}{\nu_E} \left(\frac{S^{bm}}{S_o^{bm}} - 1 \right), \tag{8.65}$$

where ν_E is the interspace compliance. In practice, P^E is determined to satisfy the water balance (i.e., the volume conservation equation), and S^{bm} is subsequently calculated using Eq. (8.65). Note that the interspace volume is taken to vary in proportion with S^{bm}, that is, $V^E/V_o^E = S^{bm}/S_o^{bm}$.

8.4.2 Determinants of Solute Flux

We have seen in section 8.2 how to compute solute fluxes across specific types of transporters. More generally, the flux of solute S from compartments M to N is written as:

$$\begin{aligned} J_S^{MN} = \left(1 - \sigma_S^{MN}\right) \overline{C}_S^{MN} J_V^{MN} + h_S^{MN} \zeta_S^{MN} \left(\frac{C_S^M - C_S^N \exp\left(-\zeta_S^{MN}\right)}{1 - \exp\left(-\zeta_S^{MN}\right)} \right) \\ + J_S^{MN}(coupled) + J_S^{MN}(\text{ATP-driven}). \end{aligned} \tag{8.66}$$

8.4 Full Model Specification

The first term represents convective transport: $\overline{C}_S^{MN} = (C_S^M - C_S^N) / (\ln C_S^M - \ln C_S^N)$ is the mean membrane solute concentration. The second term denotes passive diffusion driven by the electrochemical potential gradient; h_S^{MN} is the permeability of the membrane to solute S (this symbol is chosen instead of P_S^{MN} to avoid confusion with the pressure P), and ζ_S^{MN} is a non-dimensional electric potential difference, defined as:

$$\zeta_S^{MN} = \frac{z_S F}{RT} \left(\psi^M - \psi^N \right). \tag{8.67}$$

In the absence of an electric field, the passive diffusion term reduces to the well-known form (see Eq. 2.15):

$$J_S^{passive\ diffusion} = h_S^{MN} \left(C_S^M - C_S^N \right). \tag{8.68}$$

The third term in Eq. (8.66) accounts for the coupled transport of S and other solutes (across cotransporters and exchangers), and the last term for primary active transport (across ATPases). Examples of both were provided in Sect. 8.2.

8.4.3 Numerical Solution

As a last step, the initial and boundary conditions need to be specified. To date, most models of transepithelial transport have focused on steady-state conditions; the time derivatives in the conservation equations are thus set to zero. As for boundary conditions, concentrations in the peritubular solution are fixed, and the luminal fluid composition, pressure and flow rate at the tubule inlet are specified. The conservation equations are then integrated to yield the steady-state solute concentrations, volume, pH, and electrical potential in the cell cytosol, lateral space, and tubular lumen as a function of position along the tubular axis. These differential equations are typically discretized, and the resulting set of algebraic equations can be solved with Newton's method.

8.4.4 A Simple Cell Model

We now develop a simple epithelial cell model to illustrate the concepts presented above. We consider the transport of water and three solutes (Na^+, K^+, Cl^-) across the hypothetical epithelial cell depicted in Fig. 8.5. As shown, the apical membrane of this cell expresses Na^+, K^+, and Cl^- channels, and the basolateral membrane expresses Na^+,K^+-ATPase pumps, K^+ channels, and KCl cotransporters. For simplicity, we assume that the contribution of paracellular pathway corresponds to 233 pmol/min/cm^2 epithelium of negative charge moving from the lumen to the

Fig. 8.5 Schematic representation of an epithelial cell that transports Na^+, K^+, and Cl^-. In this simplified model, the tight junctions are taken to be impermeable to water. Conversely, the lateral space between cells exchanges freely with the peritubular space, and these two compartments are not distinguished

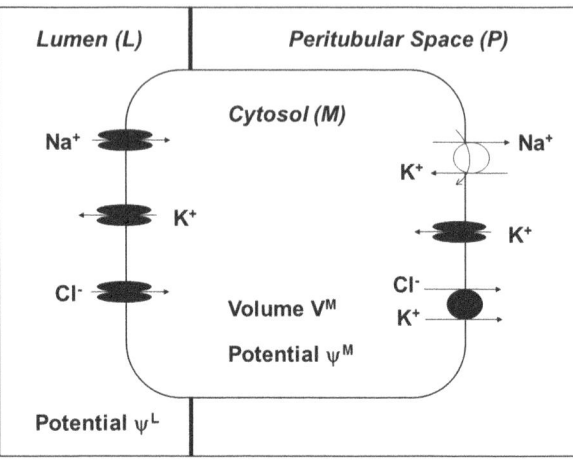

Table 8.1 Epithelial cell parameters

	Apical	Basolateral
Membrane surface area (cm^2/cm^2 epith)	1.2	6.0
Water permeability (cm/s)	0.20	0.10
Na$^+$ channel permeability (cm/s)	0.2×10^{-5}	0
K$^+$ channel permeability (cm/s)	0.8×10^{-5}	0.01×10^{-5}
Cl$^-$ channel permeability (cm/s)	1.0×10^{-5}	0
Maximum Na$^+$,K$^+$-ATPase flux (mmol/s/cm^2)		339.3×10^{-9}
KCl cotransporter coupling coefficient (mmol^2/J/s/cm^2)		2.47×10^{-9}

Surface areas are normalized by that of the lumen - hence the notation per cm^2 epith

peritubular space. Our objective is to determine, at steady state, the intracellular concentrations of Na^+, K^+, Cl^-, the intracellular volume, and the electric potentials in the lumen and cytosol.

The composition of the lumen and peritubular space is taken to be the same: $[Na^+] = 140$ mM, $[K^+] = 5$ mM, and $[Cl^-] = 145$ mM. The hydraulic and oncotic pressures are zero in these two compartments. The reference concentration of impermeant proteins (of valence -1) in the cytosol is 80 mM, and the reference cell volume is $V_o^M = 4 \times 10^{-4}$ cm^3/cm^2 epithelium; note that the reference epithelial surface area is based upon the inner diameter of the tubule. Other cell properties are given in Table 8.1.

The six variables to be determined are obtained by solving six conservation equations. At steady state, the conservation of volume in the cell is expressed as (see Eq. 8.46):

$$A^{LM} J_V^{LM} + A^{PM} J_V^{PM} = 0. \tag{8.69}$$

8.4 Full Model Specification

Similarly, the conservation equation for each of the three (non-reacting) solutes is expressed as (see Eq. 8.48):

$$A^{LM} J_S^{LM} + A^{PM} J_S^{PM} = 0, \quad S = \text{Na}^+, \text{K}^+, \text{Cl}^-. \tag{8.70}$$

The last two equations to be solved express the conservation of charge in the cytosol and lumen, respectively (see Eqs. 8.60 and 8.61):

$$0 = \sum_{\text{solute } S} z_S C_S^M = C_{Na}^M + C_K^M - C_{Cl}^M - C_{imp}^M, \tag{8.71}$$

$$A^{LM} F(J_{Na}^{LM} + J_K^{LM} - J_{Cl}^{LM}) + A^{LP} F(zJ)_{net}^{LP} = 0, \tag{8.72}$$

where $F(zJ)_{net}^{LP}$ denotes the net current across the paracellular pathway. To solve these equations, we must now determine volume and solute fluxes. The apical (LM) and basolateral (PM) fluxes of water into the cell are given by:

$$J_V^{LM} = -RTL_p^{LM} \left[\sum_{ss=Na,K,Cl} (C_{ss}^L - C_{ss}^M) - C_{imp}^M \right]$$

$$= -RTL_p^{LM} \left[\sum_{ss=Na,K,Cl} (C_{ss}^L - C_{ss}^M) - C_{imp,o}^M \left(V_o^M / V^M \right) \right], \tag{8.73}$$

$$J_V^{PM} = -RTL_p^{PM} \left[\sum_{ss=Na,K,Cl} (C_{ss}^P - C_{ss}^M) - C_{imp,o}^M \left(V_o^M / V^M \right) \right]. \tag{8.74}$$

The apical entry of Na$^+$ is mediated by Na$^+$ channels, and its basolateral exit by sodium pumps. The corresponding Na$^+$ fluxes are given by:

$$J_{Na}^{LM} = h_{Na}^{LM} \zeta_{Na}^{LM} \left(\frac{C_{Na}^L - C_{Na}^M \exp\left(-\zeta_{Na}^{LM}\right)}{1 - \exp\left(-\zeta_{Na}^{LM}\right)} \right), \tag{8.75}$$

$$J_{Na}^{PM} = -J_{Na}^{NaK,\max} \left[\frac{C_{Na}^M}{C_{Na}^M + K_{Na}^i} \right]^3 \left[\frac{C_K^P}{C_K^P + K_K^e} \right]^2. \tag{8.76}$$

There is a minus sign in Eq. (8.76) because J_{Na}^{PM} denotes the Na$^+$ flux from the peritubular space into the cytosol, and the Na$^+$,K$^+$-ATPase pumps sodium out of the cell. We assume for simplicity that the pump affinities are constant, with $K_{Na}^i = 4$ mM, and $K_K^e = 1$ mM. Let $\zeta_+^{LM} = (\psi^L - \psi^M)F/RT$. We then have $\zeta_+^{LM} = \zeta_{Na}^{LM} = \zeta_K^{LM} = -\zeta_{Cl}^{LM}$.

The apical entry of Cl⁻ is mediated by Cl⁻ channels, and its basolateral exit by KCl cotransporters. In the absence of kinetic parameters, the KCl cotransporter flux is computed using the non-equilibrium thermodynamic formalism. The Cl⁻ fluxes are thus given by:

$$J_{Cl}^{LM} = -h_{Cl}^{LM} \zeta_+^{LM} \left(\frac{C_{Cl}^L - C_{Cl}^M \exp(+\zeta_+^{LM})}{1 - \exp(+\zeta_+^{LM})} \right), \tag{8.77}$$

$$\begin{aligned} J_{Cl}^{PM} &= L_{KCl} (\Delta \mu_K + \Delta \mu_{Cl}) \\ &= L_{KCl} \left(RT \ln \left(\frac{C_K^P}{C_K^M} \right) - RT\psi^M + RT \ln \left(\frac{C_{Cl}^P}{C_{Cl}^M} \right) + RT\psi^M \right) \\ &= L_{KCl} RT \ln \left(\frac{C_K^P C_{Cl}^P}{C_K^M C_{Cl}^M} \right). \end{aligned} \tag{8.78}$$

Finally, the apical and basolateral fluxes of K⁺ are given by:

$$J_K^{LM} = h_K^{LM} \zeta_+^{LM} \left(\frac{C_K^L - C_K^M \exp(-\zeta_+^{LM})}{1 - \exp(-\zeta_+^{LM})} \right), \tag{8.79}$$

$$J_K^{PM} = -(2/3) J_{Na}^{PM} + J_{Cl}^{PM} + h_K^{PM} \zeta_+^{PM} \left(\frac{C_K^P - C_K^M \exp(-\zeta_+^{PM})}{1 - \exp(-\zeta_+^{PM})} \right), \tag{8.80}$$

where $\zeta_+^{PM} = -\psi^M F/RT$. As can be inferred from the flux expressions, the six conservation equations are highly coupled and non-linear, so they cannot be solved analytically. We used a numerical solver to determine the solution of this system. The predicted steady-state intracellular concentrations and transepithelial fluxes are given in Table 8.2. The electrical potential in the cytosol and lumen are $\psi^M = -70.04$ mV and $\psi^L = -25.59$ mV. The cell volume is 2.67×10^{-4} cm³/cm² epithelium, as can be inferred from the impermeant concentration given in Table 8.2.

It can be seen that our hypothetical epithelium reabsorbs a significant amount of Na⁺, 678 pmol/s/cm² epithelium, that is, 25.6 pmol/min/mm tubule assuming a tubular diameter of 20 μm. The epithelium conversely secretes K⁺ into the lumen, 14.6 pmol/min/mm. It also reabsorbs a small amount of chloride, 2.2 pmol/min/mm.

Note that in Table 8.2 fluxes are multiplied by corresponding membrane surface areas, that is, the apical flux represents $A^{LM} J_S^{LM}$ and the basolateral flux $A^{PM} J_S^{PM}$.

Following the approach outlined in previous paragraphs, this simple model could be extended (a) to include more species, such as acid-base pairs; (b) to explicitly account for the paracellular pathway and the barrier between the lateral space between cells and the peritubular space; (c) and to incorporate changes in luminal composition along the tubule.

8.4 Full Model Specification

Table 8.2 Epithelial cell concentration and fluxes

	Intracellular concentration (mM)	Apical flux (pmol/s/cm^2 epith)	Basolateral flux (pmol/s/cm^2 epith)
Na$^+$	14.4	677.7	−677.7
K$^+$	130.6	−387.1	387.1
Cl$^-$	25.0	57.2	−57.2
Impermeant	120.0	0	0

8.4.5 Current Limitations

As summarized by Weinstein (2003), recent mathematical models of renal tubular function have provided an accurate bookkeeping of solute and water transport, and they have yielded important insights into transport pathways, driving forces, and coupling mechanisms. Their main limitations can be divided into two categories: some stem from the paucity of experimental data, others are inherent to the model structure.

Model parameters are derived from in vivo and in vitro measurements. The structural properties of the epithelial barrier (i.e., morphological parameters) have overall been well characterized in rabbits and rats, but less so in mice – which is unfortunate, given the current importance of this animal model and the ease with which specific genes can be down- or up-regulated in this species. Transport parameters, such as permeability and kinetic data, are still lacking for a number of solutes, carriers, and cell types. In both cases, unknown values can generally be estimated by extrapolation or adjusted to match other experimental observations. More challenging situations arise when transport pathways remain to be fully characterized (e.g., when the transporter that mediates cell entry or exit has not been identified), or when new transporters are found to be expressed experimentally but their functional importance is unclear. Under these circumstances, mathematical models may be helpful in generating hypotheses; ultimately these will have to be validated experimentally.

Current models do not incorporate detailed intracellular signaling cascades, but could easily be expanded to do so, by adding more solutes (such as messengers) and reaction rates. A more serious limitation is that these models do not consider spatial inhomogeneities within a given compartment. The cytoplasm includes a variety of organelles, as well as sub-plasmalemma microdomains, which necessarily affect the rate of intracellular diffusion, but also play active roles in transport and trafficking. Expanding current models to account for the complexity of intracellular organization represents a difficult endeavor. Finally, we should keep in mind that renal function results from the spatial (along the nephron), but also temporal, integration of transport processes. Developing cell-based, tubular models with a dynamic dimension is ultimately essential to understand how the kidney adapts to physiological and pathological changes in its environment.

Fig. 8.6 Schematic representation of a K^+/Cl^- cotransporter, with ordered binding. The Cl^- ion (denoted by "a") binds first to the empty carrier ("x"), followed by either K^+ ("b") or NH_4^+ ("g"). After translocation across the cell membrane, Cl^- unbinds last. The superscripts i and e denote the internal and external faces of the membrane, respectively

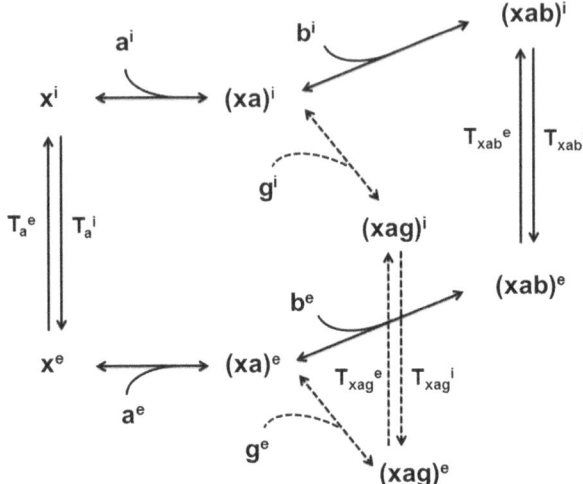

8.5 Problems

Problem 8.1. Determine the tight junction permeability of the rabbit thick ascending limb to Na^+, knowing that its resistance is 24.6 $\Omega \cdot cm^2$, and that the Na^+-to-Cl^- permeability ratio is 2.7:1.

Problem 8.2. Determinants of intracellular pH.

(a) Under physiological conditions, the intracellular pH (pH_i) is 7.2, the extracellular pH (pH_e) is 7.4, and the transmembrane voltage difference (V_m) is -60 mV. Show that protons passively diffuse into the cell.
(b) Assume that the concentration of NH_3 is the same on both sides of the membrane. Show that the Nernst potential of OH^- and NH_4^+ is the same as that of H^+. In which direction(s) do the first two ions move passively?

Problem 8.3. Explain why the Na^+/HCO_3^- cotransporter functions as an acid-extruder with a 1:2 stoichiometry, and as an acid-loader with a 1:3 stoichiometry. You may assume that the dissolved concentration of CO_2 is 1.2 mM both inside and outside the cell. State clearly your other assumptions.

Problem 8.4. Determine five relationships between rate constants, based upon the principle of detailed balance, for the thiazide-sensitive NaCl cotransporter depicted in Fig. 8.3.

Problem 8.5. Fluxes across a K^+/Cl^- cotransporter.

(a) Determine the fluxes of Cl^-, K^+ and NH_4^+ across the K^+/Cl^- cotransporter depicted in Fig. 8.6. Note that NH_4^+ competes with K^+ for the same binding sites. Assume that the internal and external binding affinities for each ion are identical. The forward and backward translocation rates differ, however.

(b) Plot the normalized outward Cl^- flux (relative to its maximal value) as a function of external Cl^- in the absence of NH_4^+. Assume that the forward and backward translocation rates are $T_x^i = 300,000\ s^{-1}$, $T_x^e = 30,000\ s^{-1}$, $T_{xab}^i = 10,000\ s^{-1}$, and $T_{xab}^e = 1,000\ s^{-1}$, and that the binding affinities for Cl^- and K^+ are 20 and 2 mM respectively. Set the cytosolic K^+ and Cl^- concentrations to 100 and 15 mM, and the external K^+ concentration to 5 mM.

Problem 8.6. Consider the Na^+/H^+ exchanger depicted in Fig. 8.2.

(a) Determine the fluxes of Na^+, H^+, and NH_4^+ across the exchanger when the internal and external binding affinities of each ion are different, and the forward and backward translocation rates for a given ion are also different.
(b) In the limiting case where there is negligible Na^+ on the internal side of the membrane, and negligible H^+ and NH_4^+ on the external side, calculate the H^+-NH_4^+ flux ratio. Express that ratio in terms of dimensional variables.

References

Boron, W.F.: Regulation of intracellular pH. Adv. Physiol. Educ. **28**(4), 160–179 (2004)
Chang, H., Fujita, T.: A kinetic model of the thiazide-sensitive Na-Cl cotransporter. Am. J. Physiol. Renal Physiol. **276**(6), F952–F959 (1999)
Garay, R.P., Garrahan, P.J.: The interaction of sodium and potassium with the sodium pump in red cells. J. Physiol. **231**, 297–325 (1973)
Job, G., Herrmann, F.: Chemical potential – a quantity in search of recognition. Eur. J. Phys. **27**, 353–371 (2006)
Koeppen, B.M.: Conductive properties of the rabbit outer medullary collecting duct: outer stripe. Am. J. Physiol. Renal Physiol. **250**(1), F70–F76 (1986)
Strieter, J., Stephenson, J.L., et al.: A mathematical model of the rabbit cortical collecting tubule. Am. J. Physiol. Renal Physiol. **263**, F1063–F1075 (1992)
Weinstein, A.M.: Nonequilibrium thermodynamic model of the rat proximal tubule epithelium. Biophys. J. **44**, 153–170 (1983)
Weinstein, A.M.: A kinetically defined Na+/H+ antiporter within a mathematical model of the rat proximal tubule. J. Gen. Physiol. **105**(5), 617–641 (1995)
Weinstein, A.M.: A mathematical model of the outer medullary collecting duct of the rat. Am. J. Physiol. Renal Physiol. **279**(1), F24–F45 (2000)
Weinstein, A.M.: Mathematical models of renal fluid and electrolyte transport: acknowledging our uncertainty. Am. J. Physiol. Renal Physiol. **284**(5), F871–F884 (2003)

Chapter 9
Solutions to Problem Sets

Chapter 2

Problem 2.1

Based on Eq. (2.11), K_f can be calculated as:

$$K_f = \frac{GFR}{<\Delta P> - <\Pi_{pr}^P>} = \frac{FF \cdot Q^A}{<P^P> - <P^B> - <\Pi_{pr}^P>}. \quad (9.1)$$

We assume that $<\Delta P> \approx P^{GC} - P^T$. The average oncotic pressure along the capillary can be estimated as the arithmetic average between the afferent and efferent values:

$$<\Pi_{pr}^P> = \frac{\Pi_{pr}^A + \Pi_{pr}^E}{2} = \frac{a_1(C_{pr}^A + C_{pr}^E) + a_2\left[(C_{pr}^A)^2 + (C_{pr}^E)^2\right]}{2}, \quad (9.2)$$

where we have used Eq. (2.27) to relate oncotic pressures to protein concentration. Intermediate and final results are tabulated in Table 9.1.

These results indicate that enalapril raised K_f nearly twofold in treated vs. untreated animals. This difference is mostly due to the reduced value of P^{GC} in treated animals (see Table 2.2), which itself stems from the vasodilatation induced by enalapril, leading to a reduction in efferent arteriolar resistance and in P^{GC}.

Problem 2.2

As stated above, the constant a_s can be obtained relatively easily from an overall mass balance equation. The molar flow of solute at the capillary outlet must equal that at the inlet minus that in Bowman's space. The volume flow rates at the outlet

Table 9.1 Ultrafiltration coefficient calculations

	$FF \cdot Q^A$ (nl/min)	$<\Delta P>$ (mmHg)	$<\Pi_{pr}^P>$ (mmHg)	K_f (nl/min/mmHg)	K_f (nl/s/mmHg)
Group 1	72.5	50	24.9	2.88	0.048
Group 2	67.8	36	23.6	5.46	0.091

and in Bowman's space are respectively given by $(1 - FF)Q^A$ and $(FF)Q^A$. The concentration of solute in Bowman's space is equal to $\theta_s C_s^A$, and that at the capillary outlet is given by:

$$C_s^P(x = L) = C_s^A [1 + a_s(1 - \exp(-b))]. \tag{9.3}$$

The mass balance equation can thus be written as:

$$Q^A C_s^A = (FF \cdot Q^A)(\theta_s C_s^A) + (1 - FF)Q^A C_s^A [1 + a_s(1 - \exp(-b))], \tag{9.4}$$

which after rearrangement yields:

$$a_s = \frac{FF(1 - \theta_s)}{(1 - FF)(1 - \exp(-b))}. \tag{9.5}$$

Problem 2.3

By definition of ω, the volume of filtrate passing through the shunts (J_V^{shunt}) can be written as:

$$J_V^{\text{shunt}} = \frac{\omega}{1 - \omega} J_V^{ro}, \tag{9.6}$$

where J_V^{ro} is the volume of filtrate passing through the population of small pores of radius r_o. As noted above, the driving flux for J_V^{shunt} is ΔP, since the non-selective pores do not restrict the passage of plasma proteins, whereas that for J_V^{ro} is $\Delta P - \Pi_{pr}^P$. Hence we have:

$$J_V^{\text{shunt}} = L_p^\omega \Delta P, \tag{9.7}$$

$$J_V^{ro} = L_p^{ro}(\Delta P - \Pi_{pr}^P), \tag{9.8}$$

where L_p^ω and L_p^{ro} are the hydraulic conductivity of the non-selective and small pores, respectively. Substituting Eqs. (9.7) and (9.8) into Eq. (9.6) and rearranging yields:

$$\frac{\omega}{1 - \omega} = \left(\frac{L_p^\omega}{L_p^{ro}}\right) \frac{\Delta P}{(\Delta P - \Pi_{pr}^P)}. \tag{9.9}$$

Let's rewrite Eq. (9.9) in the absence of plasma proteins: the fraction of the filtrate volume passing through the shunts is then ω_o, also by definition, and the driving force for fluid movement through the two pathways is the same (i.e., ΔP). Thus,

$$\frac{\omega_o}{1-\omega_o} = \left(\frac{L_p^{\omega_o}}{L_p^{ro}}\right). \tag{9.10}$$

As we have seen, the hydraulic conductivity of a given population of pores is inversely proportional to the viscosity of the fluid going through this population (Eq. 2.51). In the presence of plasma proteins, the viscosity of the filtrate going through the non-selective shunts is approximately that of plasma (η_p). In the absence of plasma proteins, this viscosity is equal to that of saline (η_s). Therefore:

$$\frac{L_p^{\omega}}{L_p^{\omega_o}} = \frac{\eta_s}{\eta_p}. \tag{9.11}$$

We then combine Eqs. (9.9)–(9.11) to eliminate hydraulic conductivities:

$$\frac{\omega}{1-\omega} = \left(\frac{L_p^{\omega}}{L_p^{ro}}\right)\frac{\Delta P}{(\Delta P - \Pi_{pr}^P)} = \left(\frac{L_p^{\omega}}{L_p^{\omega_o}}\right)\left(\frac{L_p^{\omega_o}}{L_p^{ro}}\right)\frac{\Delta P}{\Delta P - \Pi_{pr}^P}$$

$$= \left(\frac{\eta_s}{\eta_p}\right)\left(\frac{\omega_o}{1-\omega_o}\right)\frac{\Delta P}{(\Delta P - \Pi_{pr}^P)}, \tag{9.12}$$

which can be rearranged to yield:

$$\omega = \frac{1}{1 + \left(\frac{\eta_p}{\eta_s}\right)\left(\frac{1-\omega_o}{\omega_o}\right)\frac{(\Delta P - \Pi_{pr}^P)}{\Delta P}}. \tag{9.13}$$

Problem 2.4

The y-component of the solute flux can be obtained from Eq. (2.88):

$$N_s^y = v_y W_s C_s - H_s D_s^\infty \frac{\partial C_s}{\partial y}. \tag{9.14}$$

At steady state, N_s^y is constant. Thus, Eq. (9.14) can be integrated over the GBM thickness (between 0 and δ^{bm}) to obtain an expression similar to Eq. (2.19):

$$C_s(y) = b_1 \exp(\text{Pe}\, y/\delta^{bm}) + b_2, \tag{9.15}$$

where b_1 and b_2 are two constants to be determined from the boundary conditions, and

$$\text{Pe} = \frac{v_y W_s \delta^{bm}}{H_s D_s^\infty}. \tag{9.16}$$

Substituting Eq. (9.15) into the expression for the solute flux yields:

$$N_s^y = b_2 v_y W_s. \tag{9.17}$$

The boundary conditions are written as:

$$C_s = C_o^{bm}, \quad \text{at } y = 0, \tag{9.18}$$

$$C_s = C_\delta^{bm}, \quad \text{at } y = \delta^{bm}. \tag{9.19}$$

However, these upstream (C_o^{bm}) and downstream (C_δ^{bm}) concentrations are not known and must be expressed in terms of other variables. The boundary condition downstream is rewritten to incorporate epithelial variables:

$$C_\delta^{bm} = \phi_s C_o^{ep} = \phi_s \frac{C_\infty^{ep}}{\theta_s^{ep}}, \tag{9.20}$$

where ϕ_s is the glomerular basement membrane-to-epithelium concentration ratio at equilibrium, C_o^{ep} is the solute concentration at the upstream edge of the slit diaphragm, and C_∞^{ep} that far downstream from the slit. We then make use of the ultrafiltration condition at the downstream end of the slit, $C_\infty^{ep} = N_s^y/v_y$, to rewrite Eq. (9.20) as:

$$C_\delta^{bm} = \frac{\phi_s N_s^y}{\theta_s^{ep} v_y}. \tag{9.21}$$

Substitution of this equation into Eq. (9.17) allows us to determine b_2:

$$b_2 = \frac{N_s^y}{v_y W_s} = \left(\frac{\theta_s^{ep}}{\phi_s W_s}\right) C_\delta^{bm}. \tag{9.22}$$

From the first boundary condition, we infer that:

$$b_1 = C_o^{bm} - b_2 = C_o^{bm} - \left(\frac{\theta_s^{ep}}{\phi_s W_s}\right) C_\delta^{bm}. \tag{9.23}$$

We may now replace the values of b_1 and b_2 into Eq. (9.15):

$$C_s(y) = \left[C_o^{bm} - \left(\frac{\theta_s^{ep}}{\phi_s W_s}\right) C_\delta^{bm}\right] \exp(\text{Pe}\, y/\delta^{bm}) + \left(\frac{\theta_s^{ep}}{\phi_s W_s}\right) C_\delta^{bm}. \tag{9.24}$$

9 Solutions to Problem Sets

Our final aim is to determine the glomerular basement membrane sieving coefficient. Setting $y = \delta^{bm}$ into Eq. (9.24), we have:

$$C_\delta^{bm}(y) = \left[C_o^{bm} - \left(\frac{\theta_s^{ep}}{\phi_s W_s} \right) C_\delta^{bm} \right] \exp(\text{Pe}) + \left(\frac{\theta_s^{ep}}{\phi_s W_s} \right) C_\delta^{bm}. \tag{9.25}$$

Dividing each side by the upstream concentration C_o^{bm} yields:

$$\theta_s^{bm} = \left[1 - \left(\frac{\theta_s^{ep}}{\phi_s W_s} \right) \theta_s^{bm} \right] \exp(\text{Pe}) + \left(\frac{\theta_s^{ep}}{\phi_s W_s} \right) \theta_s^{bm}, \tag{9.26}$$

which can be rearranged as:

$$\theta_s^{bm} = \frac{\exp(\text{Pe})}{\left(\frac{\theta_s^{ep}}{\phi_s W_s} \right)(\exp(\text{Pe}) - 1) + 1}. \tag{9.27}$$

Lastly, we multiply both the numerator and denominator of the RHS of Eq. (9.27) by the product $\phi_s W_s \exp(-\text{Pe})$ to obtain the result in final form:

$$\theta_s^{bm} = \frac{\phi_s W_s}{\theta_s^{ep}(1 - \exp(-\text{Pe})) + \phi_s W_s \exp(-\text{Pe})}. \tag{9.28}$$

Chapter 3

Problem 3.1

(a) Adding up the solute conservation equations for the collecting duct and central core, we get

$$2\pi (r_{\text{CD}} J_{\text{CD},V} + r_{\text{CC}} J_{\text{CC},V}) C + (F_{\text{CD},V} + F_{\text{CC},V}) \frac{\partial}{\partial x} C$$
$$= -2\pi r_{\text{CD}} J_{\text{CD},S} - 2\pi r_{\text{CC}} J_{\text{CC},S}.$$

Because both the descending and ascending limbs are water impermeable,

$$r_{\text{CD}} J_{\text{CD},V} + r_{\text{CC}} J_{\text{CC},V} = 0.$$

Since by assumption, $J_{\text{CD},S} = 0$, we have

$$r_{\text{CC}} J_{\text{CC},S} = -(r_{\text{DL}} J_{\text{DL},S} + r_{\text{AL}} J_{\text{AL},S}).$$

Thus,

$$C' = \frac{2\pi(r_{\text{DL}}J_{\text{DL},S} + r_{\text{AL}}J_{\text{AL},S})}{F_{\text{CD},V} + F_{\text{CC},V}} = \frac{2\pi(r_{\text{DL}}J_{\text{DL},S} + r_{\text{AL}}J_{\text{AL},S})}{\frac{1}{C}(F_{\text{CD},S} + F_{\text{CC},S})}, \quad (9.29)$$

$$\frac{C'(x)}{C(x)} = \frac{2\pi(r_{\text{DL}}J_{\text{DL},S}(x) + r_{\text{AL}}J_{\text{AL},S}(x))}{F_{\text{CD},S}(x) - 2\pi \int_x^L (r_{\text{DL}}J_{\text{DL},S}(s) + r_{\text{AL}}J_{\text{AL},S}(s)) \, ds}, \quad (9.30)$$

$$= \frac{2\pi(r_{\text{DL}}J_{\text{DL},S}(x) + r_{\text{AL}}J_{\text{AL},S}(x))}{F_{\text{CD},S}(L) - 2\pi \int_x^L (r_{\text{DL}}J_{\text{DL},S}(s) + r_{\text{AL}}J_{\text{AL},S}(s)) \, ds},$$

since $J_{\text{CD},S} = 0$. \hfill (9.31)

Solving this ODE, we obtain

$$\frac{C(L)}{C(0)} = \frac{F_{\text{CD},S}(L)}{F_{\text{CD},S}(L) - A}, \quad (9.32)$$

where A is given in Eq. (3.51).
(b) The answer can be seen by taking the limit $A \to F_{\text{CD},S}(L)$ in Eq. (9.32).
(c) Consider $A = F_{\text{CD},S}(L)$. Since only the collecting duct is water permeable, all the water flowing up the central core must been withdrawn from the collecting duct. Since we assume $C_{\text{CC}}(0) = C(0)$, the amount to be withdrawn is $|F_{\text{CC},V}| = A/C(0)$. But since $A = F_{\text{CD},S}(L) = F_{\text{CD},S}(0)$ (recall $J_{\text{CD},S} = 0$), and $C_{\text{CD}} = C(0)$ (by assumption), $|F_{\text{CC},V}(0)| = F_{\text{CD},V}(0)$. Thus, when $A = F_{\text{CD},S}(L)$, all the water in the collecting duct, exactly, is withdrawn into the central core, leaving only (dry) solute to emerge from the collecting duct. Then clearly, $A > F_{\text{CD},S}(L)$ would require the removal of more than is available in the collecting duct.
(d) In an actual avian medulla, a large axial concentration gradient in the interstitium and vasculature would extract substantial water from the slightly water-permeable descending limbs. Also, because of imperfect counter-current exchange, the net outflow concentration through the vasculature, analogous to $C_{\text{CC}}(0)$, may (indeed, will) exceed $C_{\text{CD}}(0)$. Thus it needs not carry away all of the water flowing into the collecting duct.

Problem 3.2

(a) We will follow the derivation of Eq. (3.44). In the upper half of the outer medulla, where all the descending limbs are infinitely water permeable, Eq. (3.35) holds. In the lower half, Eq. (3.35) holds for 1/3 of the descending limbs. Then by adding up the solute conservation equations for the descending limbs, collecting duct, and central core, we get Eq. (3.37). In the upper half, Eq. (3.38) holds. In the lower half, $J_{\text{DL},V} = 0$ for 2/3 of the descending limbs

9 Solutions to Problem Sets

and $C_{DL} \neq C_{CC}$ for those limbs. Thus, we add up solute conservation equations for only the water-permeable tubules and central core:

$$2\pi \left(\frac{1}{3}r_{DL}J_{DL,V} + r_{CD}J_{CD,V} + r_{CC}J_{CC,V}\right)C + \left(\frac{1}{3}F_{DL,V} + F_{CD,V} + F_{CC,V}\right)\frac{\partial}{\partial x}C$$
$$= -2\pi r_{AL}J_{AL,S}. \tag{9.33}$$

It follows that

$$\frac{C'(x)}{C(x)} = \frac{2\pi r_{AL}J_{AL,S}(x)}{\delta(x)F_{DL,S}(0) + F_{CD,S}(L) - 2\pi r_{AL}\int_x^L J_{AL,S}(s)\,ds}, \tag{9.34}$$

where

$$\delta(x) = \begin{cases} 1, & 0 \leq x \leq L/2, \\ \frac{1}{3}, & L/2 < x < L. \end{cases}$$

Thus,

$$\frac{C(\frac{L}{2})}{C(0)} = \exp\left[\int_0^{L/2} \frac{2\pi r_{AL}J_{AL,S}(x)}{F_{DL,S}(0) + F_{CD,S}(L) - 2\pi r_{AL}\int_x^L J_{AL,S}(s)\,ds}\,dx\right] \tag{9.35}$$

$$= \left[F_{DL,S}(0) + F_{CD,S}(L) - 2\pi r_{AL}\int_x^L J_{AL,S}(s)\,ds\right]_0^{L/2}. \tag{9.36}$$

Similarly,

$$\frac{C(L)}{C(\frac{L}{2})} = \left[\frac{1}{3}F_{DL,S}(0) + F_{CD,S}(L) - 2\pi r_{AL}\int_x^L J_{AL,S}(s)\,ds\right]_{L/2}^L. \tag{9.37}$$

So

$$R = \frac{C(\frac{L}{2})}{C(0)} \times \frac{C(L)}{C(\frac{L}{2})},$$

which can be obtained by multiplying the right-hand-sides of Eqs. (9.36) and (9.37).

(b)

$$\frac{C(\frac{L}{2})}{C(0)} = \frac{M + \frac{M}{10} - \frac{M}{4}}{M + \frac{M}{10} - \frac{M}{2}} = \frac{1 + \frac{1}{10} - \frac{1}{4}}{1 + \frac{1}{10} - \frac{1}{2}} = \frac{17}{12}, \tag{9.38}$$

$$\frac{C(L)}{C(\frac{L}{2})} = \frac{\frac{M}{3} + \frac{M}{10} - 0}{\frac{M}{3} + \frac{M}{10} - \frac{M}{2}} = \frac{\frac{1}{3} + \frac{1}{10}}{\frac{1}{3} + \frac{1}{10} - \frac{1}{4}} = \frac{26}{11}, \qquad (9.39)$$

$$\frac{C(L)}{C(0)} = \frac{17}{12} \times \frac{26}{11} = \frac{221}{66} \approx 3.3,$$

nearly twice the value for the case where all the descending limbs are water permeable.

Chapter 4

Problem 4.1

We begin by combining Eqs. (4.2) for DVR, and (4.4) for AVR:

$$\frac{dC_S^D}{dx} = -\frac{P_S S^P}{LQ^P}(C_S^D - C_S^I) = -\frac{\Omega}{L}(C_S^D - C_S^I), \qquad (9.40)$$

$$\frac{dC_S^A}{dx} = +\frac{P_S S^P}{LQ^P}(C_S^A - C_S^I) = \frac{\Omega}{L}(C_S^A - C_S^I). \qquad (9.41)$$

In addition, given the assumption of a linear interstitial concentration profile, we have:

$$\frac{dC_S^I}{dx} = \frac{C_L - C_0}{L}. \qquad (9.42)$$

Subtracting Eq. (9.42) from the two previous equations yields:

$$\frac{d(C_S^D - C_S^I)}{dx} = -\frac{\Omega}{L}(C_S^D - C_S^I) - \frac{(C_L - C_0)}{L}, \qquad (9.43)$$

$$\frac{d(C_S^A - C_S^I)}{dx} = +\frac{\Omega}{L}(C_S^A - C_S^I) - \frac{(C_L - C_0)}{L}. \qquad (9.44)$$

This system is easily solved for $(C_S^D - C_S^I)$ and $(C_S^A - C_S^I)$, yielding:

$$C_S^D - C_S^I = A \exp(-\Omega x/L) - \frac{C_L - C_0}{\Omega}, \qquad (9.45)$$

$$C_S^A - C_S^I = B \exp(+\Omega x/L) + \frac{C_L - C_0}{\Omega}, \qquad (9.46)$$

9 Solutions to Problem Sets

where A and B are constants to be determined using the boundary conditions. At $x = 0$, we have:

$$C_S^D(0) - C_S^I(0) = 0 = A - \frac{C_L - C_0}{\Omega}. \tag{9.47}$$

Substituting the value of A into Eq. (9.45), we obtain the desired expression for the DVR solute concentration profile:

$$C_S^D(x) = C_S^I(x) - \frac{(C_L - C_0)}{\Omega}[1 - \exp(-\Omega x/L)]. \tag{9.48}$$

At $x = L$, there is continuity between DVR and AVR, so that:

$$C_S^A(L) - C_S^D(L) = 0 = B\exp(+\Omega) + \frac{(C_L - C_0)}{\Omega} - A\exp(-\Omega) + \frac{(C_L - C_0)}{\Omega}. \tag{9.49}$$

The constant B is thus equal to:

$$B = -\frac{2(C_L - C_0)}{\Omega}\exp(-\Omega) + A\exp(-2\Omega)$$

$$= \frac{(C_L - C_0)}{\Omega}[\exp(-2\Omega) - 2\exp(-\Omega)]. \tag{9.50}$$

Substituting this value into Eq. (9.46) yields the full AVR concentration profile:

$$C_S^A(x) = C_S^I(x) + \frac{(C_L - C_0)}{\Omega}[1 + \exp(-\Omega(2 - x/L)) - 2\exp(-\Omega(1 - x/L))]. \tag{9.51}$$

Problem 4.2

The DVR water fluxes via the shared pathway and AQP1 are respectively given by (Eqs. 4.27 and 4.29):

$$J_{V,p}^{DVR} = L_{p,p}^{DVR}(\Delta P - \sigma_{pr}\Delta\Pi_{pr}), \tag{9.52}$$

$$J_{V,t}^{DVR} = L_{p,t}^{DVR}(\Delta P - \Delta\Pi_{pr} - RT\sum_{ss}\gamma_{ss}\Delta C_{ss}), \tag{9.53}$$

where

$$\Delta P - \sigma_{pr}\Delta\Pi_{pr} = (P^P - P^I) - \sigma_{pr}(\Pi_{pr}^P - \Pi_{pr}^I), \tag{9.54}$$

$$\Pi_{pr} = 2.1 C_{pr} + 0.16(C_{pr})^2 + 0.009(C_{pr})^3. \tag{9.55}$$

- As described above, $L_{p,p}^{DVR}$ and $L_{p,t}^{DVR}$ were respectively estimated as 1.75×10^{-6} cm·s^{-1}·mmHg^{-1} (assuming that $\sigma_{alb} = 0.89$) and 1.02×10^{-7} cm·s^{-1}·mmHg^{-1}.
- Based on the data given in Sect. 4.4.1, we assume that the hydraulic pressure is 10 mmHg in DVR lumen, and 5 mmHg in the interstitium. Thus, $\Delta P = 5$ mmHg.
- The plasma protein concentration in DVR is taken as 6.8 g/dl (Table 4.1), which yields $\Pi_{pr}^P = 24.5$ mmHg. Assuming that the reflection coefficient of the shared pathway to albumin and other proteins is 0.89, we estimate $\sigma_{pr}\Pi_{pr}^P$ as 21.8 mmHg for the shared pathway.
- As stated below Table 4.1, $\gamma_{sodium} = 1.86$ and $\gamma_{urea} = 0.90$. In addition, $R = 62.36$ mmHg·K^{-1}·M^{-1}. Hence:

$$RT \sum_{ss = sodium, urea} \gamma_{ss} \Delta C_{ss}$$
$$= (62.36)(37 + 273)[1.86(-10 \times 10^{-3}) + 0.9(-10 \times 10^{-3})]$$
$$= -533.6 \text{ mmHg}. \tag{9.56}$$

Note that RT equals 19.3 mmHg/mM at 37 °C; in other words, a 1 mM concentration gradient exerts an osmotic pressure of 19.3 mmHg across the transcellular pathway. We may now calculate the transcapillary fluxes for both limiting cases.

Case (a)

$$J_{V,p}^{DVR} = L_{p,p}^{DVR}(\Delta P - \sigma_{pr}\Delta \Pi_{pr})$$
$$= (1.75 \times 10^{-6})(5 - 21.8) = -2.94 \times 10^{-5} \text{ cm/s}, \tag{9.57}$$

$$J_{V,t}^{DVR} = L_{p,t}^{DVR}(\Delta P - \Delta \Pi_{pr} - RT\sum_{ss}\gamma_{ss}\Delta C_{ss})$$
$$= (1.02 \times 10^{-7})(5 - 24.5 + 533.6) = +5.24 \times 10^{-5} \text{ cm/s}. \tag{9.58}$$

Thus, AQP1 mediates water efflux into the interstitium, whereas water enters the lumen via the shared pathway. The net flux is directed outwardly, that is, $J_{V,p}^{DVR} + J_{V,t}^{DVR} > 0$. These calculations suggest that there is net water loss from DVR, as observed experimentally.

Case (b)

$$J_{V,p}^{DVR} = L_{p,p}^{DVR}(\Delta P)$$
$$= (1.75 \times 10^{-6})(5) = +8.75 \times 10^{-5} \text{ cm/s}, \tag{9.59}$$

$$J_{V,t}^{DVR} = L_{p,t}^{DVR}(\Delta P - RT\sum_{ss}\gamma_{ss}\Delta C_{ss})$$
$$= (1.02 \times 10^{-7})(5 + 533.6) = +5.49 \times 10^{-5} \text{ cm/s}. \tag{9.60}$$

In this case, the paracellular pathway is predicted to mediate water efflux. However, the assumption that the oncotic pressure is as high in the interstitium as it is in DVR may not be compatible with water uptake by AVR.

Problem 4.3

Oxygen is carried both in free form and as HbO$_2$ in DVR blood. The total amount of O$_2$ in a single DVR at $x = 0$ is thus given by:

$$S_{O2}^{DVR} = Q^P(0)C_{O2}^P(0) + Q^R(0)\left[C_{O2}^R(0) + C_{HbO_2}^R(0)\right]. \quad (9.61)$$

If the total blood flow is 9 nl/min and the hematocrit is 0.25, then $Q^P(0) = 6.75$ nl/min $= 0.1125 \times 10^{-9}$ l/s, and $Q^R(0) = 2.25$ nl/min $= 0.0375 \times 10^{-9}$ l/s.

With a solubility coefficient equal to 1.34 µM/mmHg in plasma and 1.56 in RBCs, we have:

$$C_{O2}^P(0) = 50(1.34) = 67 \,\mu\text{mol/l} = 67 \times 10^{-6} \,\text{mol/l}, \quad (9.62)$$

$$C_{O2}^R(0) = 50(1.56) = 78 \,\mu\text{mol/l} = 78 \times 10^{-6} \,\text{mol/l}. \quad (9.63)$$

The concentration of HbO$_2$ is calculated based on the equilibrium curve (Eq. 4.41), assuming a total hemoglobin concentration of 5.1 mM.

$$C_{HbO_2}^R = (C_{HbO_2}^R + C_{Hb}^R)\left[\frac{(C_{O2}^R/C_{50})^n}{1 + (C_{O2}^R/C_{50})^n}\right], \quad (9.64)$$

$$C_{HbO_2}^R = (5.1 \times 10^{-3})\left[\frac{(50/26.4)^{2.6}}{1 + (50/26.4)^{2.6}}\right] = (5.1 \times 10^{-3})\left[\frac{5.26}{1 + 5.26}\right]$$

$$= 4.29 \times 10^{-3} \,\text{mol/l}. \quad (9.65)$$

Note that the RBC concentration of HbO$_2$ is about two orders of magnitude higher than that of O$_2$. We may now calculate the total amount of O$_2$ supplied to the medulla by a single DVR:

$$S_{O2}^{DVR} = (0.1125 \times 10^{-9})(67 \times 10^{-6}) + (0.0375 \times 10^{-9})(78 \times 10^{-6} + 4.29 \times 10^{-3}), \quad (9.66)$$

$$S_{O2}^{DVR} = 1.71 \times 10^{-13} \,\text{mol/s}. \quad (9.67)$$

Note that the fraction of O$_2$ that is carried as HbO$_2$ under these conditions is 93.9 %.

Problem 4.4

This problem was inspired by the elegant study of counter-current oxygen transfer in fish gills by Layton (1987).

(a) Since solubility coefficients are equal in both fluids, we may substitute O_2 tension (P) for O_2 concentration (C) in the standard conservation equations. Following the approach described in Sect. 4.2, we have:

$$\frac{dQ^F P^F(x)}{dx} = -\gamma \left[P^F(x) - P^B(x) \right], \quad (9.68)$$

$$\frac{dQ^B P^B(x)}{dx} = \pm \gamma \left[P^B(x) - P^F(x) \right], \quad (9.69)$$

where the "+" and "−" signs apply to counter-current and co-current flows, respectively. Since volume flows are constant, we may rewrite the system as:

$$\frac{dP^F(x)}{dx} = -\frac{\gamma}{Q^F} \left[P^F(x) - P^B(x) \right], \quad (9.70)$$

$$\frac{dP^B(x)}{dx} = \pm \frac{\gamma}{Q^B} \left[P^B(x) - P^F(x) \right]. \quad (9.71)$$

Using the notation given above, the differential equations are written as:

$$\frac{dP^F(x)}{dx} = -a \left[P^F(x) - P^B(x) \right], \quad (9.72)$$

$$\frac{dP^B(x)}{dx} = -\sigma b \left[P^B(x) - P^F(x) \right], \quad (9.73)$$

where $\sigma = -1$ for counter-current flow, and $+1$ for co-current flow.

(b) Equations (9.72) and (9.73) must now be solved subject to the boundary conditions

$$P^F(x = 0) = P_I, \quad (9.74)$$

$$\begin{cases} P^B(x = 0) = P_V, \text{ for co-current flow,} \\ P^B(x = 1) = P_V, \text{ for counter-current flow.} \end{cases} \quad (9.75)$$

Subtracting Eq. (9.73) from Eq. (9.72) yields:

$$\frac{d[P^F(x) - P^B(x)]}{dx} = -(a + \sigma b)[P^F(x) - P^B(x)]. \quad (9.76)$$

Co-current flow ($\sigma = +1$)
If $a = b$, then $a + \sigma b = 2a$, and integration of (9.76) yields:

$$P^F(x) - P^B(x) = D \exp(-2ax), \tag{9.77}$$

where D is an integration constant, which can be solved using the boundary conditions at $x = 0$:

$$P^F(0) - P^B(0) = D = P_I - P_V. \tag{9.78}$$

Knowing the value of D, we now substitute Eq. (9.77) into Eq. (9.72). After integrating the resulting equation and taking into account the boundary condition (9.74), we obtain:

$$P^F(x) = P_I - \frac{(P_I - P_V)}{2}[1 - \exp(-2ax)]. \tag{9.79}$$

The O_2 tension profile in blood is derived in a similar manner:

$$P^B(x) = P_I - \frac{(P_I - P_V)}{2}[1 + \exp(-2ax)]. \tag{9.80}$$

Or equivalently,

$$P^B(x) = P_V + \frac{(P_I - P_V)}{2}[1 - \exp(-2ax)]. \tag{9.81}$$

Counter-current Flow ($\sigma = -1$)
If $a = b$, then $a + \sigma b = 0$, and integration of (9.76) yields:

$$P^F(x) - P^B(x) = D. \tag{9.82}$$

The constant D can be evaluated using the boundary conditions at $x = 0$:

$$P^F(0) - P^B(0) = D = P_I - P_A. \tag{9.83}$$

Note that P_A, the value of which is a priori unknown, will be subsequently replaced with known parameters. Substituting Eq. (9.82) into Eqs. (9.72) and (9.73) yields:

$$\frac{dP^F(x)}{dx} = -a(P_I - P_A), \tag{9.84}$$

$$\frac{dP^B(x)}{dx} = -a(P_I - P_A). \tag{9.85}$$

Thus, in the counter-current arrangement, P^F and P^B vary linearly with x. Integrating these two equations, we obtain:

$$P^F(x) = P_I - a(P_I - P_A)x, \tag{9.86}$$

$$P^B(x) = P_A - a(P_I - P_A)x. \tag{9.87}$$

We must now eliminate P_A from both equations. At $x = 1$, we have:

$$P^B(x = 1) = P_V = P_A - a(P_I - P_A). \tag{9.88}$$

Hence,

$$P_A = \frac{P_V + aP_I}{1 + a}. \tag{9.89}$$

After some rearrangement, the O_2 tension profiles for counter-current flow are written as:

$$P^F(x) = P_I - (P_I - P_V)\frac{ax}{1+a}, \tag{9.90}$$

$$P^B(x) = P_V - (P_I - P_V)\frac{a(x-1)}{1+a}. \tag{9.91}$$

(c) The rate of oxygen removal from the fluid F is given by:

$$R_{O2} = Q^F[P^F(0) - P^F(1)]. \tag{9.92}$$

For co-current flow, we have:

$$R_{O2}^{co} = Q^F(P_I - P_V)\left[\frac{1 - \exp(-2a)}{2}\right]. \tag{9.93}$$

For counter-current flow:

$$R_{O2}^{cr} = Q^F(P_I - P_V)\left[\frac{a}{1+a}\right]. \tag{9.94}$$

(d) The counter-current to co-current ratio of O_2 removal rate thus equals:

$$R_{O2}^{cr}/R_{O2}^{co} = \left[\frac{2a}{1+a}\right]\left[\frac{1}{1-\exp(-2a)}\right]. \tag{9.95}$$

The ratio R_{O2}^{cr}/R_{O2}^{co} is plotted as a function of the parameter a in Fig. 9.1. It is always greater than 1.0, which means that the counter-current configuration is more efficient than the co-current one, in that it allows more O_2 to be absorbed from the surrounding fluid into blood. It can easily be shown that the maximal value of R_{O2}^{cr}/R_{O2}^{co} is 2.

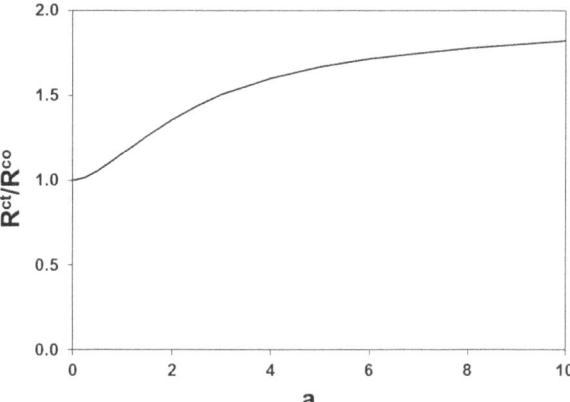

Fig. 9.1 Counter-current to co-current ratio of the rate at which O_2 is removed from fluid F, as a function of $a = \gamma Q^F$ (see text). The ratio is >1, which means that counter-current O_2 transfer is more efficient than co-current transfer

Chapter 5

Problem 5.1

We will compute the solution to the delayed differential equation

$$\frac{dx}{dt} = -2x(t-1), \tag{9.96}$$

with initial history

$$x(t) = 1, \quad t \leq 0. \tag{9.97}$$

We consider time intervals $(0, 1]$, $(t, 2]$, $(2, 3]$, etc. Over the interval $t \in (0, 1]$, $x(t-1) = 1$ as given by the initial history. Thus, we have

$$\frac{dx}{dt} = -2, \quad t \in (0, t], \tag{9.98}$$

with initial condition $x(0) = 1$. Hence,

$$x(t) = 1 - 2\int_0^t 1\, ds = 1 - 2t. \tag{9.99}$$

Over the next interval $(1, 2]$, with initial condition $x(1) = -1$, we have

$$x(t) = -1 - \int_1^t 1 - 2(s-1)\, ds = -1 - \left(3t - t^2\right)\Big|_1^t = t^2 - 3t + 1. \tag{9.100}$$

At $t = 2$, $x(2) = -1$. In the interval $(2, 3]$,

$$x(t) = -1 - \int_2^t (s-1)^2 - 3(s-1) + 1 \, ds \qquad (9.101)$$

$$= -\frac{(t-1)^3}{3} + \frac{3(t-1)^2}{2} - t - \frac{1}{6}. \qquad (9.102)$$

Problem 5.2

(a) Linearize $\mathscr{C}$ about the steady-state TAL transit time T_{MD}:

$$\mathscr{C}(T_{MD}(t)) \approx \mathscr{C}(1) + (T_{MD}(t) - 1)\mathscr{C}'(1). \qquad (9.103)$$

(b) Substituting the above linearization into Eqs. (5.16) and (5.48), we obtain

$$\mathscr{F}(t) \approx 1 + K_1 \tanh\left(\frac{\gamma}{K_1}(T_{MD}(t-\tau) - 1)\right), \qquad (9.104)$$

where $\gamma = -K_1 K_2 S'(1)$ and $S(x)$ denotes the steady-state concentration profile.

(c) Consider Eq. (5.50) as an implicit equation for transit time T_x. Set $x = 1$, so that $T_x = T_{MD}$, and linearize x by expanding in a Taylor series to first order about $T_{MD} = 1$:

$$1 \approx \int_{t-1}^t \mathscr{F}(s) \, ds + (T_{MD}(t) - 1)\mathscr{F}(t-1). \qquad (9.105)$$

By solving this equation for T_{MD}, we obtain

$$T_{MD}(t) \approx 1 + \frac{1 - \int_{t-1}^t \mathscr{F}(s) \, ds}{\mathscr{F}(t-1)} = 1 + \frac{\int_{t-1}^t (1 - \mathscr{F}(s)) \, ds}{\mathscr{F}(t-1)}. \qquad (9.106)$$

(d) The expression can be obtained by considering the linearizations to be exact and substituting.

Problem 5.3

Expand the following expressions around their steady-state values:

$$F(S(L) + \epsilon c_\epsilon(L, t - \tau)) = F(C_{op}) + \epsilon F'(C_{op}) c_\epsilon(L, t - \tau) + \mathcal{O}(\epsilon^2), \qquad (9.107)$$

$$K(S(x) + \epsilon c_\epsilon(x, t)) = K(S(x)) + \epsilon K'(S(x)) c_\epsilon(x, t) + \mathcal{O}(\epsilon^2). \qquad (9.108)$$

9 Solutions to Problem Sets

We then substitute the above expressions into Eq. (5.21), allow the steady-state terms from (5.17) to drop out, and keep only the remaining $\mathcal{O}(\epsilon)$ terms to arrive at Eq. (5.23).

Chapter 6

Problem 6.1

We begin by rewriting Eq. (6.17) for unidirectional transport:

$$J_s = -D_s \left(\frac{dC_s}{dx} + \frac{z_s F}{RT} C_s \frac{d\psi}{dx} \right), \qquad (9.109)$$

where J_s is the outward solute flux, and the axial coordinate x goes from 0 (at the cytosol-membrane interface) to L_m (at the outer edge of the membrane). Assuming that the electrical field is constant across the membrane (i.e., $d\psi/dx = -V_m/L_m$), Eq. (9.109) becomes

$$J_s = -D_s \left(\frac{dC_s}{dx} - \frac{z_s F V_m}{L_m RT} C_s \right). \qquad (9.110)$$

Let $\xi = z_s F V_m / RT$. At steady state, J_s is constant across the membrane, and Eq. (9.110) can be first transformed, then integrated, to determine $C_s(x)$:

$$\frac{dC_s}{dx} - \frac{\xi}{L_m} C_s + \frac{J_s}{D_s} = 0, \qquad (9.111)$$

$$C_s(x) = a \exp(\xi x / L_m) + \frac{J_s L_m}{\xi D_s}. \qquad (9.112)$$

To determine the integration constant a and the unknown J_s, we use the two boundary conditions:

$$C_s(0) = a + \frac{J_s L_m}{\xi D_s} = C_s^i, \qquad (9.113)$$

$$C_s(L_m) = a \exp(\xi) + \frac{J_s L_m}{\xi D_s} = C_s^e. \qquad (9.114)$$

We obtain:

$$a = \frac{C_s^i - C_s^e}{1 - \exp(\xi)}, \qquad (9.115)$$

$$\frac{J_s L_m}{\xi D_s} = C_s^i - a = \frac{C_s^e - C_s^i \exp(\xi)}{1 - \exp(\xi)}. \tag{9.116}$$

Rearranging Eq. (9.116) yields:

$$J_s = \frac{D_s}{L_m} \xi \frac{C_s^e - C_s^i \exp(\xi)}{1 - \exp(\xi)} = \frac{D_s}{L_m} \xi \frac{C_s^e \exp(-\xi) - C_s^i}{\exp(-\xi) - 1}. \tag{9.117}$$

Substituting the definition of ξ into Eq. (9.117), we finally obtain the flux equation that leads to the GHK current equation:

$$J_s = \frac{D_s}{L_m} \frac{z_s F V_m}{RT} \frac{C_s^i - C_s^e \exp(-z_s F V_m/RT)}{1 - \exp(-z_s F V_m/RT)}. \tag{9.118}$$

Problem 6.2

The temporal variation in the fraction of open channels obeys the following equation:

$$\frac{dn}{dt} = \frac{n_\infty - n}{\tau}, \tag{9.119}$$

where the equilibrium fraction at a given V_m is given by:

$$n_\infty = \frac{1}{1 + \exp(-F V_m/RT)}. \tag{9.120}$$

Assuming that the channel operates at 37 °C, $RT/F = 26.73$ mV, so that:

$$n_\infty(V_m = -60) = \frac{1}{1 + \exp(+60/26.73)} = 0.0958, \tag{9.121}$$

$$n_\infty(V_m = +60) = \frac{1}{1 + \exp(-60/26.73)} = 0.9042. \tag{9.122}$$

The time course of n between 0 and 10τ is therefore determined by integrating Eq. (9.119) in two steps:

- $0 \le t \le 5\tau$ (depolarization phase): the initial condition is $n(t < 0) = 0.0958$, and $n_\infty = 0.9042$;
- $5\tau \le t \le 10\tau$ (repolarization phase): the initial condition is $n(t = 5\tau)$, and $n_\infty = 0.0958$.

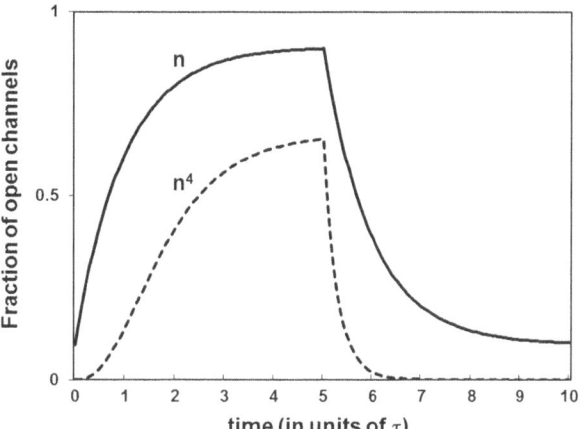

Fig. 9.2 Time course of the fraction of open channels, following a step increase in V_m from -60 to $+60\,\mathrm{mV}$ at $t = 0$, and a step decrease from $+60$ to $-60\,\mathrm{mV}$ at $t = 5\tau$. The channel consists of either one unit (n) or four identical subunits (n^4)

Results for n and n^4 are shown in Fig. 9.2. Upon depolarization, the 4-subunit channel opens more slowly than the one-unit channel; conversely, the 4-subunit channel closes faster upon repolarization.

Problem 6.3

The internal and external electrochemical potentials of solute S are given in Eqs. (6.5) and (6.6) and reproduced below:

$$\mu_s^i = RT \ln C_s^i + z_s F \psi^i, \tag{9.123}$$

$$\mu_s^e = RT \ln C_s^e + z_s F \psi^e. \tag{9.124}$$

Thus, the internal-to-external electrochemical potential difference equals:

$$\Delta \mu_S = RT(\ln C_s^i - \ln C_s^e) + z_s F(\psi^i - \psi^e)$$
$$= RT \ln(C_s^i / C_s^e) + z_s F V_m. \tag{9.125}$$

NCX, which exchanges 1 Ca^{2+} ion for 3 Na^+ ions, is at equilibrium when $\Delta \mu_{Ca} = 3\Delta \mu_{Na+}$, that is:

$$[RT \ln(C_{Ca}^i / C_{Ca}^e) + z_{Ca} F V_m] = 3[RT \ln(C_{Na}^i / C_{Na}^e) + z_{Na} F V_m]. \tag{9.126}$$

Since $z_{Ca} = 2$ and $z_{Na} = 1$, this equation can be rewritten as:

$$RT[\ln(C_{Ca}^i / C_{Ca}^e) - 3 \ln(C_{Na}^i / C_{Na}^e)] = F V_m. \tag{9.127}$$

Rearranging Eq. (9.127), we obtain:

$$\ln\left(\frac{C_{Ca}^i (C_{Na}^e)^3}{C_{Ca}^e (C_{Na}^i)^3}\right) = V_m F/RT. \tag{9.128}$$

This equilibrium relationship can also be expressed as:

$$\frac{C_{Ca}^i}{C_{Ca}^e} = \frac{(C_{Na}^i)^3}{(C_{Na}^e)^e} \exp(V_m F/RT). \tag{9.129}$$

This equation is identical to Eq. (6.38), in which the superscript "i" denoting the internal compartment has been replaced with "cyt" for cytosol.

Problem 6.4

The kinetic scheme shown in Fig. 6.10 yields the following mass balance equations:

$$\frac{dP_{C1}}{dt} = k_a^- P_{O1} - k_a^+ (C_{Ca}^{cyt})^4 P_{C1}, \tag{9.130}$$

$$\frac{dP_{O2}}{dt} = k_b^+ (C_{Ca}^{cyt})^3 P_{O1} - k_b^- P_{O2}, \tag{9.131}$$

$$\frac{dP_{C2}}{dt} = k_c^+ P_{O1} - k_c^- P_{C2}, \tag{9.132}$$

$$P_{O1} = 1 - P_{O2} - P_{C1} - P_{C2}. \tag{9.133}$$

Assuming that the kinetic steps a and b equilibrate rapidly compared with step c, we have $dP_{C1}/dt \approx 0$, $dP_{O2}/dt \approx 0$ on the slow time scale of changes in P_{C2}. Hence:

$$P_{C1} = \frac{k_a^- P_{O1}}{k_a^+ (C_{Ca}^{cyt})^4} = (K_a/C_{Ca}^{cyt})^4 P_{O1}, \tag{9.134}$$

$$P_{O2} = \frac{k_b^+ (C_{Ca}^{cyt})^3 P_{O1}}{k_b^-} = (C_{Ca}^{cyt}/K_b)^3 P_{O1}. \tag{9.135}$$

The fraction of channels not in state C_2, $\omega \equiv 1 - P_{C2}$, is thus equal to:

$$\omega = P_{O1} + P_{C1} + P_{O2} = P_{O1}\left[1 + (K_a/C_{Ca}^{cyt})^4 + (C_{Ca}^{cyt}/K_b)^3\right]. \tag{9.136}$$

That is,

$$P_{O1} = \frac{\omega}{1 + (K_a/C_{Ca}^{cyt})^4 + (C_{Ca}^{cyt}/K_b)^3}. \tag{9.137}$$

The probability that the channel is in an open state is given by the sum of $P_{O1} + P_{O2}$. Thus combining Eqs. (9.135) and (9.137), we obtain the first desired equation:

$$P_{RyR} = P_{O1} + P_{O2} = \frac{\omega[1 + (C_{Ca}^{cyt}/K_b)^3]}{1 + (K_a/C_{Ca}^{cyt})^4 + (C_{Ca}^{cyt}/K_b)^3}. \tag{9.138}$$

To obtain the second equation, we take the time derivative of ω:

$$\frac{d\omega}{dt} = -\frac{dP_{C2}}{dt} = -k_c^+ P_{O1} + k_c^- P_{C2} = -k_c^+ P_{O1} + k_c^-(1 - \omega). \tag{9.139}$$

Substituting Eq. (9.137) into Eq. (9.139) yields:

$$\frac{d\omega}{dt} = -k_c^+ \omega \left(\frac{1}{1 + (K_a/C_{Ca}^{cyt})^4 + (C_{Ca}^{cyt}/K_b)^3} \right) + k_c^-(1 - \omega). \tag{9.140}$$

By definition of K_c, we have:

$$\frac{d\omega}{dt} = -k_c^- \omega \left(\frac{1/K_c}{1 + (K_a/C_{Ca}^{cyt})^4 + (C_{Ca}^{cyt}/K_b)^3} + 1 \right) + k_c^-(1 - \omega). \tag{9.141}$$

After a few algebraic manipulations, we find that:

$$\frac{d\omega}{dt} = k_c^- \left[1 - \omega \left(\frac{1 + (1/K_c) + (K_a/C_{Ca}^{cyt})^4 + (C_{Ca}^{cyt}/K_b)^3}{1 + (K_a/C_{Ca}^{cyt})^4 + (C_{Ca}^{cyt}/K_b)^3} \right) \right]. \tag{9.142}$$

If we define ω^∞ as

$$\omega^\infty \equiv \frac{1 + (K_a/C_{Ca}^{cyt})^4 + (C_{Ca}^{cyt}/K_b)^3}{1 + (1/K_c) + (K_a/C_{Ca}^{cyt})^4 + (C_{Ca}^{cyt}/K_b)^3}, \tag{9.143}$$

then Eq. (9.142) can be rewritten as the desired result:

$$\frac{d\omega}{dt} = k_c^- \left(1 - \frac{\omega}{\omega^\infty} \right) = \frac{k_c^-(\omega^\infty - \omega)}{\omega^\infty}. \tag{9.144}$$

Note that in the original Keizer and Levine article, this equation was written as:

$$\frac{d\omega}{dt} = -(\omega - \omega^\infty)/\tau, \tag{9.145}$$

where the time constant was defined as $\tau \equiv \omega^\infty/k_c^-$.

Problem 6.5

(a) The differential equations governing the rate of change of x (or C_{Ca}^{cyt}) and y (or C_{Ca}^{SR}) are:

$$\begin{cases} \frac{dx}{dt} = -\beta x - \gamma x + k_o + k_s y + f(x)y, \\ \frac{dy}{dt} = +\gamma x - k_s y - f(x)y. \end{cases} \quad (9.146)$$

The steady-state values are found by setting the time derivatives in Eq. (9.146) to zero:

$$x_{ss} = k_o/\beta, \quad (9.147)$$

$$y_{ss} = \frac{\gamma x_{ss}}{k_s + f(x_{ss})}. \quad (9.148)$$

More specifically,

$$y_{ss} = \frac{\gamma k_o/\beta}{k_s + \frac{k_o^n}{k_o^n + (a\beta)^n}} = \frac{\gamma k_o(k_o^n + (a\beta)^n)}{\beta[k_o^n(k_s+1) + k_s(a\beta)^n]}. \quad (9.149)$$

The Jacobian matrix is given by:

$$J = \begin{bmatrix} a_{11} & a_{12} \\ a_{21} & a_{22} \end{bmatrix} = \begin{bmatrix} \frac{\partial}{\partial x} & \frac{\partial}{\partial y} \\ \frac{\partial}{\partial x} & \frac{\partial}{\partial y} \end{bmatrix} = \begin{bmatrix} -\beta - \gamma + \frac{na^n x_{ss}^{n-1} y_{ss}}{(x_{ss}^n + a^n)^2} & k_s + \frac{x_{ss}^n}{x_{ss}^n + a^n} \\ \gamma - \frac{na^n x_{ss}^{n-1} y_{ss}}{(x_{ss}^n + a^n)^2} & -k_s - \frac{x_{ss}^n}{x_{ss}^n + a^n} \end{bmatrix}. \quad (9.150)$$

The characteristic equation is then written as:

$$\det(J - \lambda I) = (a_{11} - \lambda)(a_{22} - \lambda) - a_{12}a_{21} = 0. \quad (9.151)$$

Thus, if we define $b = a_{11} + a_{22}$ and $c = a_{11}a_{22} - a_{12}a_{21}$, Eq. (9.151) can be rewritten as:

$$\lambda^2 - b\lambda + c = 0. \quad (9.152)$$

Substituting the Jacobian matrix elements into the definitions of b and c yields:

$$b = -\beta - \gamma - k_s - \frac{x_{ss}^n}{x_{ss}^n + a^n} + \frac{na^n x_{ss}^{n-1} y_{ss}}{(x_{ss}^n + a^n)^2}, \quad (9.153)$$

$$c = \beta\left(k_s + \frac{x_{ss}^n}{x_{ss}^n + a^n}\right). \quad (9.154)$$

Fig. 9.3 Values of the characteristic equation parameter b, as a function of the constant a. The steady-state values of the cytosolic and SR concentration of Ca^{2+} are stable if and only if $Re(b) < 0$

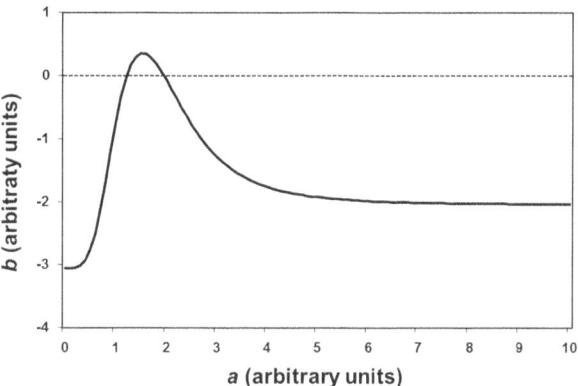

We now substitute Eqs. (9.147)–(9.149) into the latter two equations. After some algebraic manipulations, we obtain:

$$b = -\beta - \gamma - k_s - \frac{k_o^n}{k_o^n + (a\beta)^n} + \frac{n\gamma a^n k_o^n}{[k_o^n + (a\beta)^n][k_o^n(1+k_s) + k_s(a\beta)^n]}, \tag{9.155}$$

$$c = \beta\left(k_s + \frac{k_o^n}{k_o^n + (a\beta)^n}\right). \tag{9.156}$$

(b) Whereas c is positive for all parameter values, the sign of b is less clear. As described in Sect. 6.4, given that $c > 0$, the system will be stable if $b < 0$, and unstable if $b > 0$. If $n = 4$, $\beta = 1$, $\gamma = 1$, $k_s = 0.05$, and $k_o = 1$, we have:

$$b = -2.05 - \frac{1}{1+a^4} + \frac{4a^4}{(1+a^4)(1.05 + 0.05a^4)}. \tag{9.157}$$

Shown in Fig. 9.3 is a plot of b as a function of $a (0 \le a \le 10)$. These results indicate that b is positive over the interval $1.214 \le a \le 1.947$. In this interval, $Re(\lambda) > 0$ (see Eq. 6.83), i.e., the system is unstable and the model predicts C_{Ca}^{cyt} oscillations.

Chapter 7

Problem 7.1

(a) and (b) See Fig. 9.4.
   (c) See Fig. 9.5.

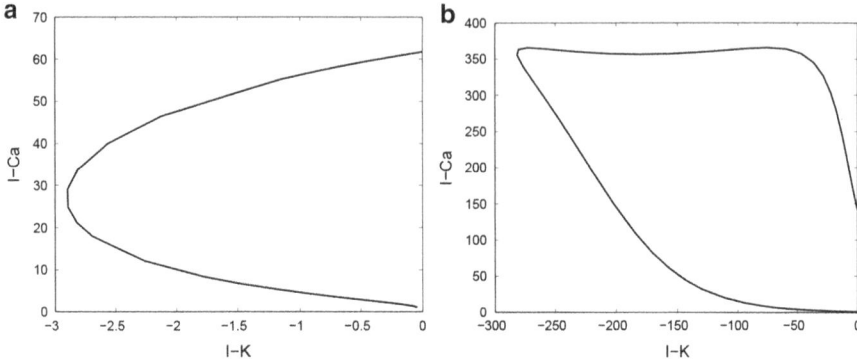

Fig. 9.4 Solution to Problem 7.1. I_{Ca}–I_K phase-plane plots. (**a**) $v(0) = -20\,\text{mV}$. (**b**) $v(0) = -10\,\text{mV}$

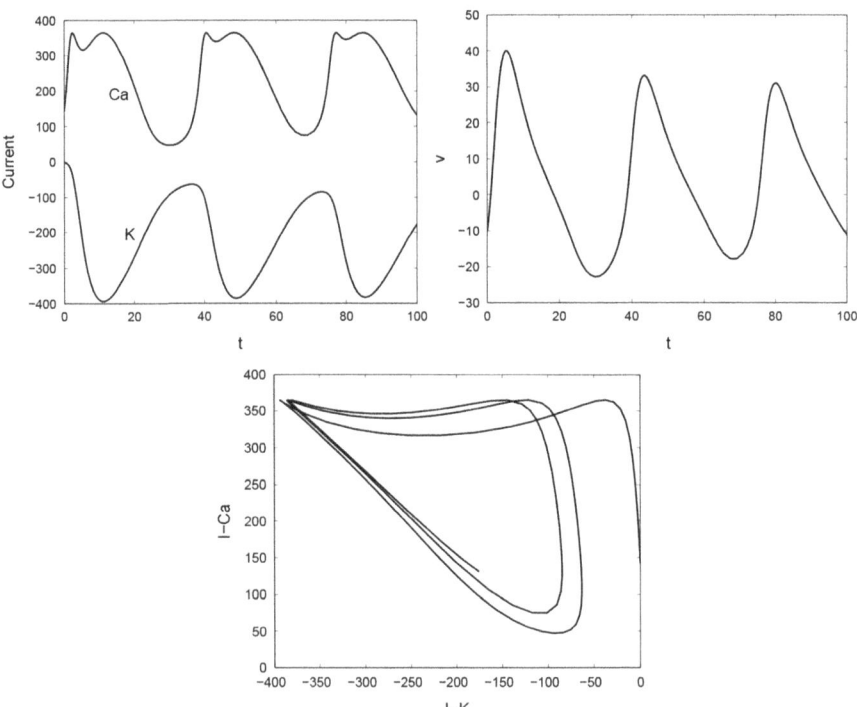

Fig. 9.5 Solution to Problem 7.1 (c). An oscillatory solution obtained with $I = 120$ and $v(0) = -10\,\text{mV}$

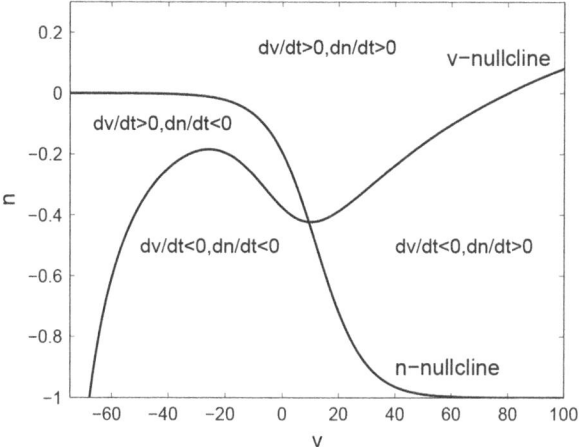

Fig. 9.6 Solution to Problem 7.2 (a). Nullclines with $I = 120$

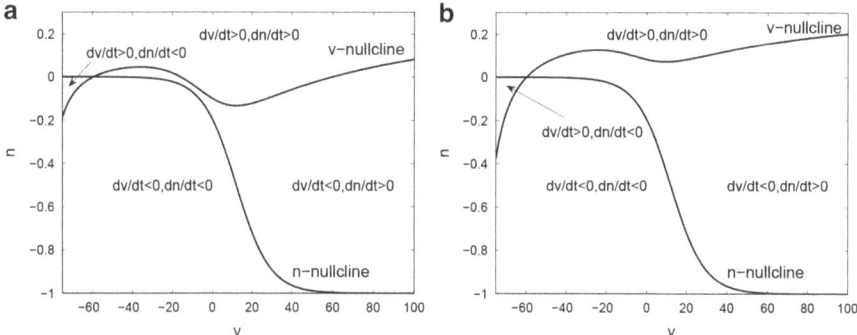

Fig. 9.7 (a) With $g_K = 16$, (b) with $g_{Ca} = 1$

Problem 7.2

(a) The nullclines are shown in Fig. 9.6. The point $(v, n) = (-10, 0)$ lies in the region where $dv/dt > 0$ and $dn/dt > 0$. Thus, we expect v to exhibit an initial rise, which is consistent with results in Problem 7.1 (c).
(b) v will exhibit an initial rise.
(c) Values of g_{Ca} and g_K that yield only one intercept and corresponding nullclines are shown in Fig. 9.7.

Problem 7.3

Results shown in Fig. 9.8.

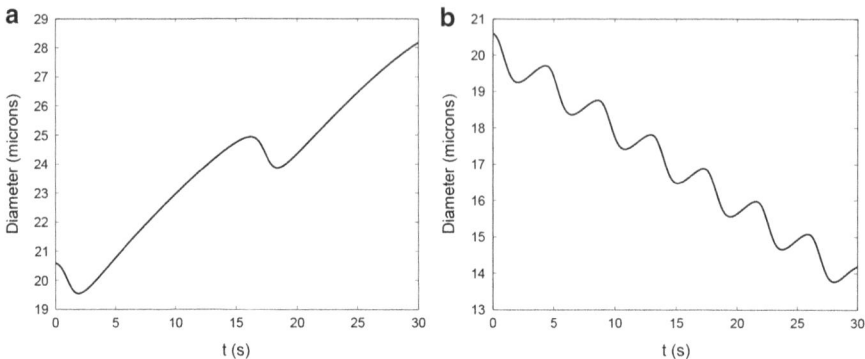

Fig. 9.8 (a) With $v_1 = -20.5\,\text{mV}$, (b) with $v_1 = -24.5\,\text{mV}$

Chapter 8

Problem 8.1

The TJ conductance equals $1/R_{TJ} = 40.7\,\text{mS/cm}^2$. It is related to TJ solute permeability as follows (Eq. 8.3):

$$G_{TJ} = \frac{F^2}{RT} \sum_{i=1\ldots n} z_i^2 P_i \bar{C}_i. \tag{9.158}$$

Since the extracellular concentration of K^+ ($\sim 5\,\text{mM}$) is much smaller than those of Na^+ ($\sim 140\,\text{mM}$) and Cl^- ($\sim 120\,\text{mM}$), we may neglect the contribution of ions other than Na^+ and Cl^- to G_{TJ} and write:

$$G_{TJ} = \frac{F^2}{RT}\left[P_{Na}\bar{C}_{Na} + P_{Cl}\bar{C}_{Cl}\right] = \frac{F^2 P_{Na}}{RT}\left[\bar{C}_{Na} + \bar{C}_{Cl}/2.7\right]. \tag{9.159}$$

The Na^+ permeability of the tight junction is therefore computed as:

$$P_{Na} = \frac{(2.57\,\text{J/mmol})(40.7\times 10^{-3}\,\text{S/cm}^2)}{(96.5\,\text{C/mmol})^2[(140 + 120/2.7)\times 10^{-3}\,\text{mmol/cm}^3]} = 6.1\times 10^{-5}\,\text{cm/s}. \tag{9.160}$$

Problem 8.2

(a) The direction of passive electrodiffusion can be inferred from the electrochemical potential gradient. For protons, the cell-to-external medium difference is given by:

$$\mu_{H+}^i - \mu_{H+}^e = RT \ln(C_{H+}^i/C_{H+}^e) + z_{H+}FV_m, \qquad (9.161)$$

$$\mu_{H+}^i - \mu_{H+}^e = 2.303 RT \log_{10}(10^{-pH_i+pH_e}) + FV_m, \qquad (9.162)$$

$$\mu_{H+}^i - \mu_{H+}^e = (2.303)(2.57)(-7.2+7.4) + (96.5)(-0.060) = -4.61 < 0. \qquad (9.163)$$

The electrochemical potential difference is negative, which means that passive diffusion carries H^+ into the cell (down the gradient).

(b) The Nernst potential of an ion S is given by:

$$E_s = \frac{RT}{z_s F} \ln\left(\frac{C_s^e}{C_s^i}\right). \qquad (9.164)$$

Thus, we have

$$E_{OH-} = -\frac{RT}{F} \ln\left(\frac{C_{OH-}^e}{C_{OH-}^i}\right) = -\frac{RT}{F} \ln\left(\frac{10^{-14+pH_e}}{10^{-14+pH_i}}\right)$$

$$= -\frac{RT}{F} \ln\left(10^{pH_e-pH_i}\right) = +\frac{RT}{F} \ln(10^{pH_i-pH_e}) = E_{H+}. \qquad (9.165)$$

At equilibrium, the concentrations of NH_4^+ and NH_3 are related as (see Eq. 8.50):

$$\frac{C_{NH3} C_{H+}}{C_{NH4+}} = K_a. \qquad (9.166)$$

If the internal and external concentrations of NH_3 are the same, we have:

$$\frac{C_{H+}^i}{C_{NH4+}^i} = \frac{C_{H+}^e}{C_{NH4+}^e}, \qquad (9.167)$$

$$E_{NH4+} = \frac{RT}{F} \ln\left(\frac{C_{NH4+}^e}{C_{NH4+}^i}\right) = \frac{RT}{F} \ln\left(\frac{C_{H+}^e}{C_{H+}^i}\right) = E_{H+}. \qquad (9.168)$$

Since V_m is more negative than $E_{H+} = E_{OH-} = E_{NH4+}$, the currents of H^+, NH_4^+ and OH^- are all negative (see Chap. 6). Recall that by convention, a negative current carries negative charge out of the cell. Thus, the negatively charged OH^- tends to passively diffuse out of the cell, whereas the positively charged ions H^+ and NH_4^+ are passively carried in.

Problem 8.3

As in Problem 8.2, we take $pH_i = 7.2$, $pH_e = 7.4$, and $V_m = -60\,mV$. As a simple hypothesis, we use the Henderson-Hasselbalch equation to estimate HCO_3^- concentrations (Eq. 8.52). We thus have:

$$C^i_{HCO3-} = (C^i_{CO2})(10^{pH_i - pK_a}) = (1.2\,mM)(10^{7.2-6.1}) = 15.1\,mM, \quad (9.169)$$

$$C^e_{HCO3-} = (C^e_{CO2})(10^{pH_e - pK_a}) = (1.2\,mM)(10^{7.4-6.1}) = 23.9\,mM. \quad (9.170)$$

We also assume that the intracellular and extracellular Na^+ concentrations are 10 and 150 mM, respectively. The electrochemical potential gradient of each ion is then calculated as:

$$\mu^i_{HCO3-} - \mu^e_{HCO3-} = RT\ln(C^i_{HCO3-}/C^e_{HCO3-}) + z_{HCO3-}FV_m, \quad (9.171)$$

$$\mu^i_{HCO3-} - \mu^e_{HCO3-} = (2.57)\ln(15.1/23.9) - (96.5)(-0.060) = +4.61 > 0, \quad (9.172)$$

$$\mu^i_{Na+} - \mu^e_{Na+} = RT\ln(C^i_{Na+}/C^e_{Na+}) + z_{Na+}FV_m, \quad (9.173)$$

$$\mu^i_{Na+} - \mu^e_{Na+} = (2.57)\ln(10/150) + (96.5)(-0.060) = -12.75 < 0. \quad (9.174)$$

Solutes passively diffuse down their electrochemical potential gradient, which means that Na^+ tends to enter the cell whereas HCO_3^- tends to exit; the Na^+/HCO_3^- cotransporter uses the gradient of one of these ions to carry the other in the same direction. Whether transport is inward or outward can be determined using the non-equilibrium thermodynamic (NET) formalism. With a 1:2 stoichiometry, the Na^+ and HCO_3^- fluxes are calculated as:

$$\begin{bmatrix} J_{Na+} \\ J_{HCO3-} \end{bmatrix} = L_{Na-HCO3} \begin{bmatrix} 1 & 2 \\ 2 & 4 \end{bmatrix} \begin{bmatrix} \Delta\mu_{Na+} \\ \Delta\mu_{HCO3-} \end{bmatrix}. \quad (9.175)$$

In other words, the flux of each ion is proportional to $\Delta\mu_{Na+} + 2\Delta\mu_{HCO3-}$. In the outward direction (from the cell to the external medium), $\Delta\mu_{Na+} + 2\Delta\mu_{HCO3-} = -12.75 + 2(4.61) = -3.54 < 0$. Hence, the outward-directed flux is negative, which means that the transporter carries the ions into the cell, and acts as acid-extruder.

With a 1:3 stoichiometry, the flux of each ion is proportional to $\Delta\mu_{Na+} + 3\Delta\mu_{HCO3-} = +1.07$. The outward-directed flux is positive in this case, i.e., the transporter carries Na^+ and HCO_3^- out of the cell and acts as an acid-loader.

Problem 8.4

There are five loops in the state diagram of the thiazide-sensitive NaCl cotransporter: (a) the E-ENa-ENaCl-ECl-E loop; (b) the mirror E'-ENa'-ENaCl'-ECl'-E' loop; (c) the E-ED-ENaD-ENa-E loop; (d) the mirror E'-ED'-ENaD'-ENa'-E' loop; (e) and the central E-ECl-ENaCl-ENaCl'-ECl'-E'-E loop. As shown in Sect. 8.2.4, the principle of detailed balance applied to loop (a) yields the following equation:

$$k_1 k_4 k_5 k_8 = k_2 k_3 k_6 k_7. \tag{9.176}$$

Consider loop (b). The rates going clock-wise are k_9, k_{13}, k_{16} and k_{12}; the rates going counter clock-wise are k_{10}, k_{11}, k_{15} and k_{14}. The product of rates in one direction is equal to that in the other direction, hence:

$$k_9 k_{12} k_{13} k_{16} = k_{10} k_{11} k_{14} k_{15}. \tag{9.177}$$

Similarly, for loops (c) and (d), we have:

$$k_1 k_{22} k_{24} k_{25} = k_2 k_{21} k_{23} k_{26}, \tag{9.178}$$

$$k_9 k_{28} k_{30} k_{31} = k_{10} k_{27} k_{29} k_{32}. \tag{9.179}$$

The last loop (e) involves six species and rate constants, and the rule in this case yields:

$$k_4 k_8 k_{11} k_{15} k_{17} k_{20} = k_3 k_7 k_{12} k_{16} k_{18} k_{19}. \tag{9.180}$$

Those five relationships were used by Chang and Fujita (1999) to reduce the number of unknown rate constants in their model of the thiazide-sensitive NaCl cotransporter.

Problem. 8.5

(a) Let a, b and g represent Cl^-, K^+, and NH_4^+, respectively; α, β and γ denote their non-dimensional concentrations:

$$\alpha \equiv \frac{C_a}{K_a}, \quad \beta \equiv \frac{C_b}{K_b}, \quad \gamma \equiv \frac{C_g}{K_g}. \tag{9.181}$$

In the equations below, the superscript "i" and "e" denote the internal and external faces of the cell membrane. According to Fig. 8.6, Cl^- binds to the carrier before the other ion (K^+ or NH_4^+), and unbinds last. Hence, the carrier can exist under four different forms on either side of the membrane: empty (x), bound to Cl⁻ (xa), bound to KCl (xab), or bound to NH₄Cl (xag). Assuming that binding reactions are much faster than translocation rates and can be considered to be at equilibrium, the concentrations of the bound carrier species on a given side are given by:

$$C_{xa} = \frac{C_x C_a}{K_a} = \alpha C_x, \quad C_{xab} = \frac{C_{xa} C_b}{K_b} = \alpha\beta C_x, \quad C_{xag} = \frac{C_{xa} C_g}{K_g} = \alpha\gamma C_x, \quad (9.182)$$

where K_a, K_b, and K_g are the corresponding equilibrium constants. The total amount of carrier on both sides of the membrane (x_T) is conserved:

$$C_x^i(1 + \alpha^i + \alpha^i\beta^i + \alpha^i\gamma^i) + C_x^e(1 + \alpha^e + \alpha^e\beta^e + \alpha^e\gamma^e) = x_T. \quad (9.183)$$

If T_x, T_{xab} and T_{xag} represent the translocation rates of x, xab, and xag, the zero net flux condition is written as:

$$T_x^i C_x^i + T_{xab}^i C_{xab}^i + T_{xag}^i C_{xag}^i = T_x^e C_x^e + T_{xab}^e C_{xab}^e + T_{xag}^e C_{xag}^e. \quad (9.184)$$

That is,

$$C_x^i(T_x^i + T_{xab}^i \alpha^i \beta^i + T_{xag}^i \alpha^i \gamma^i) = C_x^e(T_x^e + T_{xab}^e \alpha^e \beta^e + T_{xag}^e \alpha^e \gamma^e). \quad (9.185)$$

Eqs. (9.183) and (9.185) are rewritten as:

$$\sigma^i C_x^i + \sigma^e C_x^e = x_T, \quad (9.186)$$

$$\eta^i C_x^i - \eta^e C_x^e = 0, \quad (9.187)$$

where

$$\sigma^i \equiv 1 + \alpha^i + \alpha^i\beta^i + \alpha^i\gamma^i, \quad \sigma^e \equiv 1 + \alpha^e + \alpha^e\beta^e + \alpha^e\gamma^e, \quad (9.188)$$

$$\eta^i \equiv T_x^i + T_{xab}^i \alpha^i \beta^i + T_{xag}^i \alpha^i \gamma^i, \quad \eta^e \equiv T_x^e + T_{xab}^e \alpha^e \beta^e + T_{xag}^e \alpha^e \gamma^e. \quad (9.189)$$

Solving Eqs. (9.186) and (9.187) for C_x^i and C_x^e yields:

$$C_x^i = \frac{\eta^e x_T}{\sigma^i \eta^e + \sigma^e \eta^i}, \quad C_x^e = \frac{\eta^i x_T}{\sigma^i \eta^e + \sigma^e \eta^i}. \quad (9.190)$$

The net outward flux of K⁺ is given by:

$$J_b = T_{xab}^i C_{xab}^i - T_{xab}^e C_{xab}^e$$

$$= T_{xab}^i C_x^i \alpha^i \beta^i - T_{xab}^e C_x^e \alpha^e \beta^e. \quad (9.191)$$

Let $\sum = \sigma^i \eta^e + \sigma^e \eta^i$. After substituting Eqs. (9.190) into Eq. (9.191) and rearranging, we obtain:

$$J_b = \frac{x_T}{\sum} \left[(T_{xab}^i T_x^e \alpha^i \beta^i - T_x^i T_{xab}^e \alpha^e \beta^e) \right.$$
$$\left. + (T_{xab}^i T_{xag}^e \alpha^i \beta^i \alpha^e \gamma^e - T_{xag}^i T_{xab}^e \alpha^i \gamma^i \alpha^e \beta^e) \right]. \quad (9.192)$$

By symmetry, the net outward flux of NH_4^+ is equal to:

$$J_g = \frac{x_T}{\sum} \left[(T_{xag}^i T_x^e \alpha^i \gamma^i - T_x^i T_{xag}^e \alpha^e \gamma^e) \right.$$
$$\left. + (T_{xag}^i T_{xab}^e \alpha^i \gamma^i \alpha^e \beta^e - T_{xab}^i T_{xag}^e \alpha^i \beta^i \alpha^e \gamma^e) \right]. \quad (9.193)$$

The net outward flux of Cl^- is the sum of the K^+ and NH_4^+ fluxes:

$$J_a = \frac{x_T}{\sum} \left[T_x^e \alpha^i (T_{xab}^i \beta^i + T_{xag}^i \gamma^i) - T_x^i \alpha^e (T_{xab}^e \beta^e + T_{xag}^e \gamma^e) \right]. \quad (9.194)$$

(b) In the absence of NH_4^+, $\gamma^i = \gamma^e = 0$, and the net Cl^- flux is given by:

$$J_a = \frac{x_T}{\sum} \left[T_x^e T_{xab}^i \alpha^i \beta^i - T_x^i T_{xab}^e \alpha^e \beta^e \right]. \quad (9.195)$$

More specifically, the flux is calculated as:

$$J_a = \frac{x_T (T_x^e T_{xab}^i \alpha^i \beta^i - T_x^i T_{xab}^e \alpha^e \beta^e)}{(1 + \alpha^i + \alpha^i \beta^i)(T_x^e + T_{xab}^e \alpha^e \beta^e) + (1 + \alpha^e + \alpha^e \beta^e)(T_x^i + T_{xab}^i \alpha^i \beta^i)}. \quad (9.196)$$

If the internal and external K^+ concentrations are 100 and 5 mM, and the K^+ affinity is 2 mM, then $\beta^i = 100/2 = 50$, and $\beta^e = 5/2 = 2.5$. Similarly, the non-dimensional internal Cl^- concentration is $\alpha^i = 15/20 = 0.75$. These values, and those of the translocation rates, are substituted into Eq. (9.196) to compute J_a as a function of external Cl^- (C_{Cl-}^e). The outward Cl^- flux is plotted on Fig. 9.9. Under physiological conditions, the cotransporter mediates the efflux of Cl^- and K^+ from the cytosol. Transport is driven by the electrochemical potential gradient of K^+, which favors the passive diffusion of K^+ out of the cell. The flux is maximal when there is no external chloride, and it decreases gradually as C_{Cl-}^e increases. It can easily be shown that the flux is zero when $\alpha^e \beta^e = \alpha^i \beta^i$, that is, when $C_{Cl-}^e = C_{Cl-}^i (C_{K+}^i / C_{K+}^e) = 300$ mM.

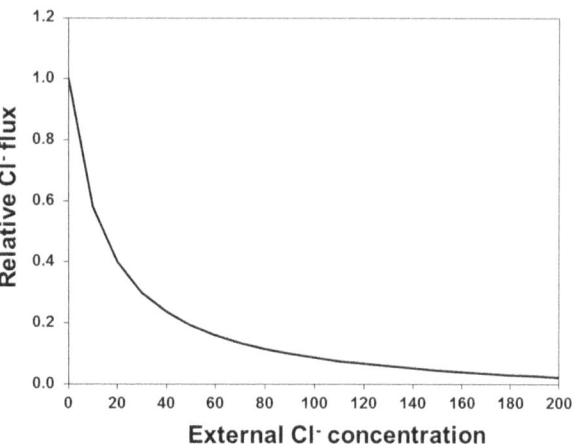

Fig. 9.9 Outward Cl⁻ flux across the K^+/Cl^- cotransporter as a function of external Cl⁻ concentration (in mM). The flux is normalized to 1.0 when there is no Cl⁻ in the external medium. As the external Cl⁻ concentration is raised, the driving force across the exchanger decreases and so does the flux

Problem 8.6

(a) We use the same notation as in Sect. 8.2.3, except that we now have to distinguish between internal and external equilibrium constants. Hence, assuming that the binding reactions are instantaneous, we have:

$$K_a^i = \frac{a^i x^i}{(ax)^i}, \quad K_a^e = \frac{a^e x^e}{(ax)^e}, \tag{9.197}$$

$$K_b^i = \frac{b^i x^i}{(bx)^i}, \quad K_b^e = \frac{b^e x^e}{(bx)^e}, \tag{9.198}$$

$$K_c^i = \frac{c^i x^i}{(cx)^i}, \quad K_c^e = \frac{c^e x^e}{(cx)^e}, \tag{9.199}$$

where the superscripts "i" and "e" refer to the internal and external sides of the membrane. Conservation of the total amount of carrier is still written as (see Eq. 8.16):

$$x^i + (ax)^i + (bx)^i + (cx)^i + x^e + (ax)^e + (bx)^e + (cx)^e = x_T. \tag{9.200}$$

With different forward and backward translocation rates, the zero net flux condition can be expressed as:

$$T_a^i(ax)^i + T_b^i(bx)^i + T_c^i(cx)^i = T_a^e(ax)^e + T_b^e(bx)^e + T_c^e(cx)^e. \tag{9.201}$$

We may define the following non-dimensional variables:

$$\alpha^i \equiv \frac{a^i}{K_a^i}, \quad \alpha^e \equiv \frac{a^e}{K_a^e}, \quad \beta^i \equiv \frac{b^i}{K_b^i}, \quad \beta^e \equiv \frac{b^e}{K_b^e}, \quad \gamma^i \equiv \frac{c^i}{K_c^i}, \quad \gamma^e \equiv \frac{c^e}{K_c^e}.$$
(9.202)

With this notation, Eqs. (9.197)–(9.199) may be rewritten as:

$$(ax)^i = a^i x^i / K_a^i = \alpha^i x^i,$$
(9.203)

$$(ax)^e = a^e x^e / K_a^e = \alpha^e x^e,$$
(9.204)

$$(bx)^i = b^i x^i / K_b^i = \beta^i x^i,$$
(9.205)

$$(bx)^e = b^e x^e / K_b^e = \beta^e x^e,$$
(9.206)

$$(cx)^i = c^i x^i / K_c^i = \gamma^i x^i,$$
(9.207)

$$(cx)^e = c^e x^e / K_c^e = \gamma^e x^e.$$
(9.208)

And Eqs. (9.200) and (9.201) can be expressed as:

$$x^i + \alpha^i x^i + \beta^i x^i + \gamma^i x^i + x^e + \alpha^e x^e + \beta^e x^e + \gamma^e x^e = x_T,$$
(9.209)

$$T_a^i \alpha^i x^i + T_b^i \beta^i x^i + T_c^i \gamma^i x^i = T_a^e \alpha^e x^e + T_b^e \beta^e x^e + T_c^e \gamma^e x^e.$$
(9.210)

That is,

$$x^i \left[1 + \alpha^i + \beta^i + \gamma^i\right] + x^e \left[1 + \alpha^e + \beta^e + \gamma^e\right] = x_T$$
(9.211)

$$-x^i \left[T_a^i \alpha^i + T_b^i \beta^i + T_c^i \gamma^i\right] + x^e \left[T_a^e \alpha^e + T_b^e \beta^e + T_c^e \gamma^e\right] = 0.$$
(9.212)

We may determine x^i and x^e by solving this 2×2 system. The determinant is given by:

$$\sum = (1 + \alpha^i + \beta^i + \gamma^i)(T_a^e \alpha^e + T_b^e \beta^e + T_c^e \gamma^e)$$
$$+ (1 + \alpha^e + \beta^e + \gamma^e)(T_a^i \alpha^i + T_b^i \beta^i + T_c^i \gamma^i).$$
(9.213)

And we have:

$$x^i = x_T (T_a^e \alpha^e + T_b^e \beta^e + T_c^e \gamma^e) / \sum,$$
(9.214)

$$x^e = x_T (T_a^i \alpha^i + T_b^i \beta^i + T_c^i \gamma^i) / \sum.$$
(9.215)

We can now calculate the flux of each ion across the carrier. The net outward flux of sodium is given by:

$$J_a = T_a^i (ax)^i - T_a^e (ax)^e = T_a^i \alpha^i x^i - T_a^e \alpha^e x^e.$$
(9.216)

After substituting Eqs. (9.214) and (9.215) into Eq. (9.216) and rearranging, the net outward flux of Na$^+$ simplifies to:

$$J_a = \frac{x_T}{\Sigma}\left[T_a^i \alpha^i (T_b^e \beta^e + T_c^e \gamma^e) - T_a^e \alpha^e (T_b^i \beta^i + T_c^i \gamma^i)\right]. \tag{9.217}$$

By symmetry, the net outward fluxes of H$^+$ and NH$_4^+$ are given by:

$$J_b = \frac{x_T}{\Sigma}\left[T_b^i \beta^i (T_a^e \alpha^e + T_c^e \gamma^e) - T_b^e \beta^e (T_a^i \alpha^i + T_c^i \gamma^i)\right], \tag{9.218}$$

$$J_c = \frac{x_T}{\Sigma}\left[T_c^i \gamma^i (T_a^e \alpha^e + T_b^e \beta^e) - T_c^e \gamma^e (T_a^i \alpha^i + T_b^i \beta^i)\right]. \tag{9.219}$$

We now consider the limiting case when the internal concentration of Na$^+$ and the external concentrations of H$^+$ and NH$_4^+$ are negligible. In other words $\alpha^i \approx 0$, $\beta^e \approx 0$, $\gamma^e \approx 0$. Under these conditions, the fluxes of H$^+$ and NH$_4^+$ are given by:

$$J_b = \frac{x_T}{\Sigma}(T_b^i \beta^i T_a^e \alpha^e), \tag{9.220}$$

$$J_c = \frac{x_T}{\Sigma}(T_c^i \gamma^i T_a^e \alpha^e). \tag{9.221}$$

And their ratio is equal to:

$$J_b/J_c = T_b^i \beta^i / T_c^i \gamma^i. \tag{9.222}$$

In terms of dimensional variables, this ratio is written as:

$$J_b/J_c = \frac{T_b^i (b^i/K_b^i)}{T_c^i (c^i/K_c^i)}. \tag{9.223}$$

This result makes intuitive sense: the flux ratio is proportional to the ratio of translocation rates and to that of "effective" concentrations. By effective concentration, we mean the concentration divided by the binding affinity.

References

Chang, H., Fujita, T.: A numerical model of the renal distal tubule. Am. J. Physiol. Renal Physiol. **276**(6), F931–F951 (1999)

Layton, H.E.: Energy advantage of counter-current oxygen transfer in fish gills. J. Theor. Biol. **125**(3), 307–316 (1987)

Index

A
Active transport, 78, 158–161, 177
Afferent arteriole, 64, 107, 122, 141, 151
Arcuate arteries, 1

B
Bayliss effect, 151
Bifurcation analysis, 96, 98
Bowman's capsule, 7
Brinkman equation, 35
Brusselator, 133

C
Central core, 53–56, 58–60
Chang–Fujita model, 165
Characteristic equation, 96, 134
Collecting duct, 5, 66, 157, 161
Concentration polarization, 38
Connecting tubule, 5, 169
Continuity equation, 34, 35
Continuously distributed loops, 57
Convection, 17, 18, 38, 74, 177
Cortex, 1, 63, 75
Countercurrent configuration, 44, 64, 66
Countercurrent exchange, 66, 68
Countercurrent multiplication, 48
Coupling, 103

D
Darcy's law, 35
Delay-differential equation, 87
Detailed balance principle, 166
De Young–Keizer model, 128
Diffusion, 17, 18, 22, 38, 74, 110, 114, 159, 177

Discrete-loop representation, 57
Distal convoluted tubule, 165
Distal tubule, 4
Distributed loops, 57

E
Efferent arterioles, 2, 64, 65, 80
Electrochemical potential, 110, 119, 121, 158, 168, 177
Endothelium, 8, 34, 36, 64, 76
Epithelium, 8, 34, 36, 155, 156

F
Fahraeus effect, 64
Feedback response, 92
Fenestra, 8, 33, 35, 63, 64, 73
Fick's law, 17, 114
Filtration fraction, 10, 14
Fractional clearance, 10, 25, 27
Fundamental mode, 100

G
Glomerular basement membrane, 8, 33, 35, 36, 38
Glomerular capillary, 7, 12, 32
Glomerular filtration rate, 10, 14, 15, 33, 85
Glomerulus, 1, 7
Goldbeter–Dupont–Berridge model, 126–127
Goldman–Hodgkin–Katz equation, 113–115, 117, 157

H
Hai–Murphy model, 136
Hindrance coefficient, 22, 23

Index

Hydraulic conductivity, 14, 15, 23, 34, 36, 71–74, 161, 175
Hydraulic pressure, 14, 15, 20, 71, 72, 75, 161, 175
Hydrostatic pressure, 46
Hypertonic, 43
Hysteresis, 144

I
Inner medulla, 44, 64, 65
Inner stripe, 64, 65
Interlobar arteries, 1
Isoporous model, 21–25, 27
Isoporous-plus-shunt model, 28, 32

K
Kedem–Katchalsky equation, 14, 17, 71
Keizer–Levine model, 130

L
Landis–Pappenheimer equation, 19, 71
Limit-cycle oscillations, 94, 95, 98, 102, 103, 153
Loop of Henle, 4, 66

M
Macula densa, 85, 92
Medulla, 1, 63, 75
Membrane potential, 108, 113, 114, 122, 143, 174
Michaelis–Menten kinetics, 47, 77, 127
Morris–Lecar model, 144, 153
Mullins model, 119
Myogenic response, 107, 142, 151

N
Navier–Stokes equation, 23, 34
Nernst Planck equation, 114
Nernst potential, 110, 111, 113, 114, 142
Non-equilibrium thermodynamics, 14, 167–168, 180
Nullcline, 147

O
Ohm's law, 113
Oncotic pressure, 13, 15, 16, 21, 46, 71, 72, 75, 161, 175

Osmolality, 46, 63, 66, 161
Osmosis, 44
Osmotic coefficient, 14, 21, 46, 71–74, 175
Osmotic pressure, 13, 46, 71, 72, 175–176
Outer medulla, 4, 64, 65
Outer stripe, 4

P
Partition coefficient, 22, 38
Passive transport, 158, 177
Patlak equation, 19
Péclet number, 18, 24, 30, 38, 74
Pericyte, 64, 107, 109, 122, 126
Podocyte, 8
Poiseuille flow, 23, 26, 176
Proximal tubule, 4, 10, 40, 63, 155, 156, 160, 163

R
Renal arteries, 1
Renal plasma clearance, 9
Renal plasma flow, 10, 13

S
Saddle-nodes bifurcation, 144
Sieving coefficient, 10, 25, 30, 31, 37, 39
Slit diaphragm, 8, 33, 34, 37, 38
Solute conservation, 16–17, 20, 38, 45, 70, 76, 80, 90, 111–112, 131, 132, 171, 172, 174
Solute diffusivity, 17, 18, 22, 74, 114
Solute permeability, 17, 18, 21, 37, 47, 67, 74, 114, 157, 168, 177
Spontaneous vasomotion, 148
Static head, 94
Stokes equation, 34, 35

T
TGF delay, 93, 95, 99, 104
TGF gain, 94, 95, 98
Thick ascending limb, 72, 76, 78, 165
Tubuloglomerular feedback (TGF), 85, 107

U
Ultrafiltration coefficient, 15, 21, 23–24
Ultrafiltration pressure, 15

V
Vasa recta, 2, 64–66, 69–74, 78, 107
Vascular bundle, 64, 65
Vasoconstriction, 133, 135, 141
Vasodilation, 107, 141
Vasomotion, 141

W
Water conservation, 12–13, 20, 45, 69, 79, 169–172
Water permeability, 54. *See also* Hydraulic conductivity

The manufacturer's authorised representative in the EU is Springer Nature Customer Service Centre GmbH, Europaplatz 3, 69115 Heidelberg, Germany. If you have any concerns regarding our products, please contact ProductSafety@springernature.com

Printed and bound by CPI Group (UK) Ltd, Croydon, CR0 4YY

23/03/2026

02076666-0014